YOGA for AMPUTEES

YOGA for AMPUTEES

THE ESSENTIAL GUIDE TO FINDING WHOLENESS AFTER LIMB LOSS

FOR YOGA STUDENTS AND THEIR TEACHERS

MARSHA THERESE DANZIG, C-IAYT, RYT 500, M.ED

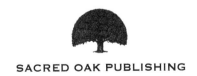

SACRED OAK PUBLISHING

Cover and interior design: Emilia Ryan

Photographs of the author:
Amanda Barbosa - cover and pages: xi, 233, 234, 306, 366
Rebecca Brown, page 86
Jamie Baird, page 132

Photographs of amputees: Augusta Rose Photography

The remaining images: www.stock.adobe.com and unsplash.com

978-0-9744858-4-3

Sacred Oak Publishing
1211 Far Hills Avenue
Dayton, OH 45419
www.yogaforamputeesbook.com

First Printing, 2018
Printed in the United States of America

ACKNOWLEDGEMENTS

I would like to thank the following people for contributing to this book in so many ways: Emilia Ryan for her exquisite graphics and vision for beauty, Augusta Rose Photography for her compassionate and gorgeous photos, our amputee models: Aimee, Bug, Molly, Ray, Jenny, Kelly, Jeff, Laura and Juanita for their warmth, willingness and bravery to be seen; prosthetists who make our lives as amputees so much easier, especially Keith Cornell, and Optimus prosthetics, for their love and care, Amps4Ohio for creating a support network of amputees, many of whom modelled for this book, the Amputee Coalition for continuously advocating on behalf of amputees, Amanda Barbosa for her stunning cover photo, headshot and more, Rebecca Brown photography for finding a tree stump for me to stand on, researchers, inventors and explorers who are finding new ways through technology to help amputees thrive even more, Kripalu Center for instilling in me the gift of compassionate yoga, my beautiful students who gave me the gift of teaching, medicine, which has continued to keep me here to do my work, my family who have always had my back, my incredible father, Robert J. Danzig, who chose the magic of life every day, the yoga tradition, which has withstood the test of time, the spirit of God which infuses all living things, and all amputees everywhere for living life fully.

CONTENTS

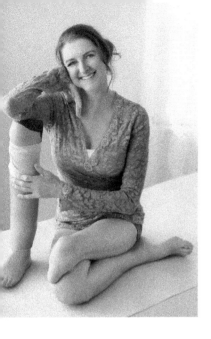

A TRAGIC LOSS BECOMES A GLOBAL MOVEMENT

Dear Friend,

It is with great pleasure that I present this book to you, over forty years in the making! I am so glad you are here.

I lost my leg in 1976, when I was a teenager whose main concern was boys, clothes and getting into a good college. Bone cancer, and the subsequent amputation of my left leg below the knee, changed all that. No longer was I worried about whether my hairstyle was trendy, I was worried about whether I'd live or die. Fortunately, I made it through, but not without many scars, both physical and emotional.

When I found yoga in my early twenties, I was desperate to feel 'normal' again. Before yoga, I lived with terror that I would be found out for the "handicapped "girl I was, and no-one would want to know me. At that time, prosthetics hadn't changed since World War II. They were cumbersome, irritating and ugly. I wore a heavy suspension belt around my waist, endured daily blisters, and worried constantly that 'this would be the day' that my residual limb gave out. Disability rights were still under the radar. The American Disabilities Act (ADA) was years away. I felt very alone as an amputee. But after yoga came into my life, I stopped hiding myself. Yoga gave me back my true self.

With yoga, I began to love and accept myself exactly as I was, after learning to embody compassion for myself. I got my confidence back. By finding ways to adapt my yoga poses, I was able to do things I used to do as a gymnast, which made me feel like me again. I developed a profound ability to listen to and work with my body, which reduced my prosthetic irritations and helped me see how much potential for movement I really had. Lastly, because yoga taught me that deep down, I was one with all of life, I stopped feeling so alone in the world. I learned to trust life again, living in connection with the world around me, rather than separate or fearful of a frightening future.

I felt like a brave pioneer, always the only amputee in yoga class. I was proud of that! To this day I still kiss myself at the end of yoga class, appreciative of the heroic journey I have taken. From battling bone cancer twice, enduring kidney failure, eleven years on dialysis, a kidney transplant, congestive heart failure and a host of physical and emotional challenges along the way, the physical strength, inner calm and mental peace that yoga has given me has made my life better .

I wrote this book for my fellow amputees, who want to learn how you, too, can benefit from yoga as I have. You, like me, want to feel whole, strong and confident on a regular basis. You want to know that your life has purpose, that you are not alone in the world and that you can gain back your independence. You want to feel good in your body, and prevent future illness or injury. You seek hope, a way out of your suffering, or a way to help other amputees who are struggling.

There is something for everyone in yoga, from quieting the stressed-out mind in meditation, to strengthening the core in an advanced yoga pose. When looked at with yoga eyes, boredom becomes a message for personal growth. Fear becomes an opportunity to break free of beliefs that have held you back. Skepticism challenges you to look deeper at old habits. Accepting your body as it is right now shows you ways your body IS working well. A deep breath grants you the optimism you have been searching for.

This book includes so much more than basic yoga techniques adapted to amputees. Amputees have a lot at stake beyond range of motion. While this book does spend significant time on adapting yoga poses and yoga techniques to amputees, it is the deeper yoga practices of inner healing from pain, grief, life changes, body image and trauma that I feel matter most to amputees.

Wholeness (feeling home within oneself body, mind and spirit) is at the core of this book. Each chapter provides a yoga solution to a common amputee challenge, with the end result that we as amputees feel whole. Throughout the book, amputees of all levels share how yoga has helped them overcome their difficulties, and how they reclaimed their wholeness.

Advancements in prosthetics, disability awareness, and a global adaptive yoga movement make this book timely for amputees. Yoga has taken a front seat in western medicine, with therapeutic yoga programs popping up at hospitals and clinics all over the world. These holistic medicine programs prove that yoga works, increasing patient wellness without invasive procedures or excessive prescriptive medications. Wholeness is not simply having four limbs. Wholeness is knowing that you are complete within yourself, just as you are.

Yoga can make that happen. The pages of this book will reveal just how.

Love, Marsha

CHAPTER ONE | WHY YOGA

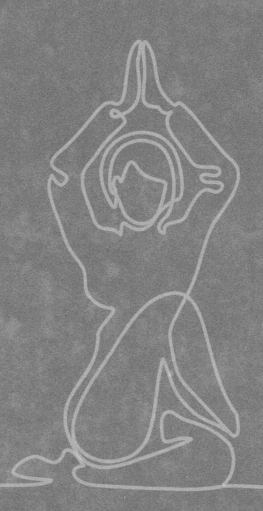

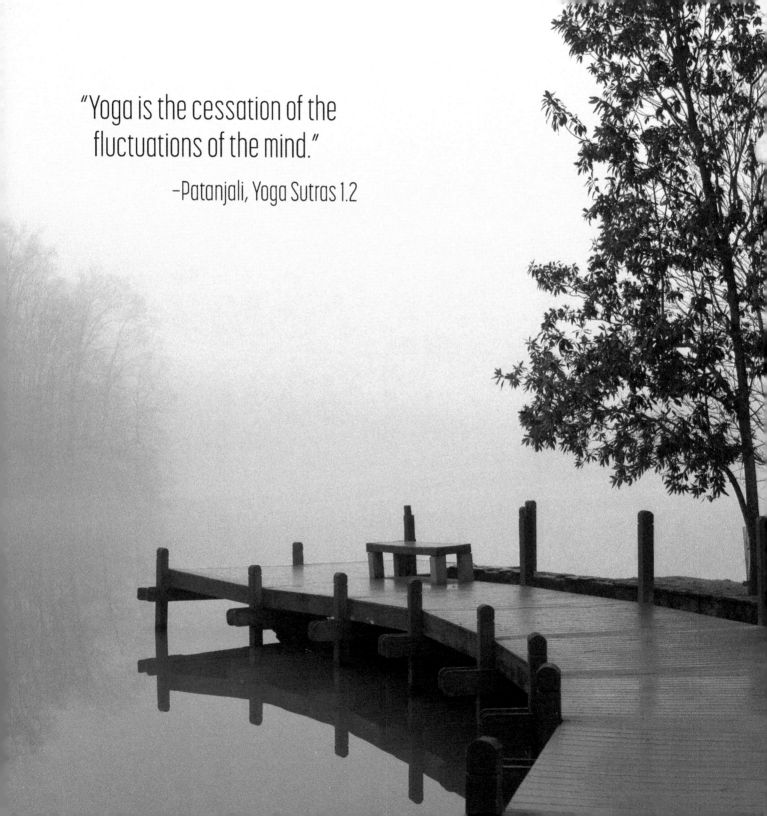

"Yoga is the cessation of the fluctuations of the mind."

–Patanjali, Yoga Sutras 1.2

What is Yoga?

Yoga is a 5,000 year plus tradition originating in India. Believed to be descended from the Indus, an advanced and technologically sophisticated civilization which thrived near the Sarasvati River, yoga was a natural extension of the spiritual roots of the culture, which sought to unite the divine with everyday life, and everyday life with the divine. The first written text about yoga, the Rig-Veda (adoration of the divine knowledge), is an exploration of life's purpose, and the quest to understand the mystery of the spiritual realms.

The Indus were a people like so many ancient cultures, who lived lives according to the rhythms of nature, and the spiritual influences that nature presented. Sacrifice, self-observation and discipline were viewed as the way to unite with the divine that permeated all of life. For the spiritual seeker, that meant stilling the mind for long periods of time, abstaining from distractions like alcohol and sex, and gaining purity of mind and body. Through these disciplines the devotee hoped to experience transcendence, timelessness and unification with the divine.

Many fundamental principles of yoga evolved from these Vedic ("from knowledge") yoga practices, including many scriptures and refined teachings on meditation and yoga techniques. The Bhagavad Gita, in particular, is a beautiful poem which tells us that, in order to unite with our blissful nature, we must also act with love, integrity, free from self-serving (or ego driven) deeds.

In the second century AD, yoga was further refined with the writings and tradition of Raja yoga (the Royal Path), prescribed by Patanjali in his Yoga Sutras (yoga threads) and his book of Ayurveda (science of life) as well as the teacher Vyasa.

Patanjali's life is both legend and tradition. It is said that he was born of Vishnu, one of the divine emanations of God, in the form of a tiny

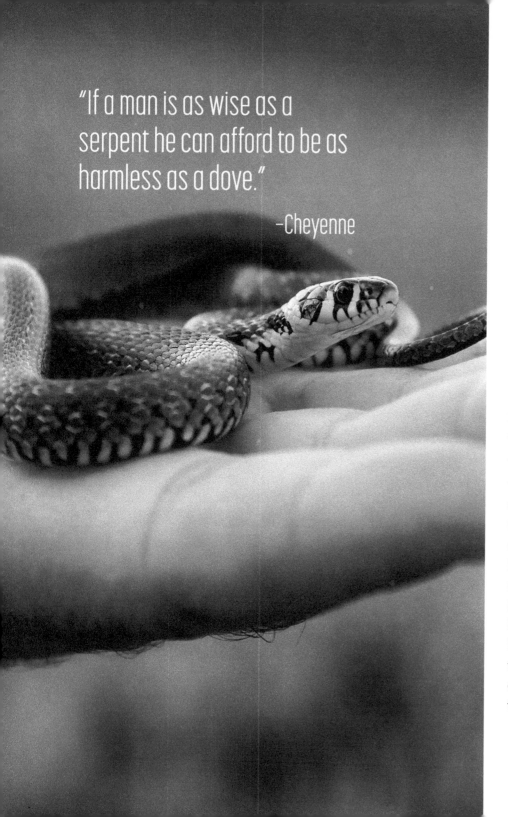

> "If a man is as wise as a serpent he can afford to be as harmless as a dove."
>
> —Cheyenne

serpent, into the palms of a devout Hindu woman named Gonika. He was a physician, scientist and author of the Yoga Sutras, short maxims for right living using the full practice of yoga, which means yoking with the divine. Patanjali proposed that we were all made up of prakriti (matter) and purusha (spirit). The purpose of yoga became the purification of prakriti (matter) so that the individual operates from pure purusha (spirit) within the context of the material world. Much of modern yoga is based on Patanjali's sutras.

Yoga continued to shift with the times. Physically based yoga, such as Tantra and eventually Hatha Yoga, which came about a number of centuries after Patanjali, brought in more advanced practices of asana (yoga poses) to support the body with better health and life fulfillment, a change from transcending the body, to celebrating the body as the temple of the divine.

Yoga is a shift in consciousness of simply 1%, to allow a new reality, new thought patterns and a new belief system to emerge that is in harmony with all of life.

Many modern yoga techniques practiced today are a result of these explorations and enhancements.

Central to most of yoga is a belief that, ultimately, we are all part of the same divine source. How we 'get back home' is multi-faceted. Yoga is a shift in consciousness of simply 1%, to allow a new reality, new thought patterns and a new belief system that is in harmony with all of life. Or, as some like to see it, yoga helps us remember our true selves. Amputation can offer a clean slate for the future, about who an amputee wants to be and how she wants to experience the fullness of life. Yoga plants new seeds of consciousness.

This brings us to now. **How can yoga, its gifts and traditions, benefit an amputee now?**

Benefits of yoga for an amputee

Yoga is a healing practice that makes life better for amputees, especially as they grapple with prosthetics, body image, pain, freedom of movement, and other residual effects of limb loss. In fact, many amputees experience yoga without even knowing it. When an amputee learns to walk or grip a cup, he is very present to the task at hand and is usually slowing down his breath to stay focused, building motor and mental control in spite of fears about falling or dropping something. This is meditation in action. Over time, that present moment awareness becomes a natural state, more solidified through an ongoing practice of yoga.

The positive mind/body connection that an amputee develops is refined, creating **new neural pathways** and often a new outlook on life. An amputee who practices yoga not only continues to build these stronger neural pathways, he also gains physical strength, flexibility and balance, and insight into the inner world of his emotions, accessing a holistic non-invasive way to heal trauma, pain , suffering and stress.

Pain is a big concern for amputees. Using yoga, an amputee is better able to recognize pain triggers, relax the mind, increase resilience and decrease reactivity to pain with yoga breathing (pranayama), poses (asana) and active rest (yoga nidra) .

Bad habits, such as smoking or spending the day glued to the couch, fall away, as an amputee begins to feel better through yoga. As health and mindset improve, more preventative actions, such as better nutrition and exercise become needed daily rituals that take over those bad habits.

Spiritually, through meditation to still the mind and contemplation on the concept of oneness with all of life, an amputee gains insight into the meaning of amputation, life purpose, and a sense of the wisdom gained from limb loss. Rather than feeling separate or isolated, an amputee, through yoga, will have a renewed sense of joy in life and a deeper connection to the world.

A person practicing yoga even for a short while sees changes almost immediately. New yoga practitioners report better sleep, better coping skills, more confidence, more energy, greater sex drive and more peace of mind. Seasoned yoga practitioners have better access to higher realms of consciousness, including fine-tuned body awareness as well as profound experiences of bliss. Long-term yoga practice evokes a deeper level of understanding about what it means to be whole, and the nature of life's purpose.

"Every living being is an engine geared to the wheelwork of the universe. Though seemingly affected only by its immediate surrounding, the sphere of external influence extends to infinite distance."
—Nikola Tesla

Strength
Stamina
Balance
Flexibility
Immunity
Energy
Confidence
Vitality
Peace
Health
Wisdom
Renewal
Creativity
Sleep
Sexuality
Restoration
Purpose
Clarity
Self-Realization
Relief
Love
Hope
Connection

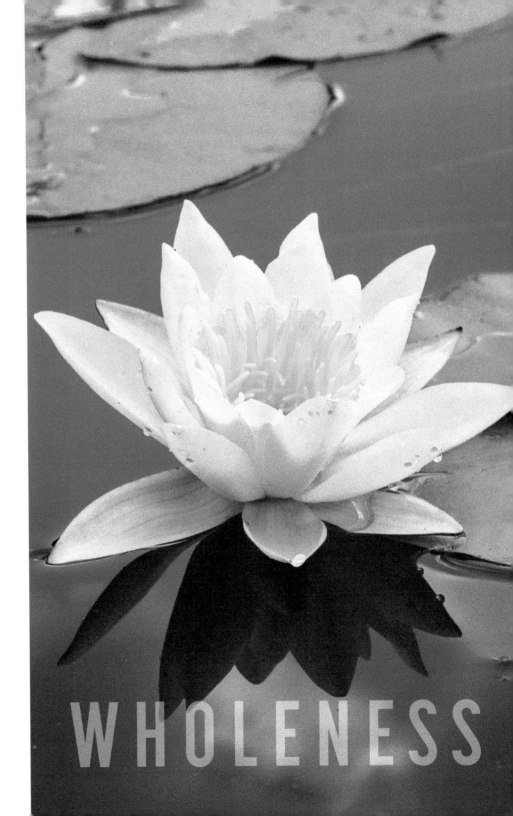

WHOLENESS

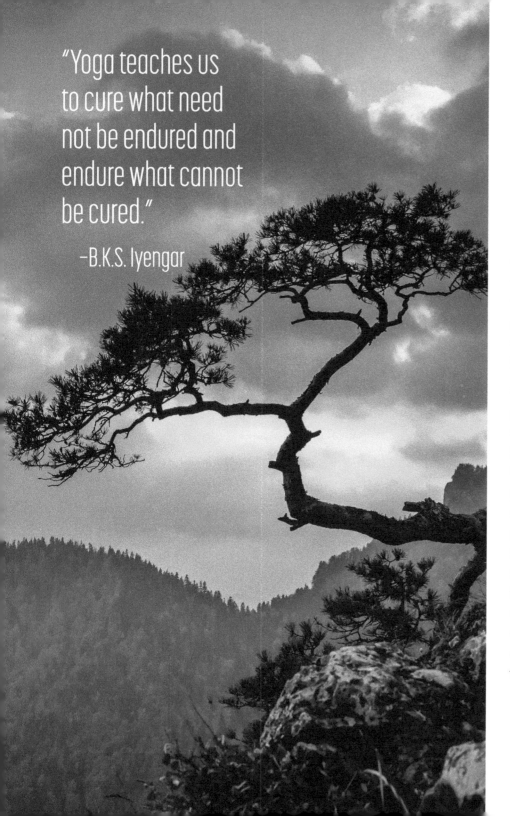

"Yoga teaches us to cure what need not be endured and endure what cannot be cured."

–B.K.S. Iyengar

What is required of an amputee to harness the benefits of yoga?

Commitment to one's own transformative joy and well-being through daily yoga practice, preferably at the same time each day, establishes a new healthy habit more fully.

When an amputee sets noble goals of health, wellness and wholeness through yoga, he becomes his own advocate, taking control of his life where possible. Life becomes more abundant when the practice of yoga is included, offering daily transformation in the body, mind and spirit. Perhaps this is the greatest benefit of yoga: **a renewed spirit of vitality, hope and health, which revolutionizes an amputee's whole being from the inside out.**

MEET JEFF

Jeff lost his lower right leg after multiple corrective surgeries from earlier injuries were unsuccessful. Given the option of leg amputation, Jeff chose to forego the risk of more surgical corrections in place of lower leg amputation.

Jeff is passionate about tennis, participating in adaptive tennis tournaments and advocating adaptive tennis to be approved as an official sport with the USTA (United States Tennis Association). Since losing his leg and increasing his commitment to fitness, Jeff has lost over 100 pounds and feels great. Once he met his 100 pound mark, he agreed to wear a tutu after being challenged by his trainer! What a brave guy.

His prosthesis, which has a Rush foot, helps him walk as if he had two legs. Because of that, he wears his prosthesis from the moment he wakes up in the morning to the moment he goes to sleep. He feels that the light weight of his prosthesis, combined with the energy feedback of his Rush foot, keeps him comfortable in his prosthesis all day. Yoga helps Jeff maintain his balance and keep up his tennis form.

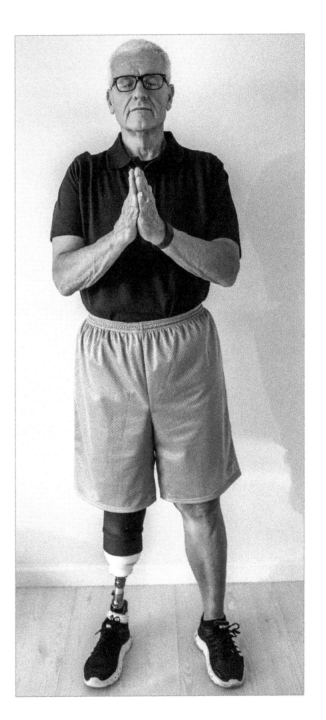

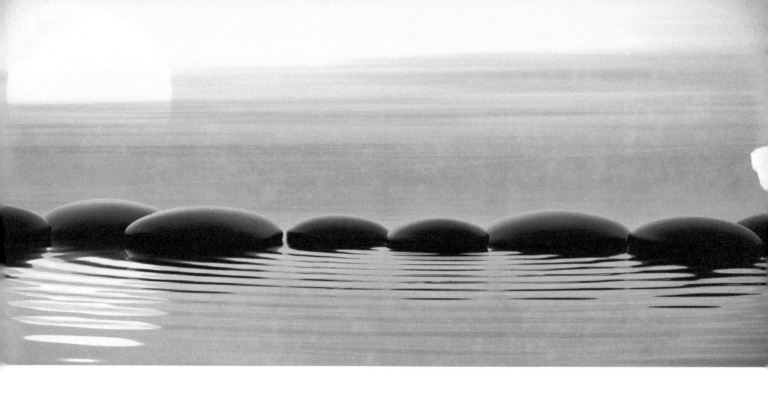

Wholeness Practice - The Royal Path

There are eight principles of the Royal Path of Yoga outlined in the Yoga Sutras (or threads), Patanjali's definitive text on yoga. These are:

YAMA (moral precepts)

NIYAMA (self-realization practices)

ASANA (yoga poses)

PRANAYAMA (yoga breathing)

PRATYAHARA (withdrawal of the senses)

DHARANA (focused concentration)

DHYANA (meditation)

SAMADHI (bliss)

Within the YAMAS and NIYAMAS there are ten sub-categories. The first five are considered 'external' practices, while the last five are considered 'internal' practices. The yamas and niyamas are personal to each practitioner. They enhance both the physical practice of yoga and the effects yoga has on an amputee's everyday life. For an amputee to best practice yoga breathing and poses, **compassion** and **self-care** play a vital role. It is far easier on the body, mind and spirit to come to yoga with no previous judgments about yoga, or about oneself, but to remain curious about the yoga journey itself.

YAMA	Social Ethics
Ahimsa	Compassion Non-violence
Satya	Truthfulness Non-deception
Asteya	Generosity Non-stealing
Aparigraha	Trust in Life Non-clinging
Brahmacharya	Moderation Non-greed

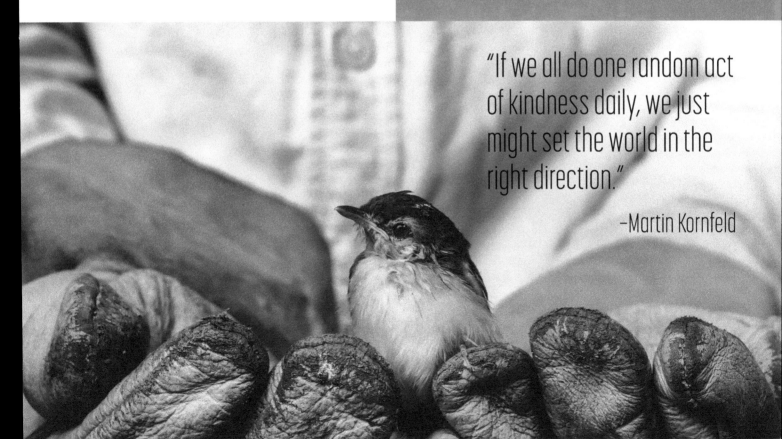

"If we all do one random act of kindness daily, we just might set the world in the right direction."

–Martin Kornfeld

NIYAMA	Personal Ethics
Shaucha	Self-care Purity
Santosha	Contentment Gratitude
Tapas	Discipline Commitment
Svadhyaya	Self-observation Study of Scriptures
Isvara Pranidhana	Surrender to God Humility

Take care of yourself.
In so doing you can change
your entire world.

NIYAMAS

Be kind to yourself.
Kindness to others
naturally follows.

YAMAS

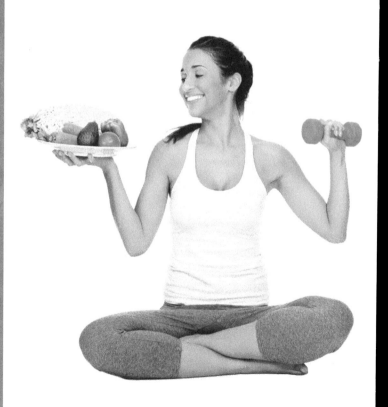

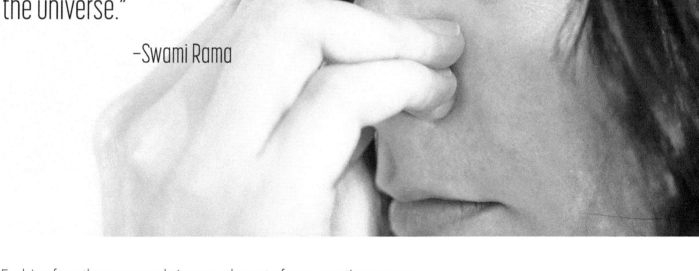

> "Pranayama literally means the ayama - the expansion or manifestation - of prana. Prana is the vital energy of the universe."
>
> –Swami Rama

Evolving from the yamas and niyamas , the rest of yoga practice emerges.

First comes PRANAYAMA, or breath control.

Yoga breathing, or pranayama, opens the door to a more relaxed, stronger, and more restful yoga practitioner. The breath is what separates yoga from stretching. Pranayama is not just a simple inhale and exhale. **Prana** means life force, while **yama** means control. Pranayama is a symbiotic relationship of give and receive, between the yoga practitioner and the life force that pervades all of life. Every yoga posture, every transition, is informed by a mindful observation of the breath. This helps the practitioner to stay present, rather than sinking into the past or over thinking the future.

When a yoga practitioner moves into a yoga pose, the breath shows her whether to go deeper into the pose, stay right where he/she is, or ease off. **Breathing (Pranayama)** in yoga has many components, and is intended to help the practitioner to regulate the breath for different effects in the body.

A Daily Yoga Ritual to Jumpstart your Day

After performing all your daily morning routines, go to a designated yoga space in your home. Set up all necessary props. **Light a candle. Read a short entry from a favorite inspirational book. Create an intention for your yoga practice.**

 Begin in a seated position with the eyes closed.
   a. Take deep inhalations and exhalations as you tune into your inner world.
   b. Focus on the moment.

 Begin pranayama.
   a. Inhale for a count of 3.
   b. Exhale for a count of 5.
   c. Do ten rounds of this breath.

 Add pratyahara.
   a. Notice the outer world falling away as you dive into your inner world.

 Begin asana.
   a. Fold forward , reaching the arms in front if available. Alternately, open the collarbone and lift the back of the heart up.
   b. Exhale. Stay in this forward fold for 3 breaths.
   c. Inhale roll up.
   d. Twist your torso to the right. Look over your right shoulder.
   e. Inhale back to center. Exhale twist to the left and look over your left shoulder.
   f. Roll onto your back.
   g. Hug your thighs, when available, into your chest. Rock side to side.
   h. Extend your right leg out as you keep the left thigh hugging in.
   i. Breathe in and out 3 times.
   j. Switch legs.

k. Roll thighs to the right as you open your arms, when available, into a 'T' position.

l. Breathe in and out 3 times.

m. Repeat on the left.

n. Roll to the side and sit up.

 Begin dharana.

a. Fix your eyes on a lit candle.

b. Continue to breathe in and out.

c. Slowly close your eyes and focus on your intention.

 Add dhyana. Let go of your focus and allow yourself to be still, without thinking of the future or the past.

 Invite samadhi, or a state of relaxed bliss as you continue to enjoy the fruits of your yoga practice.

a. Blow out your candle.

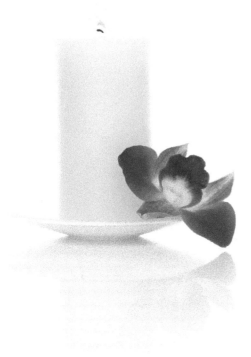 Get on with your day, peaceful, relaxed and energized.

ASANA (or yoga posture), next in the Royal Path, is translated as 'seat'. Sitting is usually comfortable for most of us. A steady easy pose is the goal in yoga postures and in life. With yoga, the pose is the seat of self-observation, mindful connection to each breath, and compassion for each sensation that arises. With increased awareness of one's physical, emotional and mental self, comes a willingness to change habits and beliefs that keep the practitioner from living in harmony and balance.

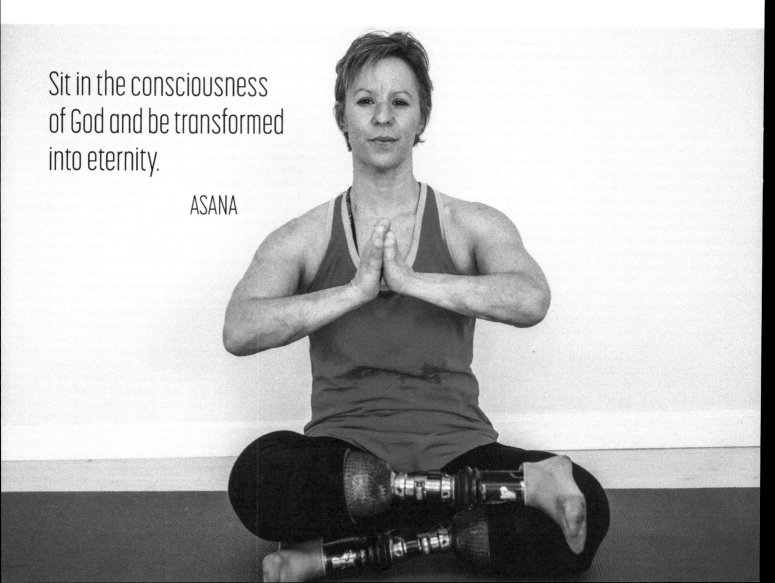

Sit in the consciousness of God and be transformed into eternity.

ASANA

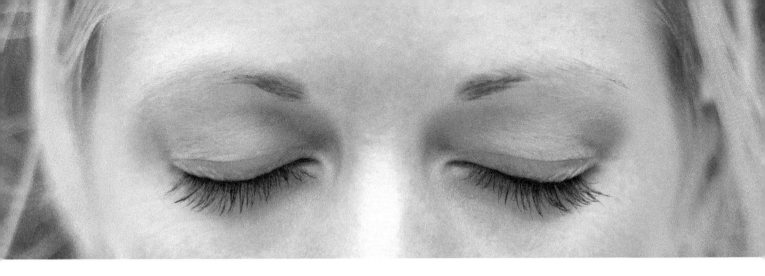

The deeper an amputee dives into her yoga practice, the more the outer world falls away. The inner world becomes alive with new awareness and vitality. Old memories, pains and clinging beliefs start to release from the system. For an amputee, this includes the release of traumas. This step in the Royal Path is called PRATYAHARA, or withdrawal of the outer world to focus on the inner world.

DHARANA, or focused attention, organically arises from the inward study of one's self. Think of dharana as the direct observance of the experiences brought on by yoga practice. Dharana gives permission for the yogi to become still in the mind.

What lies before us and what lies behind us are small matters compared to what lies within us.
—Henry David Thoreau

Dharana leads to DHYANA, or meditation, when the self begins to transform the busy thoughts of the mind and merge with simple presence. Meditation is the steady internal observance of the present moment.

At this moment of heightened meditation (dhyana), the final step on the Royal Path, that of merging with the divine nature, occurs. Known as SAMADHI or complete absorption in to the Absolute (God, Universe, Higher Power, Creative Life Force), this culminating practice is the known experience of our oneness with all that is. This blissful union with the eternal Being is limitless.

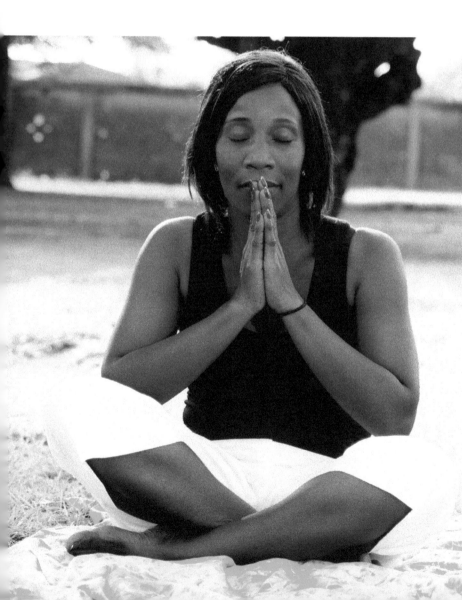

"Dhyana is retaining one's tranquil state of mind in any circumstance, unfavorable as well as favorable, and not being disturbed or frustrated even when adverse conditions present themselves one after another."

–D.T. Suzuki

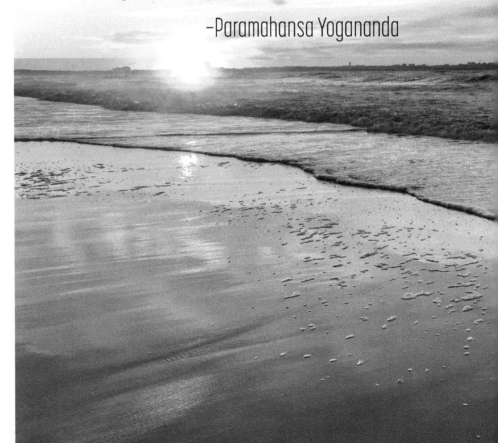

For an amputee, SAMADHI is the ultimate reminder that no matter what the body has gone through, or what was lost, the amputee is whole, ONE with all that exists and full of endless possibility.

Modern yoga has its benefits, such as improved coordination, flexibility, strength, stamina, focus and overall well-being, but the ancient roots of the Royal Path provide the wings for an amputee to live to full potential.

"Not an unconscious state or mental chloroform without wilful return, Samadhi but extends my realm of consciousness beyond the limits of my mortal frame to the bondaries of eternity, where I, the Cosmic Sea, watch the little ego floating in Me."

–Paramahansa Yogananda

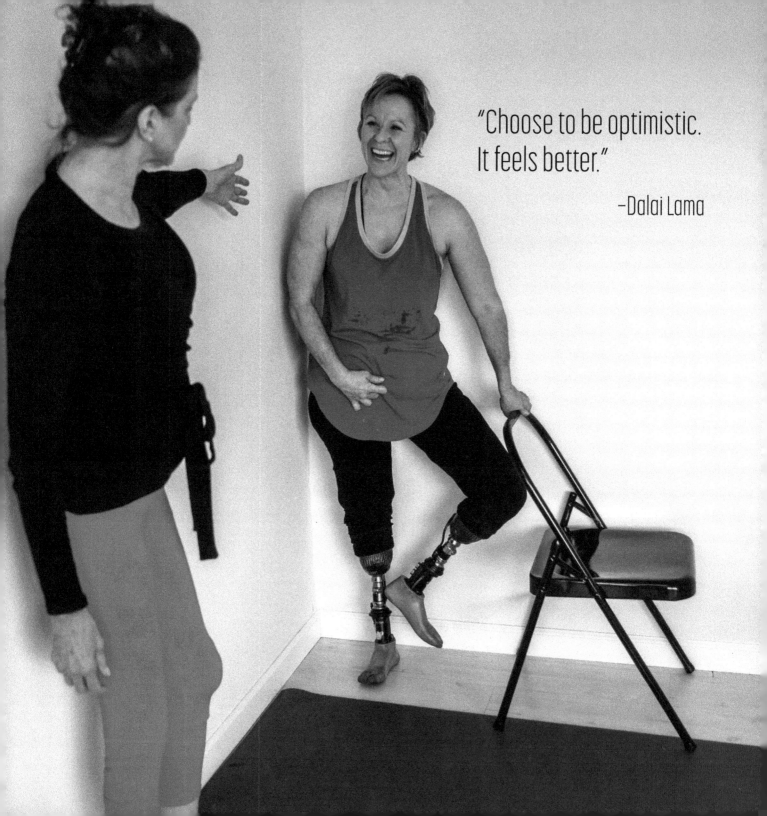

"Choose to be optimistic.
It feels better."

–Dalai Lama

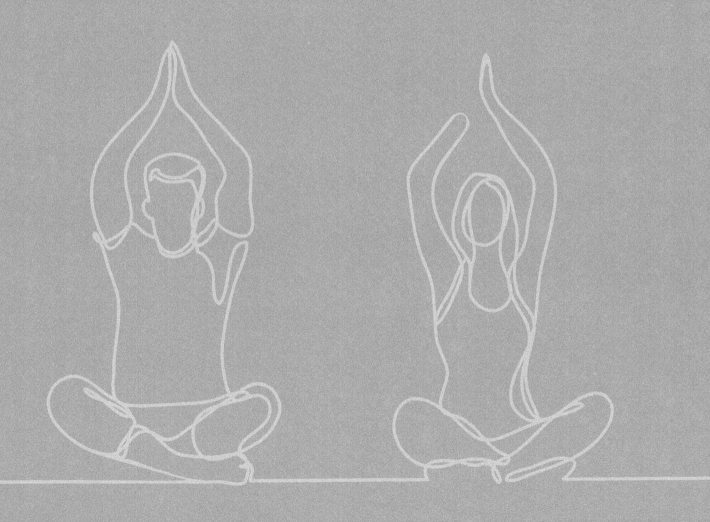

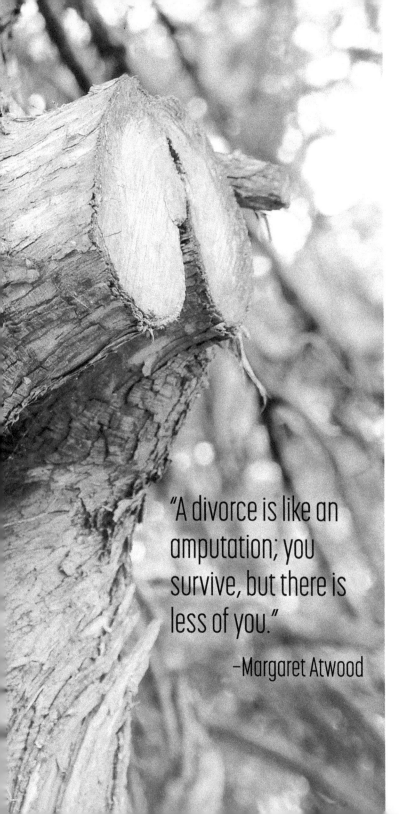

"A divorce is like an amputation; you survive, but there is less of you."

-Margaret Atwood

What is an amputation?

"An amputation is a cutting off a vital limb or limbs that contribute to the mobility of a person. Amputation includes removal of bone, muscle tissue, nerves, tendons, cartilage, veins, arteries and surrounding connective tissue. Amputations can be above or below knee, or in the upper extremities above or below the elbow." *(See resources)*

Extreme loss, for those who have not experienced amputation, can feel like an amputation, but, as any amputee can attest, the quote on this page barely scratches the surface of what it means to lose a limb or to live without limbs. The word amputation has a quality of violence, extreme pain, deformity and permanence. But for amputees, amputation can also be the beginning of a sacred journey into what it truly means to be a whole person.

Amputation can actually propel a person to become MORE of who they truly are. Tremendous loss always contains the potential to go above and beyond what was thought humanly possible. Amputees are incredible like that.

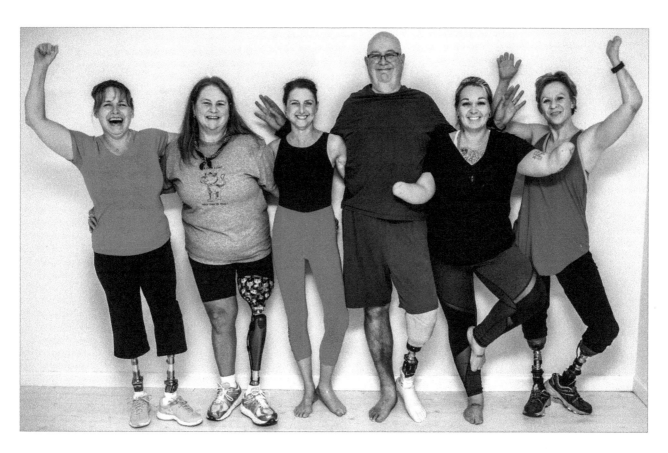

Reasons for limb loss

The majority of amputations are due to cardiovascular and diabetic illnesses (70-80%). Lower limb amputations account for most amputations. Upper limb amputation is commonly a result of work related injury (often the dominant arm), cancer and traumatic injury. Partial hand amputations are quite common as a subgroup within upper limb amputations.

According to statistics, there are at least **185,000 amputations** yearly in the United States. Globally there are over one million amputations annually.

There are six main reasons for amputation.

1. Congenital limb difference
2. Cancer
3. Traumatic injury, like war and car accidents
4. Cardiovascular and diabetic related diseases
5. Sepsis and other infections
6. Work related injury

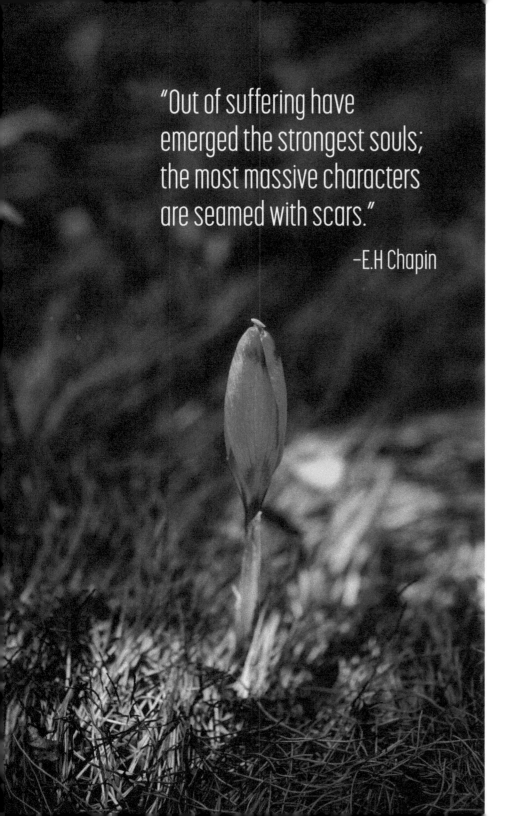

"Out of suffering have emerged the strongest souls; the most massive characters are seamed with scars."

–E.H Chapin

Additionally, almost **3,000 people lose a limb or limbs each week.** Within the United States, there are nearly two million amputees. Globally the amount keeps changing.

Amputation due to **war injury** has other referred injuries and psychological symptoms which can compound trauma. In the United States, the cost of diabetes and cardiovascular care to the medical system alone is rising to almost $10 billion annually. This means a lot more people are vulnerable to amputation, and a lot more people can learn how to fully participate in their well-being by learning yoga.

Types of amputees

Amputees come in all shapes and sizes. Depending upon the illness or injury, orthopedic surgeons will perform a variety of different types of amputations. The objectives of amputation vary as well. In most cases, amputation is performed to save a life. In other cases, the limb is simply unsalvageable due to multiple surgeries or a damaging accident. Some amputations are partial, with the insertion of a connective titanium rod directly into an exposed residual limb. This is known as **Osseointegration**. For children, surgeons may insert grow-able rods inside children's amputated bones to avoid full amputations. In all cases, amputation is a severe loss of limb with a necessary period of recovery for body, mind and spirit.

Amputations are divided into two types: *lower extremity* and *upper extremity amputations*; however, amputees can have multiple limb loss in both the upper and lower body. Those amputees are known as **bilateral** (two legs or two arms), **trilateral** (three limbs) and **quadrilateral** (four limbs). **Lower extremity amputations** include anything below the belly button, from the hips all the way down to the toes. **Upper extremity amputations** include the fingers all the way to the collarbone.

Following is a complete list of the types of amputations that occur.

Lower Extremity Amputations

Toe, foot and ankle amputations

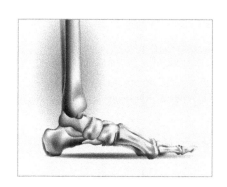

- **Trans phalangeal Amputation:** Removal of part of a toe.

- **Trans metatarsal Amputation (TMA):** Removal of all or part of the top portion of the metatarsals.

- **Lisfranc Amputation:** Removal of all or part of the mid to top portion of the foot, at the metatarsal joint.

- **Chopart Amputation:** Removal of all or part of the mid to top portion of the foot at the ankle joint.

- **Syme Amputation:** Removal of the ankle and foot, while keeping the heel pad for better weight bearing.

Toe amputation can add walking and balance issues, as can foot and ankle amputations. Foot and ankle amputees are sometimes able to wear prosthetics, depending on comfort and fit.

Leg and hip amputations

- **Transtibial Amputation:** Removal of the lower leg and ankle below the knee.

- **Knee Disarticulation:** Also known as the Callendar amputation, this procedure removes the tendon at the knee rather than the bone, for better weight bearing.

- **Supracondylar Amputation:** Also known as the Gritti- Stokes amputation, the upper leg is amputated, but the patella is surgically kept for better weight bearing.

- **Rotationplasty:** Used primarily for younger patients with cancer or injury, rotationplasty involves reattaching and revolving the lower portion of a limb to the upper limb, making the joint, such as an ankle, become a knee.

- **Transfemoral Amputation:** Removal of the leg including the knee up to the femur, with either a short or medium length femur.

- **Hip Disarticulation:** Complete removal of the lower limb at the hip.

- **Hemipelvectomy:** Removal of the pelvis and leg, sometimes including the pubic bone.

- **Internal Hemipelvectomy:** Removal of the hip with the leg remaining.

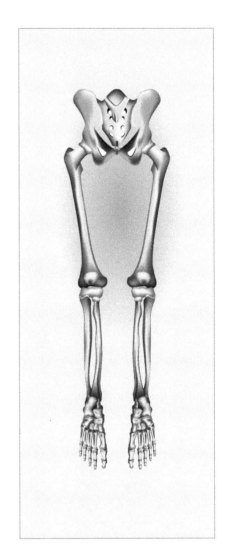

Hemipelvectomies and hip disarticulations are very rare, and are often indicated for cancer and accidents.

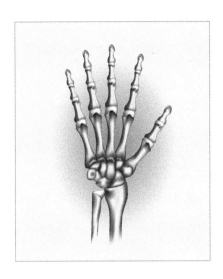

Upper Extremity Amputations

Finger and Wrist Amputations

- **Transcarpal Amputation:** Removal of fingers or portions of the hand.

- **Wrist disarticulation:** Separation of the radius and ulna from the wrist, with removal of the wrist and hand, often used for children.

Forearm to Shoulder Amputations

- **Transradial Amputation, distal and proximal:** Removal of the lower arm below the elbow joint.

- **Elbow disarticulation:** Removal of the lower arm at the joint.

- **Krunenberg procedure:** Once the lower arm and wrist have been removed, the ulna and radius are redesigned into a pincer for grasp and release.

- **Transhumeral Amputation:** Removal of the upper arm and lower arm, hand, wrist and elbow below the shoulder joint.

- **Shoulder disarticulation:** Removal of the arm from the shoulder joint.

- **Forequarter amputation:** Removal of the entire arm, shoulder joint, scapula and part of the collarbone.

With all upper extremity amputations, the goal is to maintain some level of pronation and supination in the shoulders, in addition to keeping, whenever possible, the elbow.

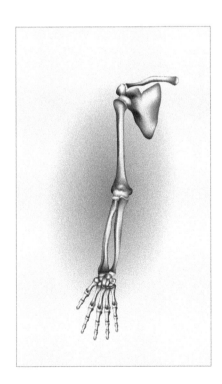

Prosthetics

What is a prosthetic?

A prosthetic is a replacement for a part of the body normally visible and/or functional, which is missing. Prosthetics include limbs, eyes, breasts, and many other body parts. In most cases, prosthetics are associated with limbs.

Types of Prosthetics

Prosthetics, for many amputees, help them feel whole again after limb loss. The ability to perform daily tasks with relative ease is well worth the added effort it takes to wear a prosthesis. When someone is limited in their ability to carry out normal daily functions, the strain and stress add up. While amputees indeed learn to adapt to their new life, prosthetics can really help make life a little easier for many amputees.

Parts of a prosthesis.

The prosthetic limb is an actual limb, made of any combination of carbon fiber, plastic, titanium, wood and foam. The socket is the fitted top in which the residual limb resides. It is the socket that makes or breaks a prosthetic limb's comfort. A plaster cast is taken of the residual limb, from which a mold is made. The mold is then filled with a plastic substance that holds the residual limb. The socket needs to fit perfectly for an amputee to avoid damage or injury to the residual limb.

The attachment holds the limb in place. Depending on the needs and comfort of the amputee the attachment may be a suction system, a pin system, a plastic or silicone suspension sleeve, or a harness. The attachment allows the amputee to feel secure.

Prosthetics fall into the following categories:

- Functional

- Cosmetic

- Robotic

- Computerized

- Athletic

Amputees wear their prosthetics based on a combination of these needs and preferences.

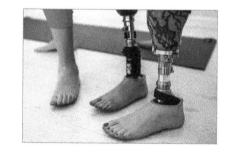

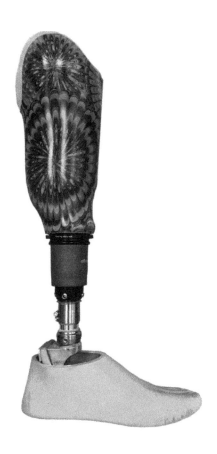

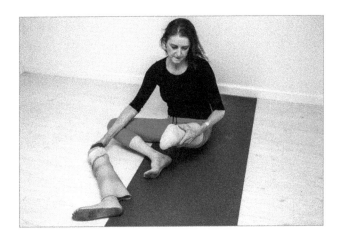

Parts of a prosthetic leg:

• Socket

• Skeleton

• Knee Joint

• Pylon

• Suspension system

• Foot

The control system for most leg amputees is the body's natural movement, and its relationship with the ground. Some leg prosthetics are battery or computer controlled, such as computerized limbs. For upper amputees, the control system ranges from a simple "claw" to the sophisticated myoelectric hand which moves based on nerve impulses of the residual limb.

There are over fifty prosthetic feet available, according to the Amputee Coalition of America. The simplest of these feet is the **Sach** foot, a non-bendable foot with some give due to its rubber heel. Mostly used by less ambulatory amputees, the Sach foot provides some stability and at least the ability to walk. More advanced prosthetic feet have single axis and multiple axis ankles which allow greater mobility and range of motion to move over various terrains, adjusting to the forward, backward and side to side weight of the gait in the amputee. Dynamic response prosthetic feet are usually open-toed and lifelike. The dynamic response foot can handle high impact, like running.

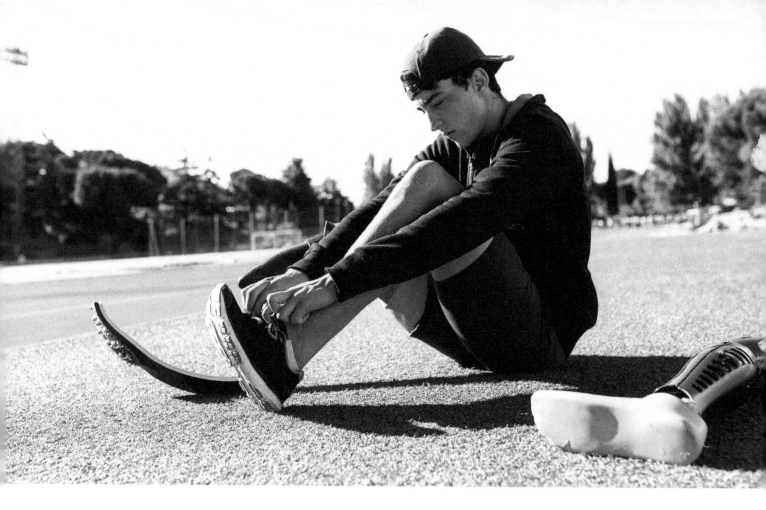

There are two important prosthetic necessities for an amputee to feel the best. The **socket** needs to fit very well, supporting the weight and pressure of the amputee, with a special focus on any unique features of the residual limb to relieve pressure and add pressure where needed to reduce breakdown of the skin. The **alignment** of the prosthetic limb to the body is of equal importance. The amputee must feel stable and balanced.

For a leg amputee, the prosthetic foot and knee influence the way she approaches yoga. A Sach foot will give an amputee grounding but it won't be flexible enough for poses that rise on to the toes, or require a turn in at the hip. Dynamic response feet are excellent for athletes who do advanced vinyasa practices, such as Astanga but may have too much bounce for the static poses in yoga. In most cases, prosthetics enhance the life of an amputee, bringing them back to a sense of normalcy and wholeness.

For arm amputees, depending on the length of the residual limb and the availability of elbows and /or shoulders, many forego prosthetics. The prosthetics can add extra weight as well as limit range of motion. If arm prosthetics are worn, they act as an additional yoga prop, along with other yoga props such as straps. Prosthetists are making arm prosthetics that have less restriction in shoulder and elbow joints , and are even innovating with what looks like a " ball and socket", or a plunger, for those arm amputees who want to practice yoga or other weight bearing exercise with a prosthesis. Newer arm prosthetics, such as the **VECTR** "vector-enhanced compression and tissue relief", which compress the residual limb in order to distribute tissue and bone more evenly, and the motion control upper arm prosthetic, which allows bending of the wrist through nerve impulses, are helping to change the way arm amputees can do yoga. Arm prosthetics , in some cases, can add more balance to an amputee's yoga practice, and protect remaining limbs from overuse.

Prosthetic innovation is often the result of patient demand. More amputees are finding yoga, and wanting to use their prosthetics as an integral part of their yoga practice. Prosthetics are making waves in the world, enhancing the way amputees live life.

What an exciting time for technology, science, and spirituality to merge!

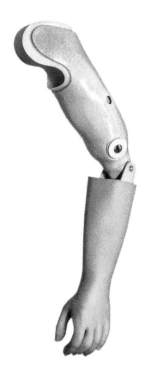

Parts of a prosthetic arm:

- Socket

- Harness

- Elbow

- Wrist

- Hand

Basic needs for amputees

All humans, to live a fulfilling healthy life, thrive best when six basic needs are met. For any amputee, when any of those needs are not met, imbalance in the physical, mental, emotional and spiritual realms can take place, each affecting the whole of the person.

The six basic needs are physical, emotional, social , intellectual, spiritual and creative.

Below is a chart showing how Yoga meets these basic needs.

Physical	YOGA	Emotional	YOGA	Social	YOGA
Air	Breathing techniques	Peace	Being in the moment	Friendship	Non competitive learning environment
Water	Balancing body fluids through movement	Compassion	Heart centered	Companionship	Camaraderie
Sleep	Harmonizing nerves helps insomnia	Belief in possibility	Trying new poses	Trust	Yoga therapy
Rest	Relaxation of mind and body	Self Esteem	Loving your body	Peer Support	Support and experience of other amputees
Exercise	Yoga Poses	Security	Yoga Props	Fun	Group Yoga activities

Intellectual	YOGA	Spiritual	YOGA	Creative	YOGA
Challenge	Problem solving with postures	Higher purpose	Connecting to wholeness	Self expression	Developing emotional vocabulary by befriending the body
Motivation	Increased physical freedom	Awareness of soul	God is in all of us	Inspiration	Breathing increases vitality
Learning new things	New neural pathways	Bliss and joy	Healing limb loss	Improvisation	Creative thinking
Developing different parts of the brain	L/R brain activation through crossing the midline in poses	Inner peace consciousness	Establishing equanimity	Imagination	Limitless potential

It is my belief that amputees have additional basic needs, which will be explored in more depth throughout this book.

These include:

• Grief and recovery

• Trauma recovery

• Personal hygiene and self care

• Empowerment

• Self acceptance and vulnerability

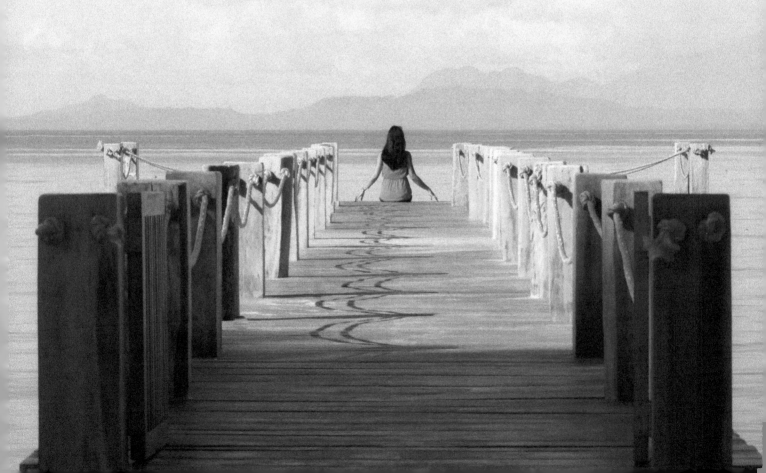

"Contentment does not mean
I desire nothing; but rather,
it's the simple decision to be
happy with what I have."

–Paula Rollo

Yoga practices to feel secure

Prosthetics can make an amputee feel more secure when practicing yoga.

The following yoga practices will support you to feel secure, confident and at peace with your life right now. For each practice, check in using this chart before and after to see how yoga has improved your body, mind and spirit.

Check In	Body	Mind	Spirit
How I feel *before* yoga			
How I feel *after* yoga			

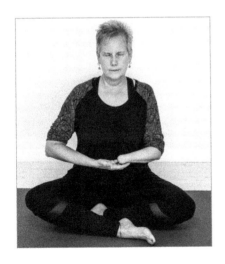

PRACTICE ONE: Just Breathe

1. Sit, in a chair or on the floor, and breathe.

2. Close your eyes.

3. Notice your breath.

4. Where is it beginning?

5. Where is it ending?

6. What is the quality of your breath?

7. Does it have a texture?

8. If you are a visual person, your breath may conjure up an image, or a color.

9. Ask yourself "how do I feel about my breath?" "Am I okay with being here right now?"

10. What are the sensations in my body? Notice where you are drawn to in your body.

11. Open your eyes, look around and come back to the present moment, noticing how you feel.

Even in the space of a few breaths, profound awareness can emerge. You might recall a memory from childhood, an ache from an old wound, a person long forgotten. Usually, memories are telling you something. The body has a way of storing information until you are ready to hear.

PRACTICE TWO: The Mindful Moment

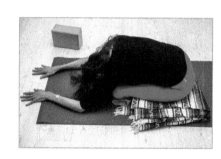

1. Breathe in.

2. As you breathe in, say to yourself silently,' I am breathing in."

3. Breathe out.

4. As you breathe out, say to yourself "I am breathing out."

5. Do this for five to ten rounds of breath.

Notice your sensations and feelings as you feel the echo of the practice in your body, mind and spirit. This "I am "breath teaches the practice of mindfulness. Note that we do not fill in the blanks with "I am ____". Being mindful of the moment is enough.

PRACTICE THREE: Relax your grip

1. Relax your hands in your lap. Or, relax your shoulders.

2. Breathe in.

3. As you do so, gently curl your fingers in and say to yourself "I am curling my fingers in." Or, shrug your shoulders to your ears and say to yourself "I am shrugging my shoulders to my ears."

4. Breathe out. As you do so, gently uncurl your fingers and say to yourself "I am uncurling my fingers." Or, say to yourself "I am relaxing my shoulders "

5. Do this five to ten times.

What do you notice? How can you carry this technique of mindful action into your day?

This simple exercise can help you get back to the present moment any time of the day.

PRACTICE FOUR: Release your stress

1. Stand or sit.

2. Inhale.

3. Lengthen your spine. Exhale.

4. Tuck the chin in as you roll down towards the floor, vertebra by vertebra.

5. If standing, keep the knees softly bent as you roll down to rest your belly on or towards your thighs.

6. Breathe out completely until you feel you have released all the stale air.

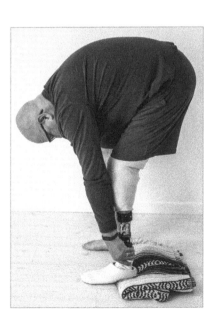

7. Stay in a forward fold for a few breaths. Sway your torso from side to side as your head, neck and shoulders completely succumb to the forward bend.

8. Feel as if all the "shoulds" and "have-tos" roll off your shoulders and float away.

9. Keeping the tailbone slightly tucked under, stack your vertebrae as you roll up to standing or sitting, inhaling on your way up.

10. Exhale. Repeat this sequence three to five times.

This moving posture is cooling and calming to the body. It shows you how to stay in tune with your body, mind and emotions in each moment.

When confronting limb loss and its effect on basic needs, these four simple yoga practices can change your mindset and reduce your tension rapidly. If a short five-minute yoga technique can do that for you, imagine what a full hour of yoga every day can do for your life?

Find your inner mountain

The home base for all yoga poses is Mountain Pose or Tadasana. A mountain is solid, strong, immovable, and magnificent. Mountains uplift and inspire us. And, they give us hope. For amputees, mountain pose is an inner experience of profound possibility as well as an outward physical journey of strength and stability. The qualities of a mountain are qualities that amputees possess in truckloads, although they might not always know that. Amputees must pull up every ounce of bravery,

While we may be wobbly on the outside, our inner resolve is immovable, our vision for ourselves magnificent once we choose to thrive in spite of our limb loss.

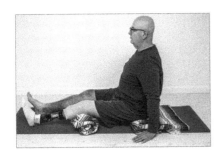

commitment, love and focus they possess to recover from amputation. When we get to know our inner mountain, retrieving it when we need it, we feel protected, empowered and confident.

Let's explore seated mountain pose.

1. Sit in an upright chair or on the floor with legs extended.

2. Take a deep breath.

3. As you breathe in draw your navel back towards your spine.

4. As you exhale expand your collar bones and relax your shoulders.

5. Continue breathing this way as you settle into your pelvis and lengthen your spine.

6. Feel the power of your spine as you continue deep breathing.

7. Allow the head to relax on the neck as you press into your sitz bones to keep the spine strong.

"Wholeness is not simply having four limbs. Wholeness is knowing that you are complete within yourself, just as you are."

–Marsha T Danzig

8. Close your eyes. Imagine that you are a strong, immovable mountain.

9. What is possible?

10. Open your eyes when you are ready.

11. Bring your inner mountain into your day.

12. Know that you are whole, strong and confident.

As you learn more about adapting yoga to your specific type of amputation, remember that *each yoga pose begins with your inner mountain and evolves from there.*

MEET AIMEE

"It's amazing, the people you meet." —Aimee

Aimee was in a terrible car accident that damaged her left leg. She had an elective amputation and is now thriving as a below knee amputee. Her amputation opened her eyes to a whole new group of people - **amputees** *- which led her to her current career as a patient advocate for a prosthetist. Her own experiences of amputation and rehabilitation help her help other amputees navigate the new terrain of living as an amputee. While her knee seal system prosthetic with detachable feet for different activities is quite functional, it is the different lace sockets that she wears that make a fashion statement. She feels that lace, combined with the industrial look of the prosthesis, is a great balance of femininity and strength. Says Aimee "I just love it."*

Aimee was in a wheelchair for nearly two years. Having an amputation and subsequent prosthesis were certainly life changers, but, in her case, her prosthesis restored her independence and sense of wholeness. For Aimee, feeling whole has everything to do with being able to function like she did before her limb loss. **She wouldn't change a thing about what happened to her.** *The people she has met, both*

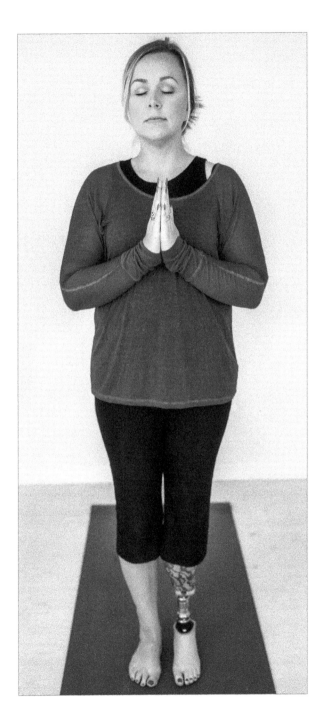

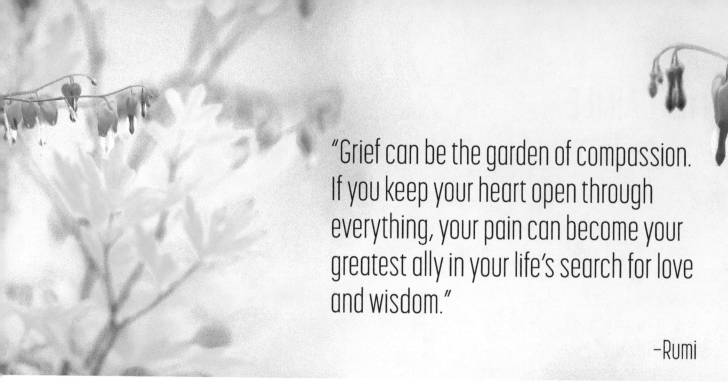

"Grief can be the garden of compassion. If you keep your heart open through everything, your pain can become your greatest ally in your life's search for love and wisdom."

–Rumi

amputees and the support team that help them, are amazing. The spirits of the people she has met inspire her.

Aimee's experience of yoga began with her introduction to me and this book. Yoga, she feels, tests her limits while also relaxing her. It has caused to her to be more health conscious and take better care of herself.

Aimee remarks "Amputation is probably one of the worst days of your life, comparable to losing a loved one because you are losing a part of yourself. And there's a grieving process to that. Every amputee is at a different stage in their grieving process. A lot of people don't make it past the initial shock, getting depressed. Yoga is so helpful for people to move through their grief. Yoga shows other amputees that it is possible to get back to a good life."

CHAPTER THREE | A FULFILLING LIFE WITH YOGA

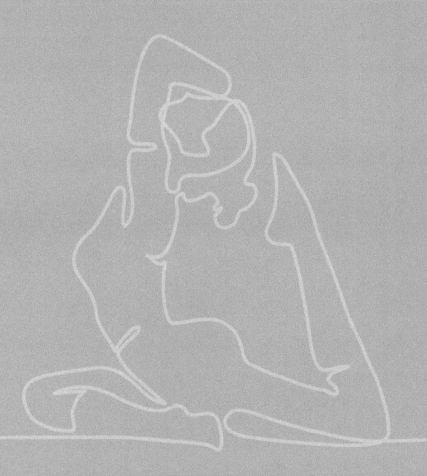

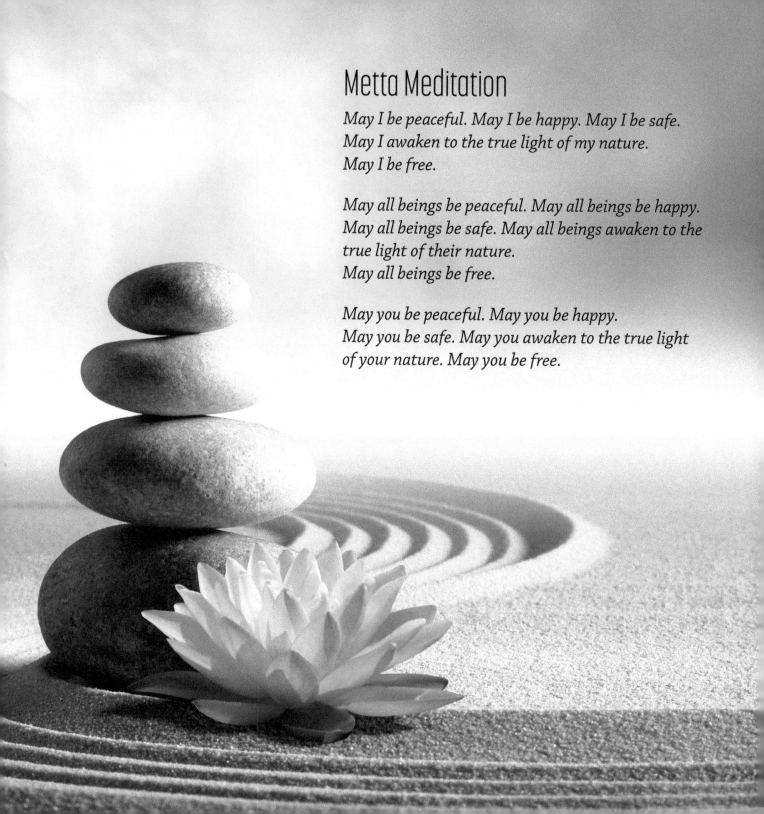

Metta Meditation

May I be peaceful. May I be happy. May I be safe.
May I awaken to the true light of my nature.
May I be free.

May all beings be peaceful. May all beings be happy.
May all beings be safe. May all beings awaken to the
true light of their nature.
May all beings be free.

May you be peaceful. May you be happy.
May you be safe. May you awaken to the true light
of your nature. May you be free.

Love Yourself

Metta, which means loving-kindness, is an ancient compassion practice, older than Buddhism (2500 years), from India, which teaches us to wish well to all living beings, including ourselves. Metta meditation is a stand-alone practice, but can easily be added to a yoga practice at the beginning or end. Research shows that **metta meditation** reduces anxiety, depression, lower back pain and stress. In addition, metta meditation invites deep, uninterrupted sleep, excellent mental focus and radiant skin.

Below is a simple **metta** meditation practice to enjoy.

1. Inhale and exhale three times.

2. Begin this meditation by saying metta meditation to yourself. After saying the prayer to yourself, say it to all living beings, and finally anyone with whom you have a conflict.

   May I be peaceful. May I be happy. May I be safe. May I awaken to the true light of my nature. May I be free.

   May all beings be peaceful. May all beings be happy. May all beings be safe. May all beings awaken to the true light of their nature. May all beings be free.

   May you be peaceful. May you be happy. May you be safe. May you awaken to the true light of your nature. May you be free.

3. End the practice with three inhalations and exhalations.

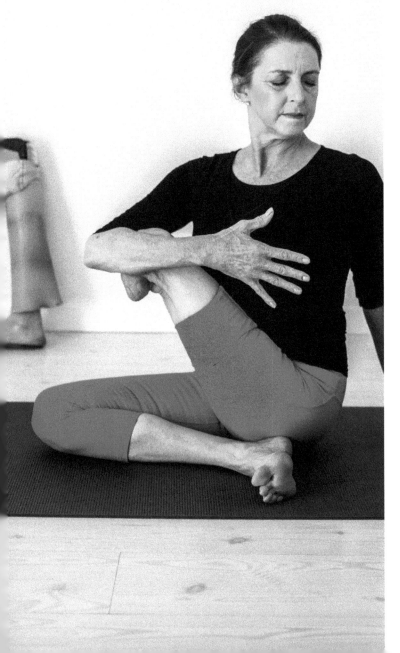

I learned to re-direct my thoughts towards who I have become now because of my limb loss, rather than what I might have been.

Making peace with your amputation through Yoga

Self-Acceptance and Compassion

Self-acceptance is so important for amputees' recovery.

How does **yoga** help amputees find self-acceptance? The eight-limbed path: yama, niyama, asana, pranayama, pratyahara, dharana, dhyana, and samadhi, provides some clues. As a reminder, the two foundational steps of yoga are the **yamas and niyamas**. The yamas prepare our hearts and minds not only for our exploration of yoga, but also for our daily lives. The niyamas keep us committed to our spiritual growth and well-being. The yamas and niyamas, like all of yoga, are there to help us reclaim our wholeness.

Self-acceptance came late to me. I had an extreme fear of being visible and stared at. I was constantly on guard, and at times I still revert to my former ways when I am feeling too vulnerable. My commitment to yoga has taught me to stay focused, that small changes make big differences, and strong emotions need to be respected rather than suppressed.

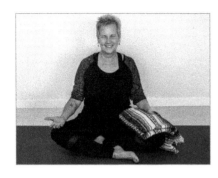

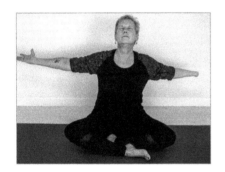

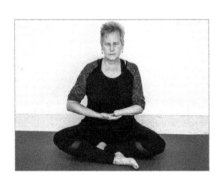

The Gentle Approach: A Self-Acceptance Yoga Practice

Breathe

1. Sit in a comfortable position.

2. Close the eyes.

3. Take seven deep breaths in and out.

4. Circle the arms above the head and back down. Alternately lift the sternum up.

5. With each circle or lift of the sternum say to yourself 'I accept myself exactly as I am'.

6. Do this three times.

7. Bring the arms back to the center.

8. Close the eyes.

9. Breathe in and out seven times.

10. Say silently to yourself 'I accept myself exactly as I am'.

11. Notice any sensations you have.

12. Complete your practice by stretching.

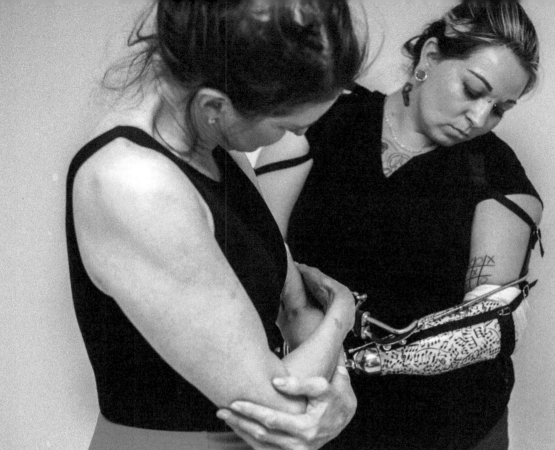

Love always heals.

Compassion in Action

Compassion is an act of love. Pain, anxiety, stress and suffering produce so many negative effects on the body, mind and spirit that the simple act of compassion can become a catalyst for health. Compassion produces the relaxation response in a person's body. This means that elevated hormone levels normalize when a person practices compassion. Pain is alleviated; joy and happiness increase. Vitality is renewed. Gratitude is restored which in turn enhances feel good hormones in the brain. Compassion for yourself and others gives you greater ability to accept yourself, missing limb/s and all.

Compassion Practice: Welcome your body

1. Close your eyes.

2. Scan your entire body slowly, beginning at the head and going all the way down to the floor.

3. With each part of the body that you focus on, say to that body part "I love you. I accept you. You are whole."

4. Include your residual limb/s and scars.

5. You may want to linger at certain spots, and pass over others. Take note, without judgment.

6. Absorb the experience.

7. Practice as often as you need.

This practice helps amputees lovingly come to accept their new body and develop a healthy relationship with the body they now have.

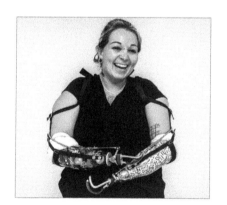

Ahimsa practice with Juanita

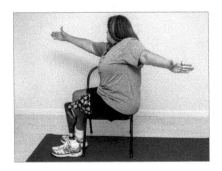

1. Sit comfortably in a chair.

2. Inhale stretch one arm forward and the other arm back. Or, press the right side of the chest forward and the left side of the chest back.

3. Exhale.

4. Switch sides.

5. Pay attention to sensations.

6. Be kind to yourself.

7. Decide if you would like to transition to the floor for a deep relaxation. You can also stay seated in the chair with the eyes closed, taking ten to fifteen deep breaths as you relax.

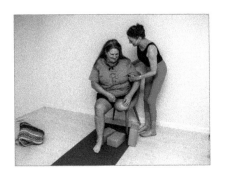

8. Ask for help if you need it!

9. If able, come onto your back.

10. If able, rest your legs on the edge of a chair.

11. Alternately extend the legs to the floor.

12. Close the eyes.

13. Relax.

14. Make sure you are comfortable. Again, be kind to yourself.

15. Take ten to fifteen deep breaths.

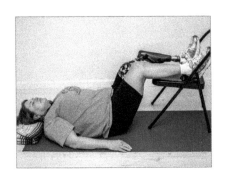

Empower yourself

Personal hygiene and self-care for amputees

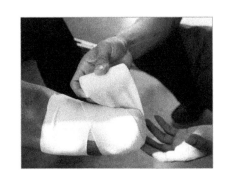

Valuing one's self-physically, emotionally and spiritually makes all the difference in an amputee's ability to thrive in life. In yoga the practice of self-care is called **Shaucha**. Shuacha is not about taking a shower and looking presentable, although that is important. Shaucha is about caring for the soul, nurturing the spirit and the mind, as well as caring for the body.

There are certain self-care techniques that are useful for amputees. Taking care of the residual limb is a vital and necessary part of living well with an amputation. The residual limb or limbs should be washed daily with mild soap and water. Drying the limb completely is essential as well, to avoid excess moisture from creeping, in which affects prosthetics and can lead to infection.

Because of issues with circulation, the amputee should never lean directly on the top of the limb, as tears in skin as well as bone spurs may occur. If swelling is a constant issue with residual limbs, the amputee should not hang the limb over chairs, pillows, beds or other objects when the prosthesis is not in use. A lot of amputees use leg shrinkers at night to avoid swelling.

For some amputees with limited mobility, elevating the residual limb too high can cause the hips or knee to lock.

Blisters and sores can develop with wear and tear on the residual limb. When possible, it is better to stay off the residual limb until sores are healed. Excess redness in an area may mean the prosthesis needs adjustment to protect from further damage.

Callouses are a part of an amputee's life. They are important for an amputee, as skin that is too soft where there is friction with the prosthesis leads to skin break down. Staying away from astringents, such as alcohol, or powders, such as corn starch, keep the limb protected.

Amputees who have gone through osseointegration must be diligent about wound and skin care as they now are living with exposed bone and other vital tissue. The possibility for infection is great, but the possibility for a new way of life with more freedom of movement is even greater!

Top Ten Shaucha (Self-Care) Routines for Amputees

1. Take deep breaths often.

2. Get enough sleep.

3. Move your body with yoga every day.

4. Practice gratitude.

5. Inspire yourself daily.

6. Drink plenty of water.

7. Choose healthy food options.

8. Wash your residual limb(s) and prosthetic liner daily.

9. Rest your leg when there is skin breakdown.

10. Be kind to yourself.

Putting on dirty liners or stump socks can cause infections. Liners that split or tear often mean the alignment or socket is off, needing to be remedied by the prosthetist. Liners should be washed daily to avoid infection.

It is not recommended to wear a prosthesis that is not designed for swimming or walking the beach or at a pool. Sand can accumulate in the prosthesis causing permanent damage. Chlorine from pool water can harm the prosthesis. For those who choose to swim with a prosthesis, a pool leg is needed. Some amputees, when walking the beach, cover their prosthesis with a plastic covering to avoid damage to the prosthesis.

Self-care rituals such as stretching and moving the body daily with yoga and pranayama, some form of cardiovascular exercise, daily personal hygiene routines, mental hygiene through inspiration, positive thinking and creativity, spiritual renewal through prayer, meditation and time in nature, will help the amputee stay healthy and whole.

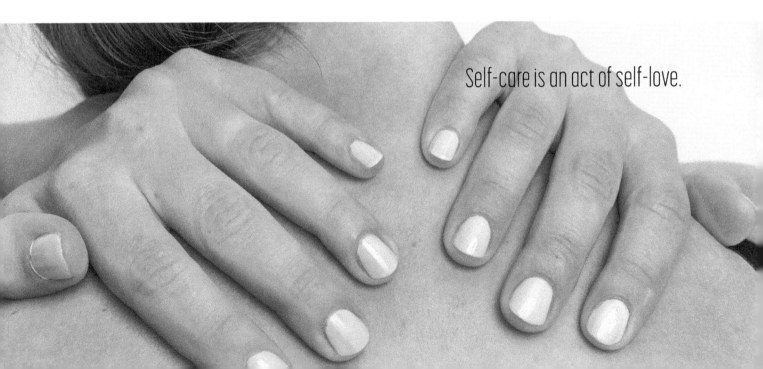

Self-care is an act of self-love.

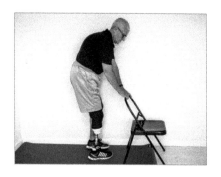

Self-Care Yoga Practice using the wall and a chair

1. Place a chair near a wall.

2. Swivel the chair so the seat is parallel to the back wall.

3. Sit on the edge of the chair.

4. Turn so the back foot presses into the back wall, the front thigh rests on the front of the seat and the front foot is underneath the front knee.

5. Lift the arms above the head in Warrior I.

6. Extend the arms.

7. Press the back hand into the wall.

8. Reach the front arm in front.

9. Look over the front arm.

10. Switch sides.

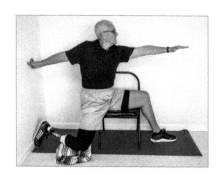

Empower yourself

What is personal empowerment?

An empowered person is confident, copes well with stress, and handles life with ease and humor. For an amputee, personal empowerment also means having a sense of purpose in life, an identity beyond limb loss, independence, financial stability, and the ability to be an active member of society. Yoga can make that happen.

Empowerment yoga practice

1. Stand in mountain.

2. Step out wide, making muscle arms if possible.

3. Bend forward at the hips.

4. Make fists if possible, placing the right hand on top of the left.

5. Imagine that these fists are holding a bat.

6. Inhale. Exhale with "Ha" imagining that you are hitting anything that is blocking your personal empowerment out of your life.

7. Switch sides and repeat to the right.

8. Return to mountain pose.

9. Feel the effects of your empowerment practice.

10. Go out and live your power.

* This pose can be done in a chair. Focus on the center of the belly, strongly pulling the abdominal muscles into the spine while at the same time, imagining the navel and the muscles all around the navel radiating like a bright sun.

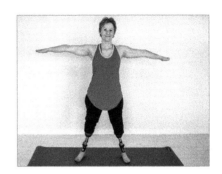

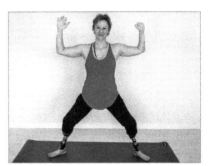

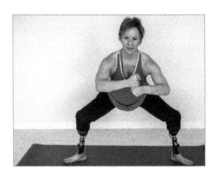

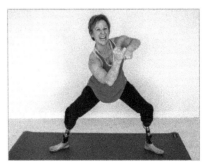

MEET JUANITA

"The best way to heal you is to help others" — Juanita

*Juanita is a former traveling nurse who was hit head on by a drunk driver. She broke both hips, femurs, knees, ankles and many other body parts. Her left foot was also crushed. Originally her left leg was salvaged, but over the years, with more than 40 surgeries and infections, she became very ill and was hospitalized. She made the elective decision to have her left leg amputated above the knee to save her life from another dangerous infection and improve her quality of life. Feeling frustrated and alone, she longed to talk to someone about it all, someone who could understand. She found that empathy with other amputees, subsequently founding a support group, now a registered non-profit, that brings resources and support to many amputees in the state of Ohio. Her decision to empower herself and advocate for her own emotional wellness has extended out into the lives of hundreds of amputees. Guiding and educating amputees about what's possible is extremely rewarding to Juanita's soul. Juanita believes that life is still amazing no matter what you are going through. She thrives on showing amputees that they are **limitless,** even with limb loss.*

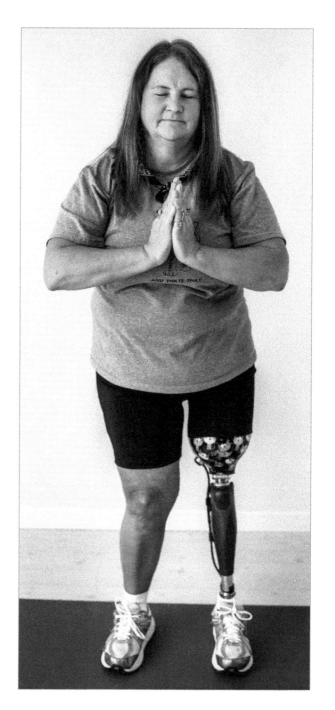

Accept yourself

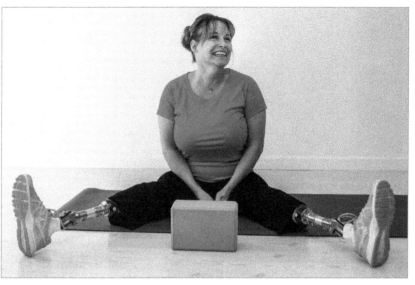

1. Sit comfortably with legs wide and spine lengthened. This can be done on the floor or in a chair.

2. Take a deep breath in.

3. Exhale with "Ha, Ha, Ha."

4. Continue to try to laugh "Ha, Ha, Ha" until you start laughing naturally.

5. Think about something you judge about yourself. Let it be part of the laugh.

6. Laughter catches on quickly.

7. Let yourself go! Laugh as long as you want.

8. End your practice by closing your eyes, feeling the echoes of the laughter in your body.

Self–acceptance is one of the biggest challenges amputees face after limb loss. Some of the blocks to self-acceptance that amputees can experience relate to survival, safety, relationships, sexuality, body image, and life purpose. Yoga can help amputees overcome those blocks and live full, whole lives once again.

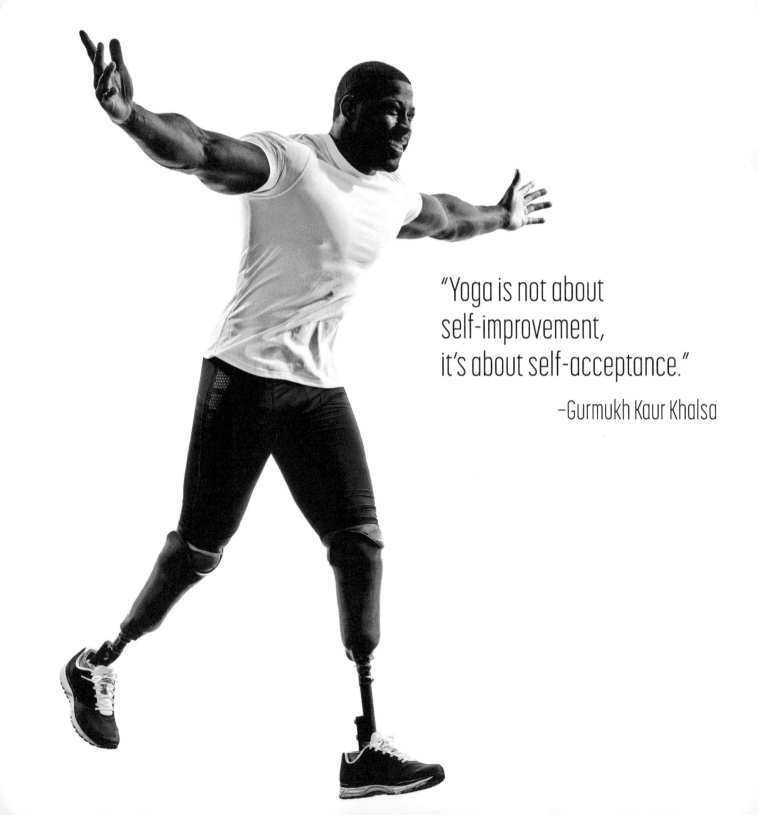

"Yoga is not about
self-improvement,
it's about self-acceptance."

–Gurmukh Kaur Khalsa

CHAPTER FOUR | HOW TO BE A YOGI

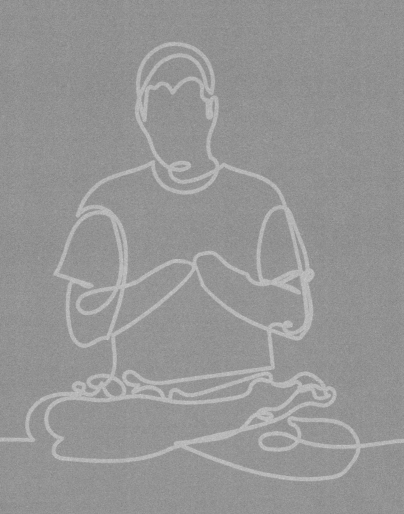

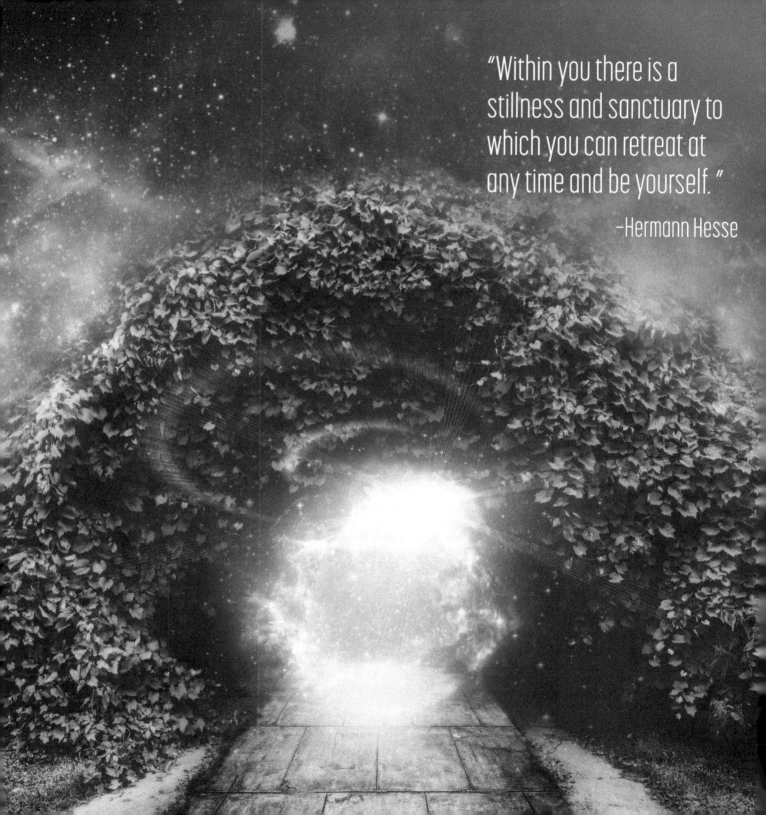

"Within you there is a stillness and sanctuary to which you can retreat at any time and be yourself."

-Hermann Hesse

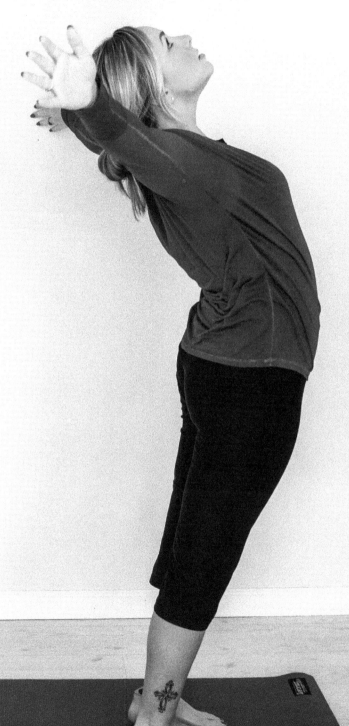

Getting to a yoga class: What you need to know

Whether you try yoga at home, or attend class at a gym or yoga studio, receiving guidance from a qualified professional will help you learn yoga correctly and safely. Coming into a yoga space is like entering a **sanctuary,** a place set apart to renew your body, mind and spirit.

How can an amputee experience this sense of sanctuary in a modern yoga class?

Initially you might go to yoga to address physical pain, build strength or gain balance. Over time, the deeper meaning of yoga rubs off. You begin to peel away old layers of resistance, grief and pain, liberating yourself from the judgments, beliefs about yourself that are not true and patterns that don't work anymore. To experience the best that yoga has to offer, amputees should feel safe. **Sanctuary** is first found in the safety you feel.

Yoga begins with an attitude in your heart. By opening your heart to a broader experience of yourself through yoga, you can find your limitless potential, as well as your highest self.

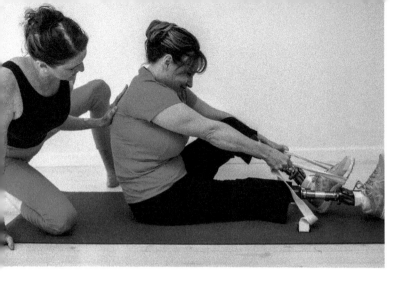

Feeling Safe

Safety for an amputee practicing yoga includes the ability to relax, to be one's self, to trust the teacher, and to move beyond fears. A person who feels safe is a person who can learn more easily. A controlled peaceful environment with a calm-voiced, knowledgeable yoga teacher invites that safety.

Learn from a qualified teacher. The best yoga teacher or yoga therapist for an amputee is someone who has a lot of experience teaching yoga, and has been trained in adaptive yoga specializing in amputees. Professionals who work with amputees and have studied yoga are also excellent. If your yoga teacher does not ask about your medical background, you may want to seek someone else. And of course, make certain your instructor is insured.

Your yoga teacher needs to care about you. That means she offers adaptive options for you, listens to you, and sees you as whole.

Seek out the best type of yoga for your body.
Power and **vinyasa** yoga are appropriate if you know your yoga poses well and can safely transition from one pose to another without the use of many props. Otherwise, seek out a **hatha yoga** class. Hot yoga, *(90 degrees or more) is not recommended* for amputees wearing a prosthesis. The heat can damage the prosthesis, and cause it to fall off. Ask your care team if there any yoga poses or practices you should avoid. *Some amputees practice hot yoga without their prosthesis.* Sweaty floors in hot yoga are slippery. Amputees with circulatory, diabetic, thyroid or high blood pressure issues should never do hot yoga.

Be honest with yourself about your capabilities and challenges. Injury is no fun for an amputee. If you are new to yoga, ask your physical therapist, prosthetist and doctor if yoga is appropriate for you before diving in full force. If you are still recovering from your amputation, an intense yoga practice, such as power yoga, may cause serious injury. If you have any medical conditions, let your yoga teacher know, so she can be prepared.

The quality and location of the yoga studio or gym are important.

These are the questions to ask when seeking a yoga studio or gym:

- Is there handicapped parking available if you need it?

- Is there an elevator if needed?

- Is the room wheelchair accessible if required?

- Is the yoga room clean, with good air circulation? Hot yoga rooms can feel stuffy and reek of sweat.

- Does the room have adequate wall space? Walls are extremely useful to lean on during yoga.

- Is the teacher audible and visible?

- Does the studio have appropriate yoga props, such as chairs, yoga blocks, bolsters, blankets, and straps? If not, the studio may still be acceptable, but the yoga practice will not be optimum.

- Is there enough room for you to practice?

- Where are the exits and bathrooms? Yoga flushes the system clean, which may lead to an urgent bathroom rush. Yoga can bring up long held traumas. Knowing your exits means reassuring yourself there is a way out of the yoga space if called for.

- *Do the studio and yoga teacher feel safe to you?*

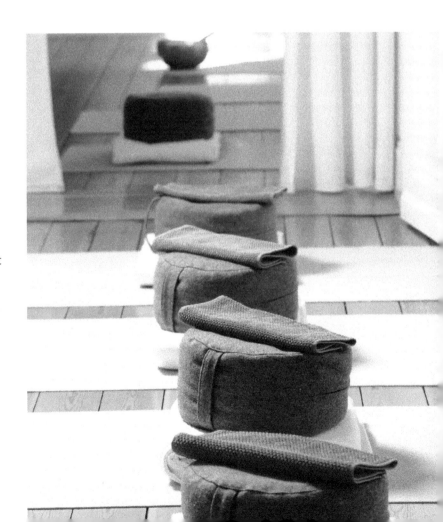

What you need to become a yogi

There are four essential elements to becoming a yogi (yoga practitioner). They are:

Awareness

Self-observation

Compassion

Intention

Awareness

Awareness is the moment to moment observation of what and how you are feeling physically, emotionally and psychologically. By bringing awareness to any given experience, you fine tune your consciousness, increasing your ability to find serenity in the here and now. You learn to release old habits, repetitive unhealthy body movements, and oppressive beliefs. Inner peace can be found anywhere when we are fully present, aware within and without.

Awareness Inquiries	
Do I have a good grasp of the steps to a yoga pose or breathing technique?	Can I differentiate pain from discomfort?
How do I feel today?	Am I willing to see what is true for me?
Are there old feelings coming up about limb loss? What are they?	Can I do more than I thought?
Do I feel balanced? If so, why? If not, how can I become more balanced?	Is my breath flowing easily or is it strained?
Do I feel secure in the pose? Why or why not? How can I become more secure?	Can I stay present when strong emotions come to the surface without pushing them away?
Do I need a yoga prop? Am I okay asking for help?	Am I present, distracted, pre-occupied, relaxed during yoga today?
Have I learned something new about myself today?	How can I apply what I've learned to my life?

Self-observation

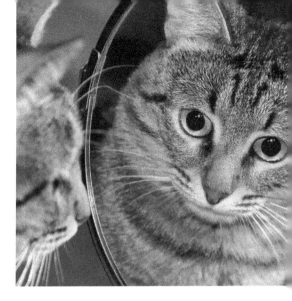

Self-observation asks us to observe ourselves with an open heart and mind before making a false judgement about ourselves. Self-observation is not self-absorption or selfishness. Self-observation is witnessing you without judgment. By "weeding out" what isn't ours and becoming AWARE of what is, our truest most magnificent self emerges. Self-observation becomes a mirror between the experience of yoga practice and the experience of everyday life.

This five-step method listed below is a foundational self-observation practice.

1. **Breathe.** *Take a deep breath in and out.*

2. **Relax.** *Relax your body. Relax your mind.*

3. **Feel.** *Feel each sensation as it arises, without judgment or expectation.*

4. **Watch.** *Watch the wave of sensations. Where are they in your body? When does a sensation start? Is there an ending to the sensation? What happens to your mind?*

5. **Allow.** *Allow your sensations to follow their natural path without directing or managing them.*

Self-Compassion

Compassion is one of the core tenets of yoga. Compassion is a deep way of understanding ourselves and each other, enlarging our capacity to embrace both mind and body exactly as they are. For an amputee, compassion heals.

When self-compassion takes precedent in a person's life, that person often becomes more motivated, less reactive and more harmonious. Active compassion reduces stress, frustration, tension and even high blood pressure! Foster compassion when you are feeling pain, discomfort, or frustration. Remind yourself that compassion is the opposite of "feeling sorry for yourself". A person who is wrapped up in self-pity is stuck in the past, rather than the present. Compassion, on the other hand, i s a present moment practice which expands your ability to see new hopeful possibilities. It is easy to have compassion on others, so why not offer some compassion to yourself too?

Intention

Often at the beginning of yoga class, yoga teachers will ask what your intention is for your practice. Creating an intention for yoga practice has an amazing way of bringing the results hoped for. The power of the positive mind to influence the body is profound.

How to create an intention

1. Take a few deep breaths.

2. Ask yourself what you really need today during yoga.

3. Be open to answers that come to you.

4. Say yes to those answers.

5. Follow through on your 'yes' with an intention.

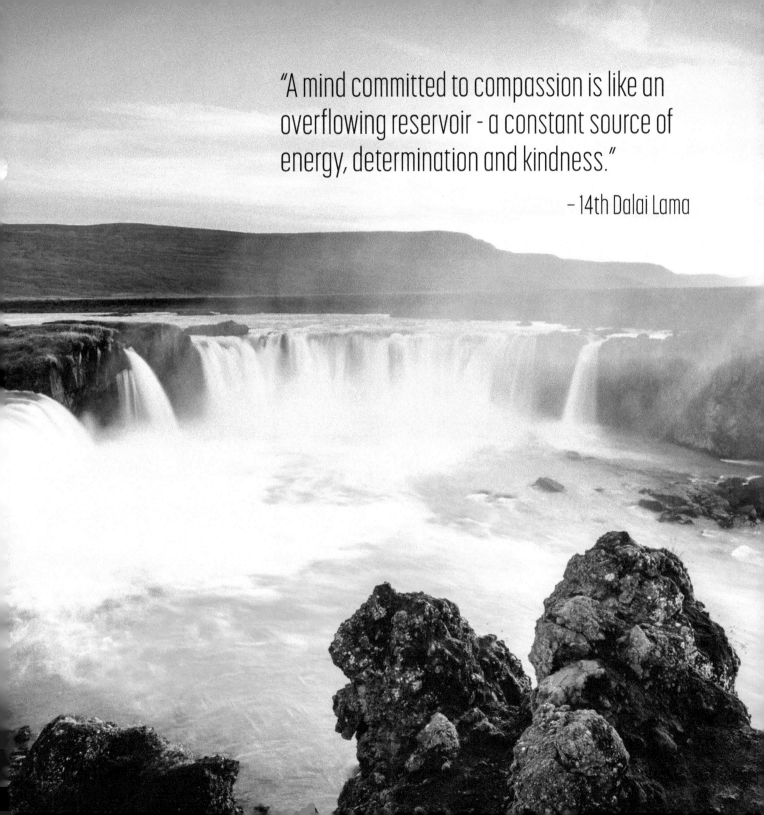

"A mind committed to compassion is like an overflowing reservoir - a constant source of energy, determination and kindness."

– 14th Dalai Lama

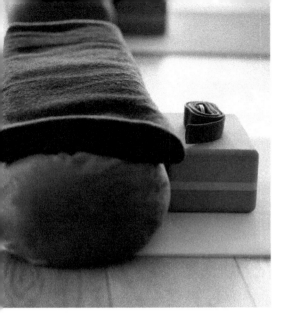

Props for Yoga

Once you have created an intention, you are ready to embark on your yoga practice. Yoga practice begins with setting up your yoga space. **Yoga props** are frequently used to support yoga practice.

Yoga props help amputees sustain postures for longer periods of time, building stamina, strength and balance. Amputees develop better range of motion and deeper stretching, important for overuse and underuse of certain muscle groups, when using props. With a yoga prop, the spine can be better aligned, the gait and balance can improve for amputees, and the breath can expand to full capacity, which helps amputees with poor circulation. Props can reduce pain and discomfort, as well as increase relaxation in the body. Yoga teachers and studios will often supply yoga props. If not, invest in some yoga props for your yoga classes or home practice. The most essential props to use in an amputee yoga practice are a *yoga mat, two yoga blocks, a yoga strap, two yoga blankets and a chair (if needed)*.

Uses for Yoga Props

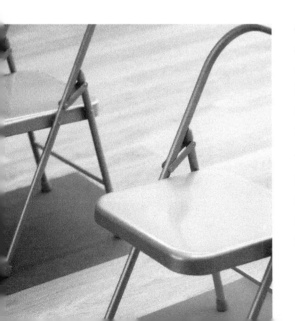

Chairs. Many amputees sit in chairs for their entire yoga practice, while others alternate between standing and sitting. Chairs can be pressed against a wall for greater stability in yoga poses, or placed below the knees for inversions such as legs up the wall or shoulderstand. For an average amputee, having a chair available is helpful if he gets tired, needs to lean on something, or needs help transitioning to the floor.

Yoga mats have a sticky texture that keeps an amputee from sliding (for the most part). Most prosthetic feet are made of a slippery material. Some amputees wear sneakers or sticky socks during yoga as well, to keep from slipping. There are amputees who have special suction feet made for yoga, while others add a non skid surface to the bottom of the prosthetic foot. A yoga mat can be rolled and placed lengthwise beneath the back in supine poses or for those seated in a chair for better spinal alignment, horizontally behind the mid-back for backbends, or underneath the buttocks to open up the hips.

Yoga blankets can be folded or rolled under the arms, lower back, bottom, knees, head, and shoulders in inversions. Blankets keep the amputee in good alignment while also protecting him from injuries. During relaxation, a yoga blanket put over the body feels comforting. The weight of the blanket invites the joints to free up and the body to settle into the floor more quickly.

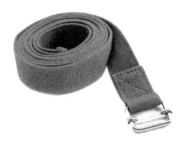

A Yoga strap helps an amputee stabilize and go further into his yoga poses. Wrapped around a foot, calf, or thigh, a strap can bring an amputee to a richer level of his yoga experience. Straps are helpful for tight hamstrings, shoulders, and hips.

Weighted bags increase body awareness. Placed on the belly in a supine pose, on the palms and wrists of the hands for relaxation, or vertically on the forehead in line with a yoga block, weighted bags aid relaxation and deep breathing. Weighted bags can be placed horizontally on the lower back or vertically on the spine in child's pose to release tension. For people suffering from PTSD, weighted bags soothe the nervous system. Some amputees hold a weighted bag in each hand during mountain pose, or place the weighted bags on the tops of the feet to teach the body to distribute weight evenly.

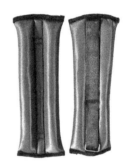

A Yoga foam wedge can be placed under the prosthetic heel or top of the foot if his hips are uneven in standing poses. The wedge is also excellent placed under the heels of the palms in downward facing dog to stabilize the body, protect sore wrists, and stretch the wrists and arms without strain.

Yoga blocks are used often in yoga practice, to open the chest in backbends, to support wrists in forward bends, to lean on in standing

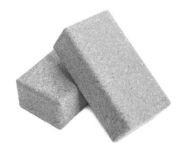

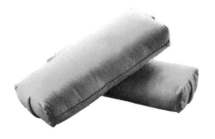

poses, to create shoulder strength when pressed between two hands, and to stand on for balance poses.

Similar to yoga blankets, **yoga bolsters** are used to lengthen the spine in supine poses, to relax the lower back in inversions or backbends, and to support forward bends for those who are less flexible. Starting with one bolster, a yoga practitioner might stack more bolsters on top of each other for a variety of restorative poses, as needed.

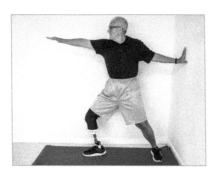

A wall with adequate wall space is very useful for an amputee. Whether the amputee is an experienced athlete or a novice, he can lose his balance. Leaning on a wall or pressing into a wall makes an amputee feel secure so he can relax into his practice without added anxiety.

A meditation pillow helps an amputee whose spine is rounding when sitting up tall. Elevating the hips on the edge of a meditation pillow tilts the sitz bones forward so an amputee can sit for longer periods of meditation.

Sticky socks are occasionally used by amputees to keep from sliding on the yoga mat, or to stabilize the feet in backbends and standing poses.

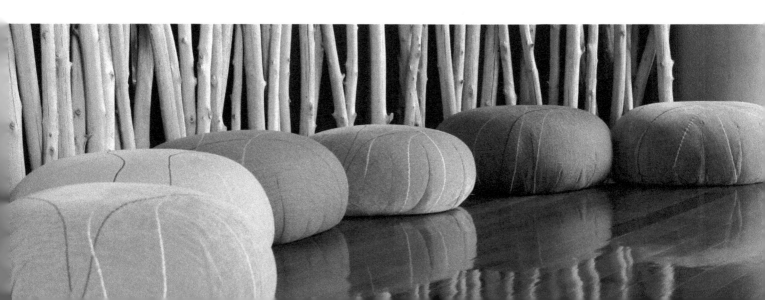

What to expect in a yoga class?

Below are the steps to a complete yoga class.

1. Set up mats and props
2. Centering
3. Pranayama
4. Warm Ups
5. Asana
6. Creative visualization
7. Relaxation
8. Closing breath
9. Mantra

Wear loose, comfortable clothing that breathes and moves easily. *Set up a yoga space* in your home or office. A yoga space is uncluttered, allowing enough room to stretch the entire body on the floor or in a standing position. Have your yoga props nearby: two yoga blocks, a chair, a yoga strap and two yoga blankets. If yoga props are not available, substitute with pillows, blankets, towels, ties, a couch, sturdy chairs and a wall. Play soothing meditative music or practice in silence. *Soft lighting* is best. Light a candle if possible, but watch for pets who may knock over candles! Keep the room *distraction free*. Turn off the cell phones, dim the computer screen, close the door and *prepare your mind, heart and body*. Follow a set series of postures

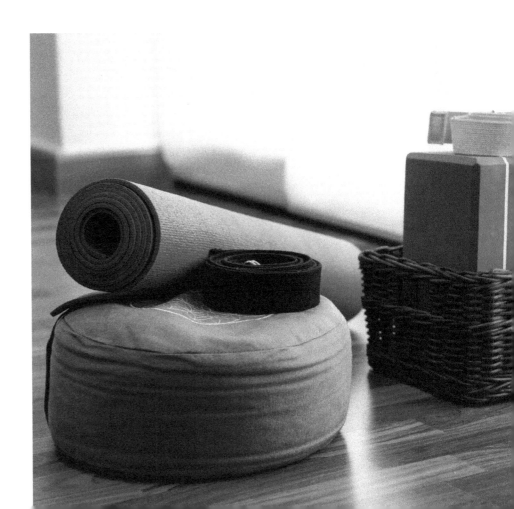

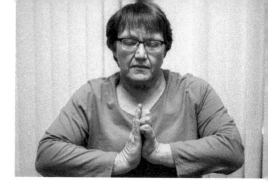

A daily yoga practice

 Seated meditation

Close your eyes. Bring all your attention to the present moment. Observe how you are feeling. Take three deep breaths. Sigh on exhale. Tell yourself "I am about to practice meditation. I will remain in the present moment." Sit in meditation for five to seven minutes.

 Centering

Focus your mind on your heart. As you breathe in and out, create an intention for your yoga practice that resonates with you. For example, you can say "My intention is to remain present during my entire yoga practice,"

 Pranayama

Do five rounds of Ujjayi breath *(see chapter on Pranayama for instructions)*

 Warm-ups

Circle all the joints, beginning at the ankles, when available, all the way up to the head and neck.

 Poses

Practice this series of yoga poses, or pick and choose from among this list. *(See Chapter Five - Bend - for instructions).*

1. Mountain
2. ½ moon
3. Tree
4. Triangle
5. Side Angle
6. Warrior I
7. Warrior II
8. Chair
9. Down Dog
10. Easy sitting
11. Bound Angle
12. Boat
13. Seated Forward Bend
14. Childs

15. Cobra

16. Locust

17. Seated Wide Angle

18. Bound Angle

19. Bridge

20. Seated Twist

21. Knees to chest

22. Legs up the wall

23. Relaxation

 Relaxation

a. Place folded blankets or a pillow under the knees, when available, or to support the residual limb.

b. Place a blanket over the body.

c. Practice relaxation for five to ten minutes.

d. When complete, roll to the side and sit up.

 Om or other closing prayer

Close your practice by chanting Om, another mantra, or repeat your intention.

 Optimize your practice by journaling about what you observed

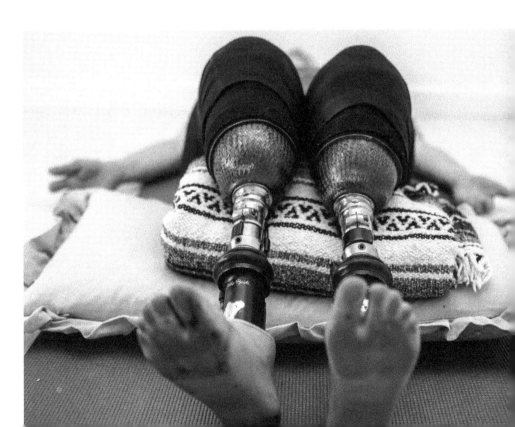

Transitions

Imagine waking up in the morning. You stretch your body, yawn, roll over to one side, swing your legs around and stand up. Simple, right? Not so for an amputee! Each daily ritual for an amputee requires adaptive thinking to move safely and avoid injury. Transitions are a constant for amputees, and while amputees become experts at adapting, they take a toll on an amputee.

Transitions and our response to them are at the heart of yoga practice. The only certainty in life is change! We practice centering, breath, warm ups, yoga poses, meditation and relaxation so that we can not only handle change, but thrive with it.

Fear of falling is very real for an amputee. Fear constricts. When we are in a state of fear, our body and mind are tight, the muscles become brittle, making movement with confidence very unlikely. On the other hand, when a person relaxes with yoga, the body tends to loosen its white-knuckle grip. Being able to balance, to find that still, centered place inside, is fundamental to an amputee building confidence as they transition throughout their day.

How to transition

In yoga practice, we are transitioning among three planes: **vertical, horizontal and sagittal**. Movement in these three planes helps an amputee expand their movement capabilities and balance their brain. In a typical yoga class, standing poses are completed first, followed by seated, prone, supine and inverted poses. For some amputees, chair adaptations are made to allow them to stay seated for their entire yoga practice. Other amputees come directly to the floor and adapt from there. In all cases, transitions from one plane to the next are an individual endeavor.

Laura transitioning from her wheelchair to the floor

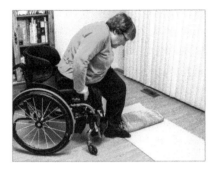 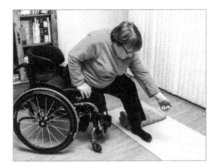 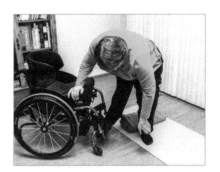

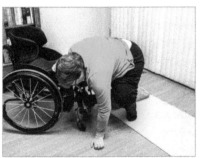 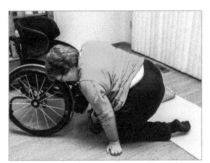 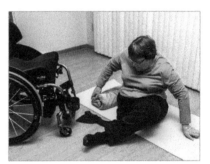

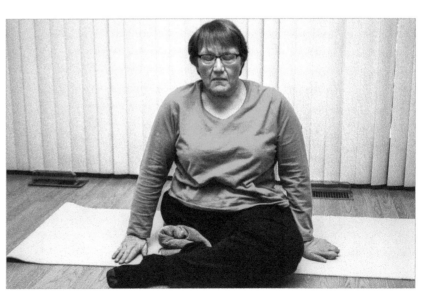

Important questions to ask an amputee who is transitioning from one plane to another.

Can they lift their body weight off a chair?	Are they within a weight range that you feel you can lift ?
Do they already know how to get up and down from the floor? If so, have them show you their approach, and only offer additional assistance when asked. It has taken them a lot of work to figure out how to transition.	Do they sit upright when in a chair? If not, they will not be able to hold themselves up in a seated floor position.
Do you have an assistant if needed?	How strong are their abdominals and upper body?
Can they get up and down from a chair?	Do they have any injuries in the shoulders, knees or hips? If so, staying in a chair or standing is the best course of action.

The "step method" is the most foolproof way to help amputees who are less mobile transition to the floor and back to a chair to standing. Starting in a chair, the amputee, with support of an assistant and wall if needed, rolls gently to the right or left from a seated position to a tiered layer of "steps", such as folded yoga blankets or a shorter sturdy stool (highly recommended, until they have reached the floor, or vice versa. A good way to test whether transitioning to the floor will work is to see if the amputee can lift her bottom off a chair without tumbling over, using the upper limbs for support if available, or the lower limbs to stand up.

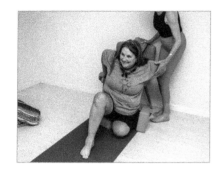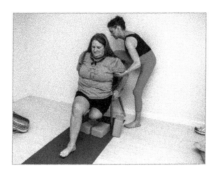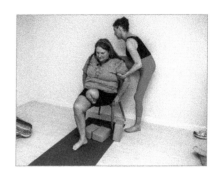
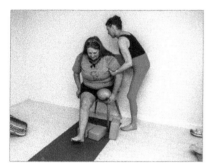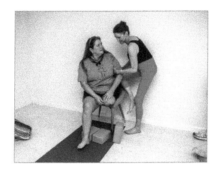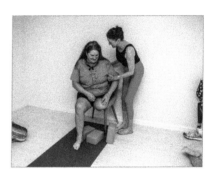

Juanita using the step method

Another way to bring an amputee to the floor is with the support of assistants who lift the amputee from a seated position using a sling under the bottom and a strong strap wrapped around the lower ribs. *This assist is only appropriate for those teachers and therapists able to lift a student or patient to the floor without personal injury.*

In addition, many amputees have a system of transition that they have mastered that works for them. Some amputees roll to one side, normally the non-amputated side, place the opposite hand in front of the pelvis, lean into both hands on that side, lift the bottom off the floor, turn and fold into a forward bend, then roll up to standing. It is a good idea to have the seat of a chair in front of the amputee to lean on, to transition to standing if needed.

Ray transitioning from the floor to standing

It is important, if the amputee is wearing his prosthesis, to involve the prosthesis as much as possible in the transition to standing. This protects the amputee from wear and tear in the remaining limb, especially around the knee or shoulder joint.

Teach an amputee to round the pelvis and back under, from the lumbar spine to the cervical spine until fully upright. This keeps the amputee from overusing joints and underusing muscles. Normally the amputee, in this case, goes to their hands (when available) and knees, rocks back into the feet, walks the hands towards the feet then rolls up one vertebra at a time. The amputee may need to lean on a wall, or stand between the backs of two chairs to stabilize themselves before moving to a seated position or another standing position.

More athletic amputees find that reversing their salutation to the sun, from plank to downward dog to standing forward bend to mountain, with a chair or wall in front to lean on if needed, is sufficient.

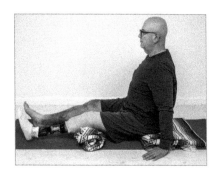
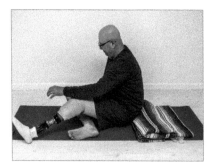
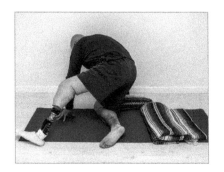
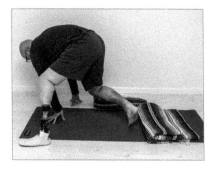
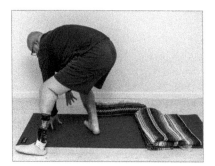

Kelly transitioning from plank pose to standing mountain

The in –between places, amid breath and asana, movement and stillness, are the moments where potential is met with possibility, meditation meets space and inner strength meets an amputee's hope. Transitions fully immerse an amputee in the deeper meaning of yoga.

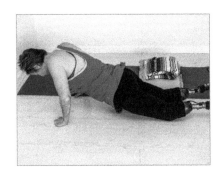
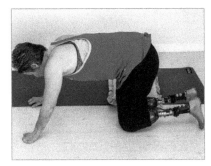
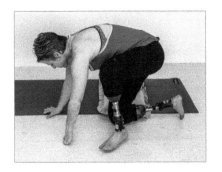
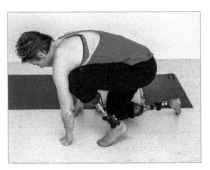
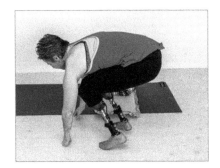
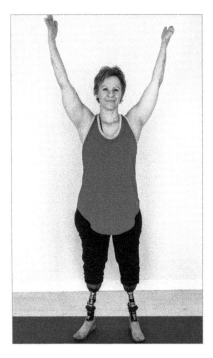

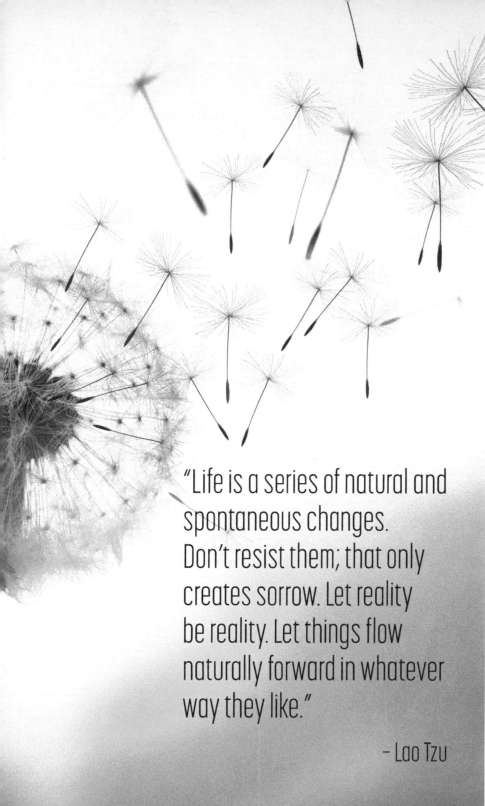

"Life is a series of natural and spontaneous changes. Don't resist them; that only creates sorrow. Let reality be reality. Let things flow naturally forward in whatever way they like."

– Lao Tzu

Jeff transitioning from a chair to standing

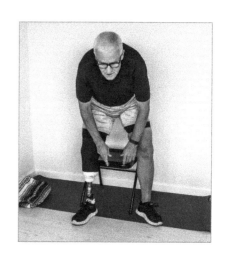

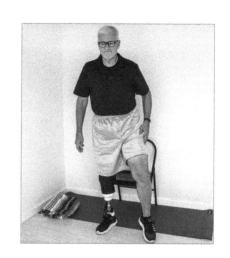

How to be even as an amputee

For many amputees, the feeling of evenness can look very different from the reality. New amputees, for example, who are re-learning proprioceptive skills, such as taking a step, standing, or being upright while wearing a man-made leg or arm, is, frankly, weird, a physically and mentally demanding task. Their version of evenness is skewed by the newness of their experience.

When new amputees being fitted for a prosthesis give feedback to the prosthetist, they don't often have the language to explain their own symmetry. As the amputee progresses, the shape of the residual limb changes, increasing or decreasing in size due to swelling, compression, or weight loss/ gain. This changes the feeling of evenness and alignment.

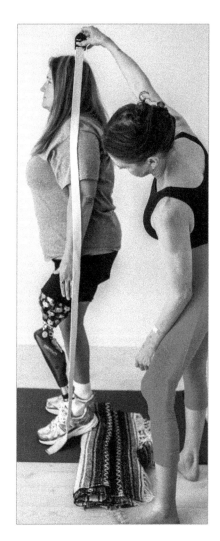

For amputees who have lived with their amputation for a while, or even their entire life, they will be accustomed to a certain way of standing that seems best and most aligned, but their habitual stance may be hurting them in the long run. New prosthetics, new prosthetists, and life changes may mean changes in alignment. The amputee may do everything possible to return to the alignment that once was. The reality is that sometimes, the "once was" can be the result of bad habits now ingrained in the body.

For example, I am most comfortable walking on tip toes, a remnant of the fit from my first prosthesis. Because of the way I walk, my step forward on my right foot is shortened. A shortened step means a tighter psoas. In addition, being a yogi, I have been barefoot most days. My prosthesis is not ideally worn barefoot, as there are always tiny alignment issues. Because of these habits, I work extra hard to keep my hips and spine in alignment. When I do, I am more grounded.

Alignment issues are quite subtle. 1/8" forward or backward in the inner structure of the prosthesis, a higher ball of the foot or heel than

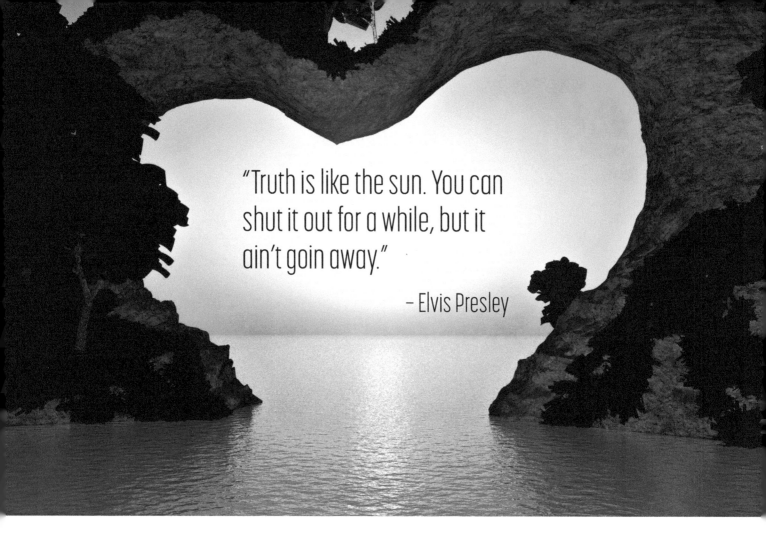

"Truth is like the sun. You can shut it out for a while, but it ain't goin away."

– Elvis Presley

needed, can cause all sorts of challenges. Therefore, when assisting and observing an amputee, or practicing yoga as an amputee, *always look at or internally feel the hips and/or ribs first.*

Evenness in yoga for the amputee is a creative process: both an external practice of body alignment, and an internal practice of balance in emotions, daily rituals, and thoughts. One thing is true: evenness creates harmony in an amputee's life. Stay open to new discoveries in your body, mind and spirit by observing how you practice being even.

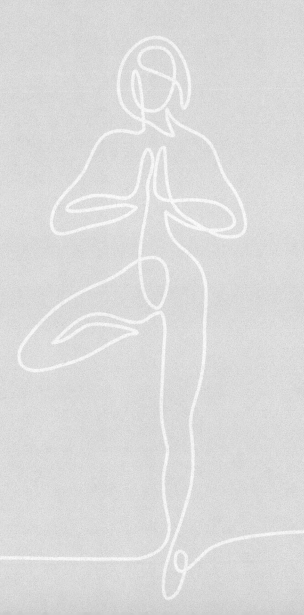

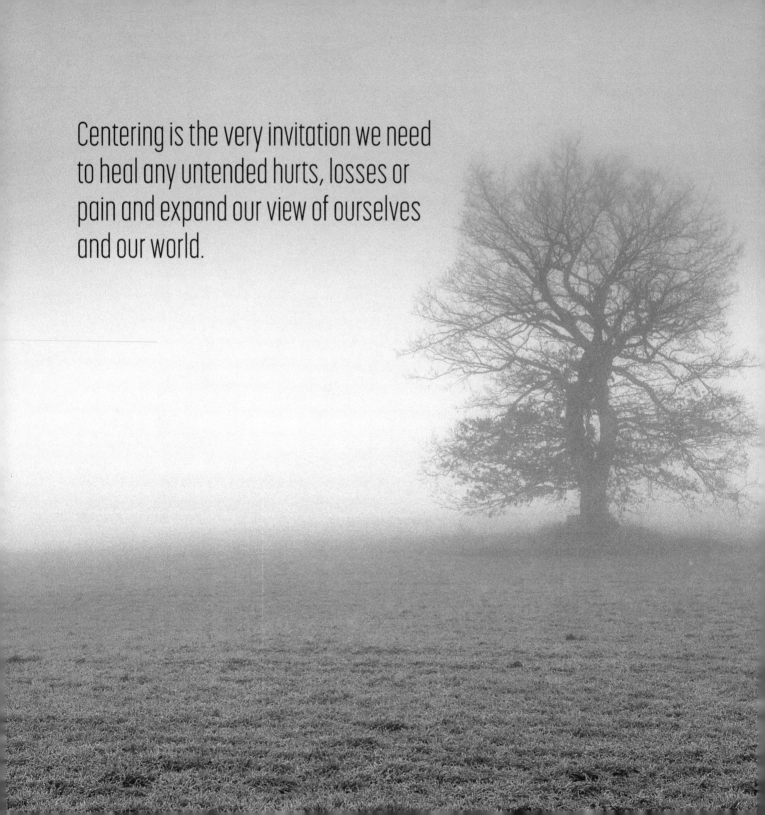

Centering is the very invitation we need to heal any untended hurts, losses or pain and expand our view of ourselves and our world.

To help an amputee remember the basics of a complete yoga practice, I created a system called 'The Five B's'. Each 'B' addresses specific techniques for that section of the practice. Within each 'B' I offer different ideas and options for developing an amputee yoga practice, based on this foundational system.

The Five B's are :

 BE

 BREATHE

 BEND

 BUILD

 BE

The first 'B' – BE - prepares the amputee yogi's body, mind and spirit. Beingness is a state of present moment awareness. There is a quality to beingness that feels expansive, a clean slate of possibility, which invites amputees and non-amputees alike to feel both whole and eternal.

The second 'B' – BREATHE - draws an amputee into the inner world of breath. Breath settles us, heals us, restores us, and helps our minds when we get distracted by past or future thoughts. Breath is essential to life and the guiding force of yoga practice. Breath is life.

The third 'B – BEND - includes the physical movements of warm ups and yoga postures. Warm ups prepare the body safely for the poses to come. Yoga postures open the rivers of energy, or prana, in the body, to prepare the body for meditation .

The fourth 'B' – BUILD - is designed to strengthen the amputee's core. Amputees need the core to not only perform everyday tasks, but to restore their sense of self after limb loss.

The fifth 'B' – BE - is the culmination of yoga practice. After a full yoga practice, an amputee's state of beingness can change dramatically for the better. The mind calms, the body feels stretched and opened and spirit feels uplifted. The fruits of yoga practice include relaxation, visualization, meditation and the sacred sound of OM, reuniting the amputee with essential wholeness, experiencing the sublime nature of the blissful body, available to all of us.

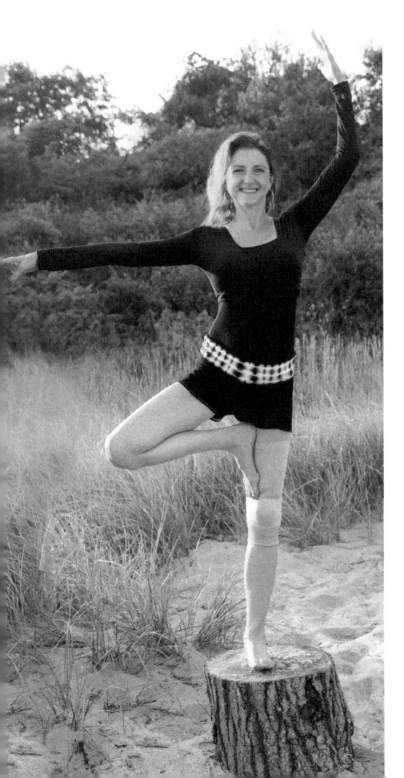

BE
BE YOU, CENTERED

Do you remember the day you lost your leg? How about the events leading up to that moment? For me, the day of my actual amputation is a blur, but the days before are clear in my memory, from the bone scan that revealed my tumor, to the office visit with the orthopedic surgeon, who placed the side of his hand, karate chop style, at the middle of my lower calf. I recoiled, pulling my leg away from him, but my amputation was inevitable.

Any memory we have is stored not just in our brains, but in our bodies, including our senses. A smell, taste, word, or sound can transport us back to a moment, whether happy or sad. *The most profound experiences we have as well as the best memories, never happen when our minds are somewhere else.* They happen when we are here, fully present.

Being present, in yoga, is a practice, an antidote to the endless chatter in our brains, and the mental sidelines we make from our real needs and feelings. For amputees, being present is not a foreign concept. Because amputees are constantly navigating spaces and situations, we have a natural ability to be present when it comes to how we move. The art of being present, or mindfulness, is a conscious practice of listening to ourselves fully in every moment. When we are present, we enter a world of new possibilities.

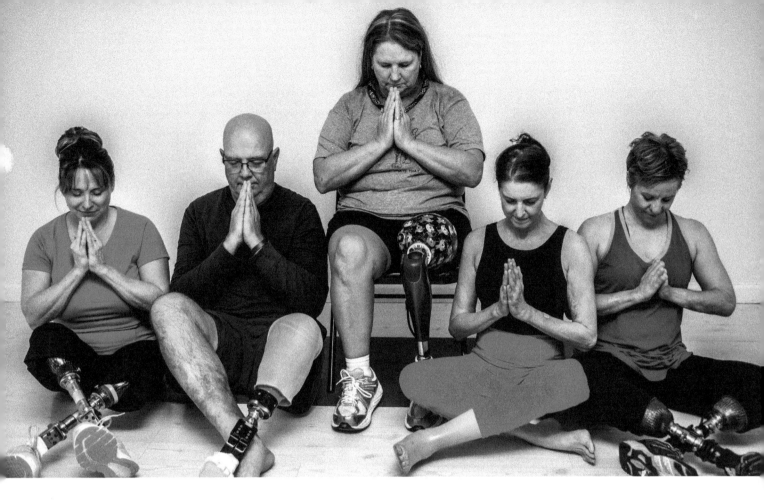

Centering is one of the simplest ways to be present in yoga. Centering teaches us how to listen more clearly to our inner voice and our body's messages. Our bodies are always giving us clues about who we are, what we need, or what will harm us. The more we practice being present through techniques like centering, the more empowered we are to live the best version of ourselves.

Center

Centering, done at the beginning of yoga practice, is a time to **tune out the world** and tune in to ourselves. Usually done seated with the spine erect and eyes closed, focus is on the breath coming and going. The act of centering is effortless. The challenge comes the moment we start to shift our focus to something outside of us, such as sounds, smells, or most often, rambling thoughts. Our bodies begin to follow our thoughts, and we lose our direct clear connection to our home base, ourselves.

Centering helps amputees re-establish a sense of ground. It has a quality of timelessness and spaciousness, which does wonders for an amputee. Amputees can feel expanded, beyond circumstances, witnessing eternal nature, inner light and unity with all of life. For amputees, that **awareness of unity** removes any notion of separation due to our limb loss.

Why practice centering?

We alone control our ability to find that still serene place inside. When we finally get to that place, we realize how much we have longed to be there. There are many reasons why this is so.

Centering relaxes the nervous system, clears the mind, and sets the mind and body to the present moment, ready for yoga poses and pranayama. Centering reminds us that there IS enough time.

Many amputees experience a need to cram in as many majestic life experiences as they can, concerned that they will "miss out" on life if they don't. However, all that cramming can elude an amputee from the very real majesty of his or her extraordinary self by simply being present.

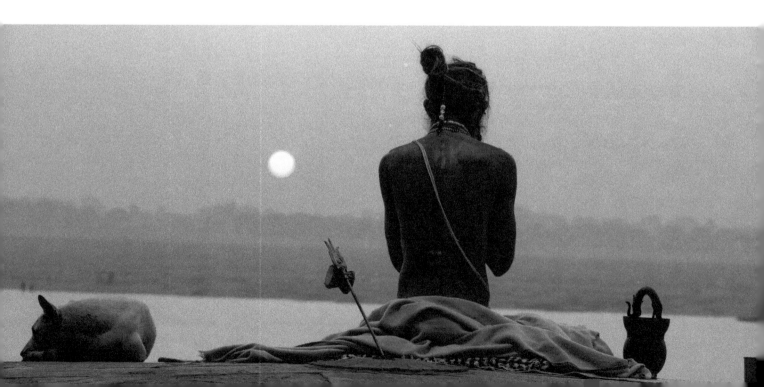

Take time for your life. Being still and mindful does not mean you are missing out on your life. It means you are tuning IN to the very magic of your life!

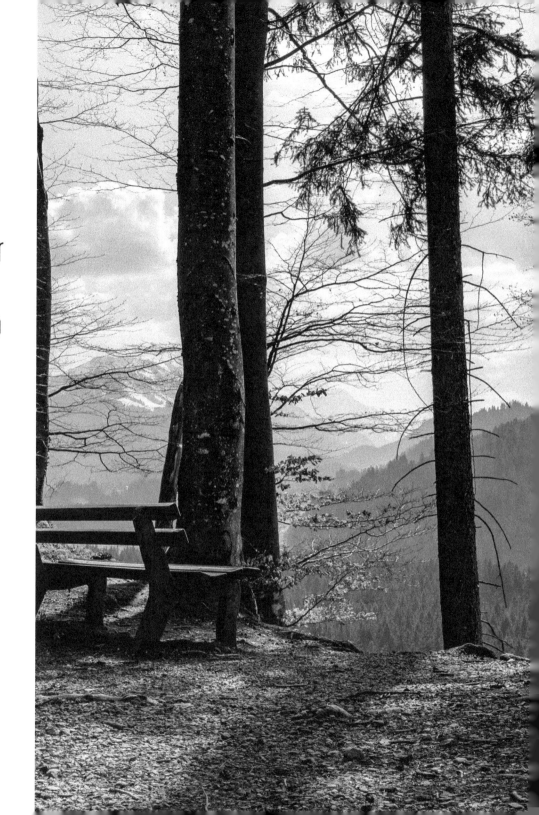

Body Scan

Observe sensations in your body from bottom to top.

What feels relaxed?

What feels tight?

Are there parts of your body you aren't aware of?

Are there parts of your body that make you feel vibrant and energized?

Tension/Release

Tighten different parts of the body as you inhale

Hold the inhale for 1-5 seconds.

Release with "AAHHH" as you exhale.

Tighten every part of your body. Start with your lower legs and travel all the way to the crown of the head.

Then close your eyes, tuning out the world, for five minutes.

"I am "Breath

As you breathe in, say to yourself "I".

As you breathe out say to yourself 'am".

Continue with this practice for 3-7 breaths.

Basic Centering Technique

1. Sit down on a mat or in a chair in a comfortable position.

2. Rock side to side until balance is achieved.

3. Relax the collarbone.

4. Lengthen the spine to allow space in the belly and ribs, to breathe.

5. Keep the eyes half open or gently closed.

6. Envision gazing inward, toward the heart or towards the floor.

7. Breathe 7-10 deep breaths.

8. Notice how you feel.

For amputees to sit comfortably, you may need to add different yoga props. Here are some adaptive versions for you to try.

- Roll a yoga mat or narrow cylinder under the bottom.

- Place blocks or blankets under the feet.

- Fold blankets under the bottom.

- Lean a chair against the wall as you sit in the chair.

MEET BUG

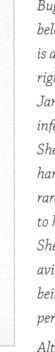

Bug is a bilateral upper extremity below the elbow amputee who is also missing three toes on her right foot and all her toenails. In January 2016, Bug got a sepsis infection after a routine surgery. She has body powered, figure 8 harness prosthetic arms which she rarely uses. She prefers to adapt to her life without her prosthetics. She is a singer/songwriter and avid yogi who finds her center by being herself, where she feels her personal power resides.

Although at times people stare at her in public, especially children, she feels strongly that her life is for her. She often uses humor to dispel people's reactions, and chooses to make light of very heavy situations.

Since her amputations, her vision for her life trajectory took a turn she, of course, was not expecting, which is why she is so committed to staying centered within herself.

There are some hidden gifts Bug has received from her limb losses. Losing her arms below the elbows has taught her patience she never knew she had. For Bug, her center is that place within her where her true essence lies. With or without arms, she is a force of life. Bug believes beauty will only be describable when she is in heaven. For the people who know and love her, Bug is heaven on earth.

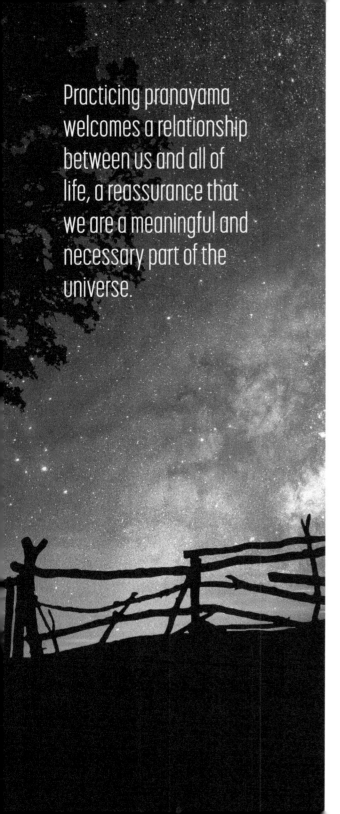

Practicing pranayama welcomes a relationship between us and all of life, a reassurance that we are a meaningful and necessary part of the universe.

PRANAYAMA

Pranayama is THE basic building block of yoga practice. Pranayama means control, or management, of prana, or life force. Pranayama provides amputees the most direct access to vitality possible. *Vitality fuels possibility and wholeness.* Prana is the life force that precedes and infuses all living things. The "breath behind the breath", which in some traditions refers to the Divine, is viewed as that which creates matter or fundamental energy as a generous gift for all living beings. By controlling our life force, we gain a more enlightened state, physiologically and spiritually.

Many of us have read about yogis who could hold their breath for extended periods of time, changing their body temperature and performing all sorts of contortions. Yes, these feats of nature are possible with years and years of yoga practice, but they are not the goal of yoga. They are a byproduct.

Restraining our life force is meant to teach us to use our energy wisely, and direct our life force towards wholeness. The more we practice pranayama, the better we feel and the more clarity of mind we enjoy.

Pranayama brings the amputee into the present moment, building him back up physically and emotionally. For example, pranayama can be used to eradicate or lessen pain. It is an intervention tool for rapid recovery, in addition to all the other benefits it provides. The breath is within any amputee's reach.

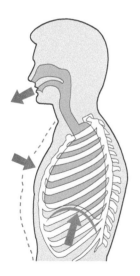

Pranayama retrains amputees with poor or inadequate autonomic breathing patterns towards more healthy breathing.

Reflexive Breathing

While you are reading this sentence, your body is actively engaged in autonomic breathing, the metabolic breath that keeps you alive, bringing vital oxygen to all body systems and tissues. Along with all the other autonomic bodily systems, such as brain function and heart beats, reflexive breathing is not something you think about. The moment you do think about your breath, you have crossed the bridge into pranayama, or, mindful control and observation of the breath.

The basics of pranayama

Autonomic breathing is an exchange of oxygen for carbon dioxide, gases for gases, toxins for purification, from bronchi to bronchioles to alveoli, from veins to arteries, from blood to brain, from nerves to blood, from blood to organs, from organs to skin, carbon dioxide to trees, trees to oxygen, oxygen to humans. Phew!

Oxygen enters the body through the nostrils, mouth and skin. The diaphragm and abdominal muscles (particularly the intercostal muscles) contract and expand to "pump" the oxygen through the body so that it properly assists the healthy functioning of all body systems. For many amputees, autonomic breathing can become difficult due to other extenuating circumstances such as pain, trauma, emotional upset, grief, injury, chronic stress and illness such as diabetes and heart disease, which can significantly alter this autonomic, reflexive process.

In its most basic form, pranayama directs mindful awareness to diaphragmatic breathing. By increasing the inhale and exhale, life force energy (or prana) increases. This relaxes the respiratory system. The lungs can then reach their natural capacity, carrying more oxygen into the body, dispelling more carbon dioxide out of the system. Because of the practice of pranayama, the lungs end up using less

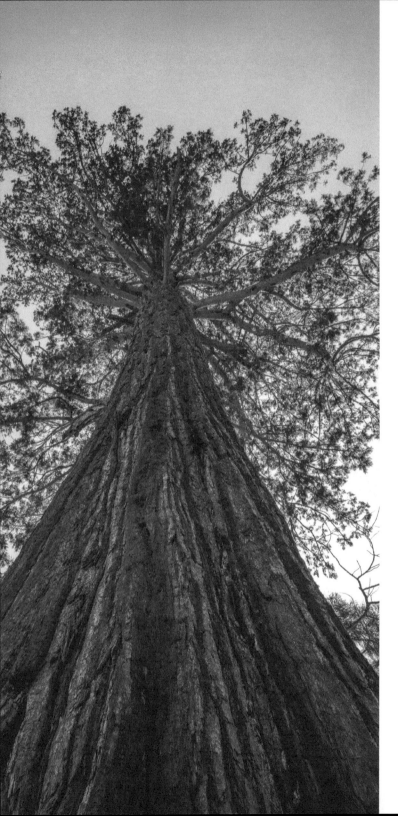

energy and effort to produce more efficient, higher volume breath. This, in turn slows down the racing mind, decreases the reactive stress response, and increases the sense of overall well-being. Emotional extremes start to subside as the body adjusts to its original peaceful state of rhythmic equilibrium.

Breath and vital life force get wasted when a person is constantly in a state of stress or overwhelm. Since the intercostals and diaphragmatic muscles are working at minimal efficiency, the body resorts to secondary means to get its breath. Hence many people use only the top portion of their lungs. Upper chest breathing tightens the muscles around the chest, neck and shoulders, which then make it even more difficult to sustain a deep breath. The diaphragm, because it is barely being used, weakens digestion and other organizing functions of the body. Upper chest breathing is meant to be used in extreme stress situations for short time periods to conserve energy.

There are three aspects to pranayama. These include **inhalation**, **retention** and **exhalation.**

As the practitioner breathes in, the lower belly

Pranayama draws the breath down to the lower belly, where amputees find their center of gravity and their ground. Awareness of the center of gravity is no longer found in the upper third of the body, but in the lower third. This is extremely important for amputees. When we are grounded, we feel part of life.

expands so the diaphragm can drop, making space for more breath. The practitioner pauses, retaining the breath for a few seconds, then exhalation begins, through the nostrils, unless otherwise specified. The lower belly draws in, the diaphragm lifting.

The pause in pranayama is as important as the inhalation and exhalation. It is in the pause that the heart rate slows, blood pumps more easily, and the brain is flooded with nourishing oxygen. The pause has emotional and psychological benefits as well. Within the pause is the opportunity for the practitioner to become comfortable with space and stillness. A longer exhalation then calms the hypothalamus, which is associated with emotional wellness.

The withdrawal of the senses, called **Pratyahara**, begins, as pranayama deepens, allowing the yogi to draw into the inner world of the heart and mind, where resilience, hope, and joy are stored.

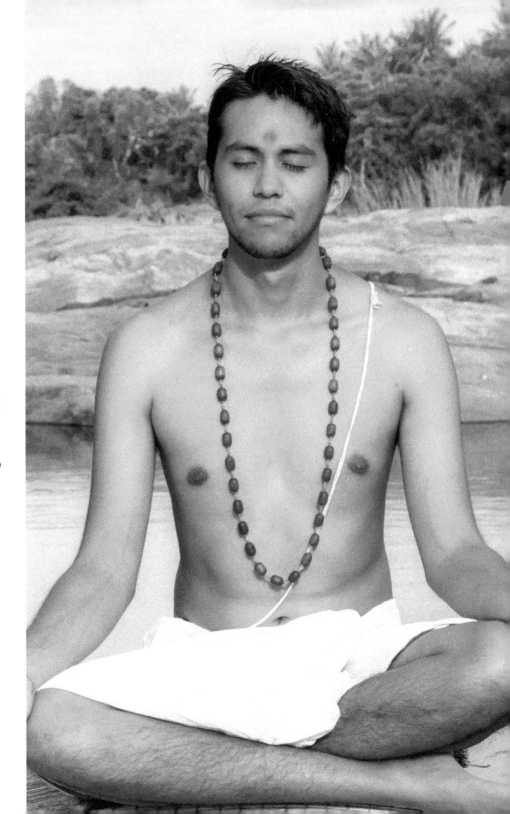

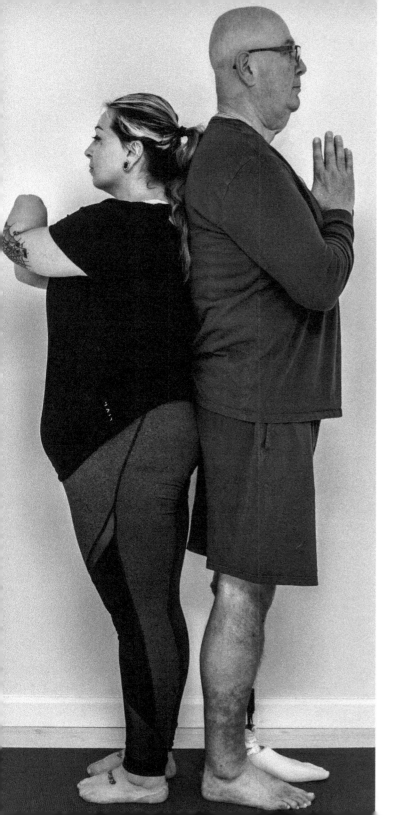

Reflective breathing

The moment an amputee begins to practice pranayama, the journey of self-inquiry has begun. Observation of the breath and the ability to control and redirect the breath, help amputees bring awareness and consciousness to any areas of the body, mind and spirit that are balanced as well as imbalanced. This is called *reflective breathing.*

Different parts of the brain are activated in reflective breathing. When a person begins to practice pranayama, or *reflective breathing*, the cerebrum, which is associated with conscious thought, perception, discernment, and acting, becomes stimulated. It has been found that the cerebrum (or cerebral cortex) begins to thicken with active yoga, pranayama and meditation practice. Reflective breathing is conscious breathing.

The importance of conscious breathing

Diaphragmatic breathing tones the *vagus nerve* which regulates our flight and fight response. Opening the throat, which happens during conscious breathing, relates to the lower portion of the brain stem, the medulla, which in turn stimulates the respiratory system. Bigger airways and more space in the lung sacs, means healthier life force flowing through the body. Nostril breathing, is unique in that it slightly constricts the airwaves, which then stimulates the vagus nerve. The chain reaction is immediate. The blood levels shift, cellular exchange and absorption of oxygen are more complete, and the brain receives even more messages to relax the body. **A relaxed amputee is an amputee who is ready for yoga!**

Pranayama works with the three main diaphragmatic muscles in the body:

- The pelvic diaphragm

- The abdominal diaphragm

- The vocal diaphragm

The **pelvic diaphragm** can carry the weight of the organs. The **abdominal diaphragm**, the one that is referred to most, expands and contracts the air entering and leaving the body. The **vocal diaphragm** at the top of the windpipe between the base of the tongue and glottis protects us from swallowing incorrectly. For an amputee, using all three diaphragms is imperative to maintaining good posture, spinal health and overall wellness.

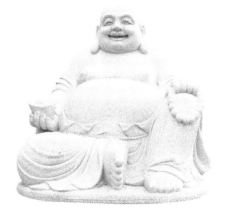

Reflect

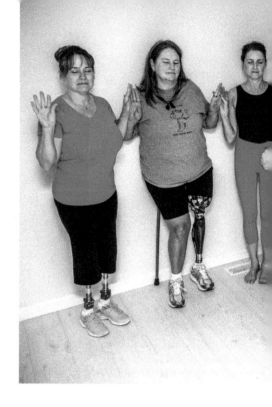

Belly Breath

1. Focus on the belly.

2. Breathe in and out.

3. Feel your belly expand on the inhale, contract on the exhale.

4. Begin to count silently on the inhale and the exhale.

5. Inhale 1-2. Exhale 1-2-3. Inhale 1-2-3. Exhale 1-2-3-4.

6. Continue until you feel complete.

Three Part Breath

1. Inhale as the breath rises from the belly through the ribs and in to the chest.

2. Exhale as the breath descends from the chest through the ribs to the belly.

3. Follow the wave of the breath until you feel complete.

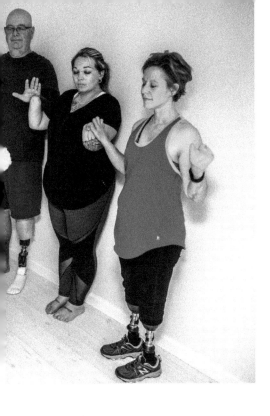

Rebuild

Ujjayi: Breath of Victory

1. With your mouth closed, whisper the word "aaahhh" as you inhale and exhale.

2. Combine the 'aaaahhh' with three-part breath to maximize your breath capacity.

3. Feel as if you are breathing through the back of the throat.

4. Complete the practice when ready.

Nadi Shodhana: Alternate Nostril Breathing

1. Take your right hand in to Vishnu mudra: thumb up, index finger and middle finger down, ring and pinky finger up. Alternately, concentrate on the breath going in through one nostril and out the other if hands are not available.

2. Inhale through both nostrils.

3. Bring the right thumb to the right nostril.

4. Exhale GENTLY through the left.

5. Inhale through the left, close off this nostril with your pinky and ring finger as you open the right nostril to exhale.

6. Exchange back and forth between left and right for eight to ten rounds, ending with an exhale on the left side.

7. Do 10-15 rounds, ending with an exhale on the left.

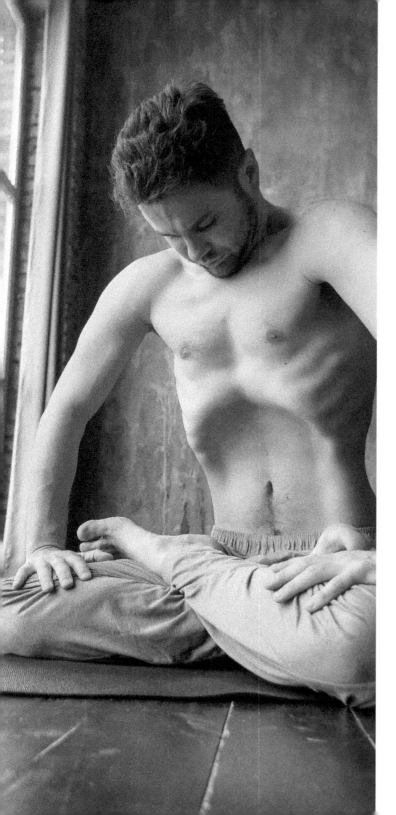

Revive

1. Begin by taking a few deep breaths.

2. Place the hands just below the ribs if able. Alternately, focus on the strong inhalation and exhalation.

3. Inhale fully.

4. Exhale briskly through the nose.

5. You will feel your belly pump inward with the forceful exhale.

6. Continue with a soft inhale and a strong, forceful exhale for ten to twenty rounds.

7. Your breath pattern will become more rapid with greater practice and proficiency.

8. Do at least 10-20 rounds.

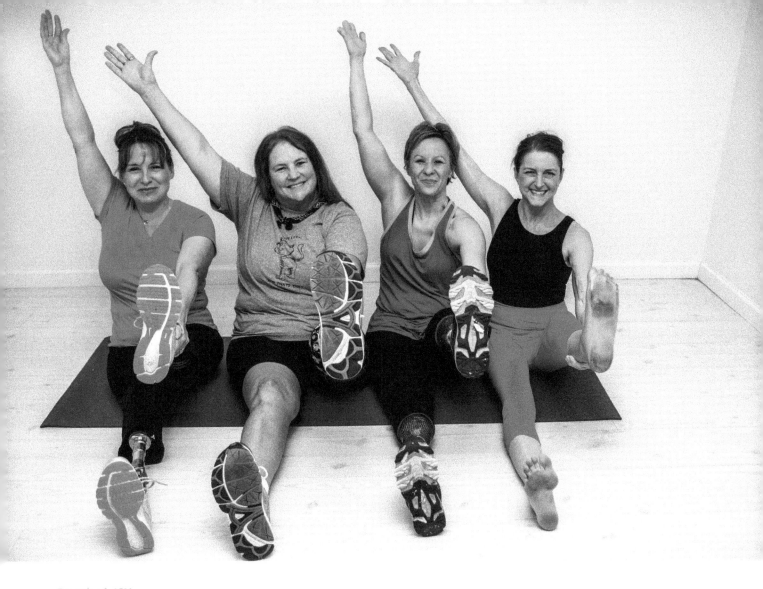

Breath of JOY

1. Stand or sit tall.

2. Inhale with three quick sniffs through the nose as you first lift your arms up over head, then out to the side, then up overhead again. If arms are not available, practice pumping the belly in with each sniff.

3. Exhale with a sigh through the mouth. Drop the arms down as you bend over slightly to release. Take a bow.

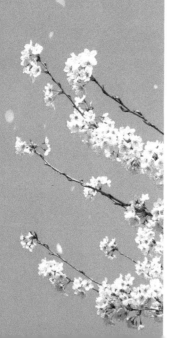

The wind of the breath carries the hope of change, of new birth, of wiping away the past. Wind is both swift action and gentle breeze.

Explore

Awareness of the Breath

1. Sit comfortably.

2. Focus on your belly.

3. Begin to breathe deeply, with the mouth closed, lips soft, allowing breath to flow through the nostrils.

4. Feel your belly rise and fall.

5. Observe your ribs.

6. Breathe in and out through both nostrils.

7. Observe your upper chest, just below the collar bone.

8. Feel the chest expand and contract with each breath.

9. Go back to your belly.

10. As you inhale, follow your breath from the belly to the ribs to the chest.

11. As you exhale, follow your breath from the chest through the ribs to the belly.

12. Repeat this pattern eight to ten times

13. Observe any shifts in your body or mind as you practice breath awareness.

BEND
PRATAPANA: WARM UPS

Each yoga pose has a focal point as well as a number of specific benefits. The best way to learn yoga poses well is to warm up the parts of the body that will be used in that pose. Warm-ups loosen up the body, bringing heat and movement to the joints and muscles. When the body and mind have a chance to loosen up, breathe, and relax, there is more room for flexibility and strength, and less room for injury. Warm ups prepare the body, mind, and spirit for yoga.

Instructions make use of the words hands, elbows, shoulders, arms, feet , knees and leg. Use what is available to you, and generate your movement from the center of the navel out through the body.

Warm the joints

Amputees' joints can get stiff and even frozen due to over and under use. Warming up the joints offers amputees more flexibility and range of motion. Gentle warm-ups soothe the body, calm the nervous system, and release toxic buildup.

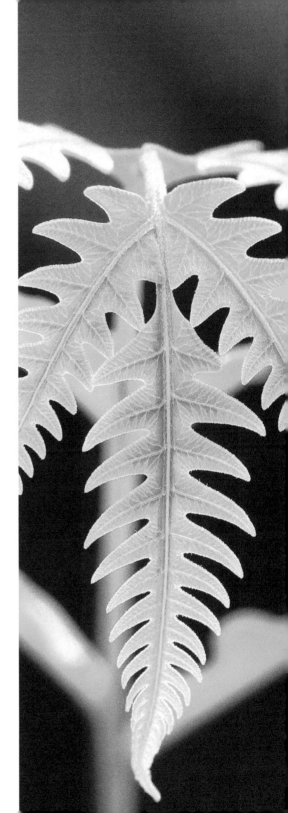

Seated Joint Opening Sequence

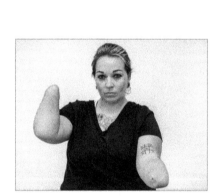

1. **Temporomandibular joint (TMJ)**

a. Open and close the jaw.

b. Stabilize the jaw and move the skull.

c. Stabilize the skull and move the jaw.

2. **Shoulder**

a. Grab the elbow, circling the head of the arm bone (humerus) in the shoulder joint.

b. Draw the elbow closer to the head and push more of the arm bone into the shoulder.

3. **Elbow**

a. Extend the arms out, shoulder height.

b. Bend the elbows, reaching the fingertips towards the top of the shoulder.

c. Release.

4. **Wrist and forearm**

a. Rotate the wrists in one direction, then the other.

b. Circle the elbow in one direction then the other.

c. Clench the hands, making fists.

d. Open the palms, spreading the fingers.

e. *If hands are not available, envision budding petals at the bottom of the residual limb.*

a. Place the left foot on the floor (if available).

b. Lift the right leg off the chair and swing the leg from left to right.

c. Repeat on the other side.

d. Roll the right hip forward then back. Repeat on the other side.

6. Ankles and feet

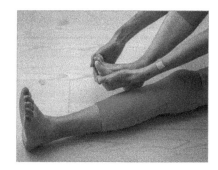

a. Flex and point each foot. *Pointing and flexing the foot can be done without a lower limb by drawing the navel into the spine, lengthening the hamstring as you stretch the residual limb out, then lengthening the top of the thigh to mimic pointing the toes.*

b. Bend the toes in toward the arches.

c. Circle the ankles in one direction then the other.

7. Knees

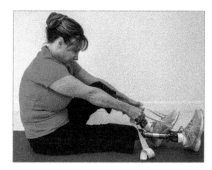

a. Inhale.

b. Straighten the knee.

c. Exhale, bend the knee.

d. Repeat three times for each leg.

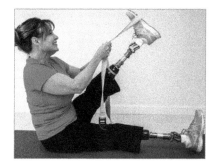

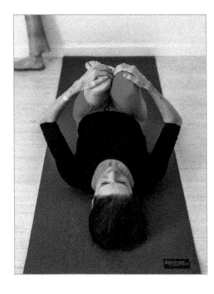

a. Laying on the back, feel the spaces between the bones of the spine.

b. Rock on the spine from side to side.

c. Move the toes, feet, ankles, knees, hips, and shoulders in circles, one joint at a time.

d. Tuck the chin in to the chest.

e. Release the chin to a neutral position.

Warm the muscles

1. Sit in a chair if able (otherwise lie on the floor with supportive props)

2. Place your hands (if available) on the hips to feel the hip flexors.

3. Tuck and release the tailbone, noticing the movement of the hip flexors.

4. Breathe in as the tailbone is released. Breathe out as the pubic bone scoops under.

5. Grab the residual limb on the outside of the thigh.

6. Roll the thigh outward as you exhale, inward as you inhale. This exercise releases the piriformis, which aids an amputee's gait.

7. Repeat on the other side.

8. Rotate both thighs inward, which draws the lower abdominals in to the spine and lengthens the psoas.

9. Grab one leg at a time to circle the hip in one direction, then the other.

10. Place the hands on the thighs and do torso circles.

11. Make figure 8's on the sitz bones.

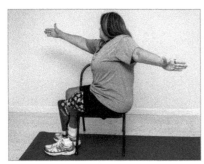

Warm ups for Lower Extremity Amputees

The focus in warming up leg amputees is releasing the hip flexors, psoas and hamstrings, as well as increasing range of motion in the pelvis. Helping leg amputees *find their tailbone* with pelvic lifting helps to ground them since the foot or feet are no longer available.

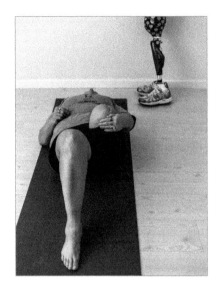

The piriformis and gluteus medius tend to be very tight, due to repetitive overuse and underuse of the corresponding limbs. By releasing these muscles, greater hip rotation and balanced gait are achieved. Leg amputees who wear prosthetics always want to improve their gait to look more natural. Strengthening and lengthening the quads through warm-ups help amputees stand tall, bringing equilibrium to the hips and a feeling of solid foundation.

Basic Warm Ups on the Floor

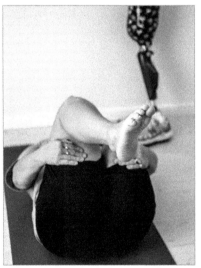

1. Lie on the back with knees bent or legs resting on a bolster.

2. Place the hands on the tops of the hips as you tuck and release the tailbone, to feel the hip flexors release.

3. Grab one leg at a time on the outside of the thigh as if placing the ankle on the opposite thigh, for an increased piriformis stretch.

4. If missing one leg, press the remaining foot into the floor as the residual limb rolls in towards the midline and the lower abdominals draw in to the spine.

5. Lie on the side. Place a yoga strap around the front of the residual limb. Lengthen the quads and hip flexors on exhale, pressing the thigh bone forward and the quads back.

6. Go on hands and knees if available. Round the back on an exhale.

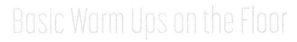

7. Reach the tailbone up to the sky as the belly drops on the inhale.

8. Repeat this sequence three times.

9. Staying on the hands and knees when available, take the hips in a circle clockwise three times, or roll hips in a circle on your back.

10. Reverse the circle.

11. Rest in a comfortable position.

Hip opener

1. Lie on the back.

2. Extend the legs straight out.

3. Bend the right knee.

4. Place a yoga strap around the right foot, calf or thigh if available.

5. Pull the right knee or residual limb into the chest, then extend it up to the sky.

6. Circle the right leg around to the right.

7. Bend the right knee.

8. Bring the left knee in to meet the right.

9. Place the strap around the left foot, calf or thigh if available.

10. Repeat the circle on the left.

11. Bring both knees into the chest.

12. Release the strap.

13. Relax the legs to the floor.

Targeted warm ups for Upper Extremity Amputees

Warm ups for upper extremity amputees release tension in the shoulders and mid back, as well as the jaw and neck. Upper extremity amputees need strengthening in the abdominals *(see below)* to maintain spinal alignment. The muscles of the shoulder girdle, such as the trapezoid, supraspinatus and sternocleidomastoid need to be stretched and fortified.

Wall clock

1. Stand within reach of the wall.

2. Place the prosthetic hand, when available, at the wall, or stretch the residual limb towards the wall.

3. If comfortable place the tip of the limb at the wall as if the wall were a clock, at 12o'clock.

4. Breathe in, then exhale as you walk the hand or limb back a few inches to 1, 2 and 3 o'clock.

5. Repeat 3-4 times, moving the arm farther and farther back, then reverse back to 12 o'clock.

6. Switch sides.

7. Circle the shoulder with deep slow breaths.

8. Roll the shoulders in towards the center of the chest, then out, away from the center.

9. Tilt the head to the right shoulder on exhale.

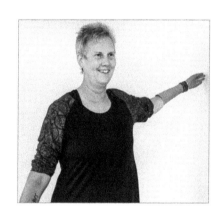

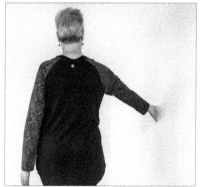

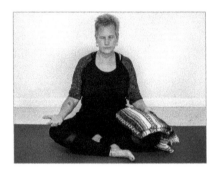

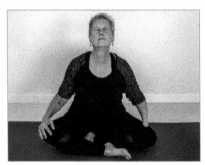

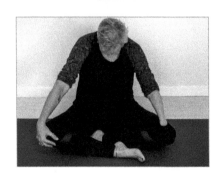

10. Inhale the head to the center.

11. Exhale the head to the left.

12. Return the head to the center.

13. Elevate and depress the shoulders, inhaling as the shoulders rise to the ears, exhaling as the shoulders drop.

14. Circle the wrist of the limb still available.

15. Alternately, circle the shoulders or ribs in, out and around.

16. Twist the torso to the right, center, left, and center.

Six Movements of the Spine

A healthy spine is a supple spine, inviting more vitality. For amputees, the health of the spine is essential to walking well and keeping an active life style. This daily warm up flexes all parts of the spine, lightens anxiety, increases clarity, and strengthens the nervous system.

Seated version of six movements of the spine: Flexion and extension

1. Sit tall in a chair or on the floor.

2. Place the hands on the floor if available or a chair beside your hips.

3. Reach the upper chest towards the ceiling as you stretch your spine (extension).

4. Inhale.

5. Round forward and exhale, pressing the chin to the chest (flexion).

Lateral stretch

1. Place your right hand to the floor or a chair beside your right hip. Or, arch the torso to the right.

2. Lift the left arm up as you inhale.

3. Exhale as you bend your left arm over to the right.

4. Inhale, come back to the center.

5. Repeat to the left.

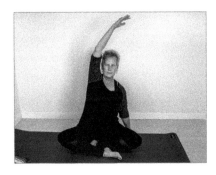

Twist

1. Sit tall.

2. Place the right hand behind your right buttock, or twist the center of the sternum to the right.

3. Inhale. Lengthen your torso.

4. Place the left hand to the right thigh or side of the chair. Exhale.

5. Twist to the right.

6. Inhale.

7. Come back to the center. Exhale.

8. Repeat to the left.

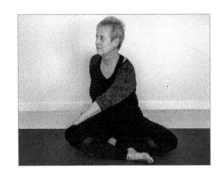

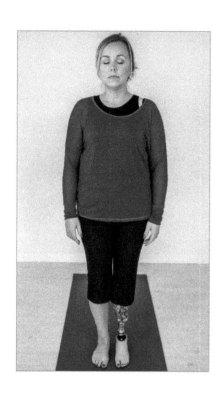

YOGA FOR STRENGTH

It takes extraordinary strength of body, mind and spirit to recover from limb loss and charge forward in life. Sometimes, an amputee has had enough, and needs the courage to move on. A yoga practice that fosters strength brings the amputee back to the truth - that she is more than a conqueror, someone who can face life head on, empowered from within.

Mountain: Tadasana

1. Stand with the feet hip width apart.

2. Reach the feet down into all four corners as you lift the crown up to the sky.

3. Lift the knee caps up.

4. Draw the belly in.

5. Lift the arms overhead on inhale, interlocking the hands, index fingers pointing to the sky.

6. Circle the arms to the side on exhale.

7. Keep the gaze at one spot 8-10 feet in front of you.

BK and AK amputees

- To be sure hips are even and there is no strain in the hamstrings, place the rolled edge of a yoga mat under the heels or toes if needed, depending on prosthetic alignment.

- Do this pose with the back to the wall.

- Place a chair in front of the body 1-2 feet to lean on for extra stability.

- Bend the prosthetic knee to keep hips even.

- Place a yoga block between the thighs to increase pelvic opening and stabilize the core.

- Place a strap under the balls of the feet. Tug on both sides of the strap to feel grounding as you press the legs down and the spine long.

UE amputees

- Draw the ribs back to stabilize the shoulders.

- Draw shoulder blades together slightly to lift the chest.

- Lift the armpits up and out.

Goddess: Utkatakonasana

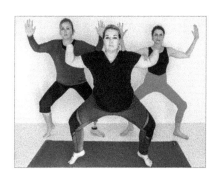

1. From Tadasana, place the hands in front of the heart and step feet wide apart about 3 - 4 feet wide. Check to see that the ankles are under the wrists, toes straight ahead, hips straight ahead.

2. Root the feet as you lengthen up through the crown and out through the fingers.

3. Breathe in to the center of the body and expand from your light in all directions. Relax the shoulders.

4. Inhale deeply into the belly and chest, exhale, and radiate out in all 5 directions.

5. Bend the knees in line with the ankles in a semi-plie.

6. Stretch your arms out from your shoulders like the letter "T".

7. Breathe in.

8. Breathe out. Bend your knees and elbows. Flex your muscles.

9. Inhale. Exhale. Jump or step back in to Mountain.

- Do this pose with the back to the wall.

- Do this sideways against a corner wall, with the top toes pressing into the side wall.

- Practice this pose seated at the edge of a chair.

- Loop a strap around the lower shins to support stability.

- Face a wall with the chair at the wall. Open the knees and press the insides of the knees into the wall. Press the palms into the wall, elbows bent, at shoulder length.

- Lay on the back with the legs lifted to the ceiling. Bend the knees out towards the shoulders. Grab hold of the calf or foot in **happy baby pose.**

- Lay on the back with the legs outstretched. Bend the knees to hip height and rest the knees on blocks, pillows, or folded blankets.

- Focus on revolving the ribs open.

- Do the pose with the back to a wall and press the shoulders into the wall.

- Practice the pose seated, with legs wide, resting elbows on vertical yoga blocks.

- Focus on opening the chest and dropping the collarbone or shoulders if available.

Chair Pose: Utkatasana:

1. Come into mountain.

2. Bend the knees as if you were about to sit in a chair.

3. Extend the arms out in front, parallel to the ground, or overhead.

4. Look straight ahead.

5. Keep heels down, knees not too far over the toes.

6. Draw the shoulder blades in towards the center.

7. Feel the mid back filling up to reduce sway back.

8. Relax the shoulders by opening through the collar bone.

9. Keep the back of the torso full and alive.

BK and AK amputees

* Roll a yoga mat under the edge of the heel/heels that may be lifting off the floor.

* Concentrate on hip alignment even if the prosthetic leg goes over the toes.

* Sit in a chair facing a wall. Press into the chair as you rise, with the tops of the toes pressing into the wall. Press the hands into the wall.

* Hold a strap between the hands or wrap a strap around the forearms or upper arms.

* Lean the bottom against a wall, facing a chair with the hands on the back edge of the chair.

* Practice sitting and getting up from a chair using abdominal muscles and quads.

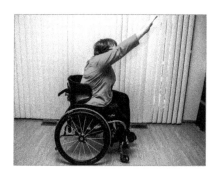

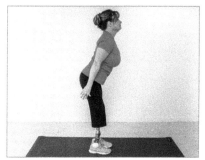

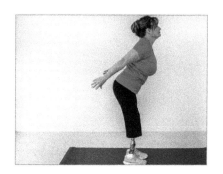

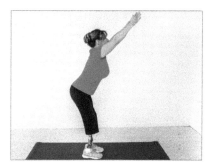

- Pull the lower belly in and up as you squat in chair pose.

- Lift the sternum towards the chin.

- When lifting the residual limb parallel to the shoulders, keep lengthening from the hips to ribs, drawing the armpit back.

Plank: Uttihita Chaturanga Dandasana

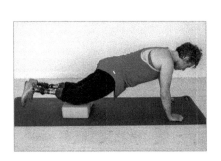

1. Start in downward dog.

2. Engage the lower belly as you press forward parallel to the floor.

3. Expand the collarbone.

4. Feel the sacrum and pubic bone draw towards each other.

5. Look towards the floor.

6. Keep the back body straight like a board.

7. To go further, bend the elbows in towards the ribs.

8. Hover the body a few inches from the ground in **chaturanga dandasana**, or four limbed pose.

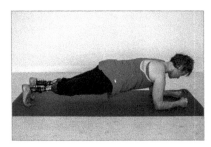

BK and AK amputees

- Begin the pose on all fours then step one leg back at a time.

- Face away from the wall, press the heels towards the wall, and place a rolled towel behind the prosthetic foot.

- Wrap a strap around the thighs to stabilize.

- Face the wall, pressing the crown of the head into the wall.

- Place yoga blocks under the knees.

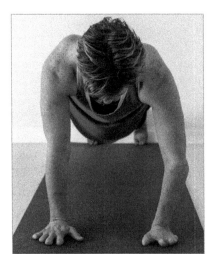

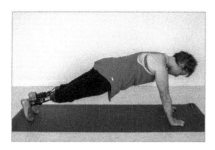

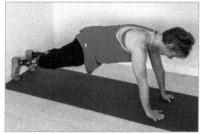

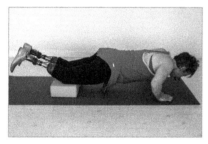

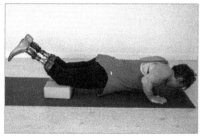

- Place a yoga block (soft only) crosswise on the upper chest, *not* directly on the sternum.

- Do the pose over a stability ball.

- Do the pose standing against the wall.

- Place a rolled blanket under the prosthetic leg and practice lifting the leg off the blanket an inch or two.

UE amputees

- Press the feet into the wall, facing away from the wall, as you draw the body toward midline.

- Wrap a strap around the thighs to create security.

- Do the pose sideways against a wall with resistance from the side of the body.

- Do the pose standing against a wall.

- Do the pose on the forearms if the elbow is available.

- Lie on the back with the feet to the wall and practice the fundamentals of the pose.

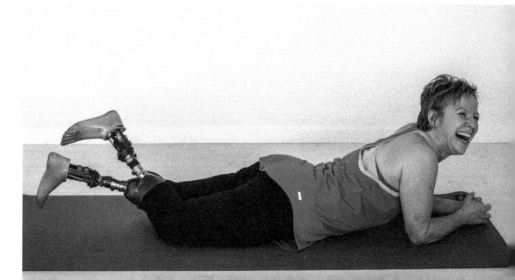

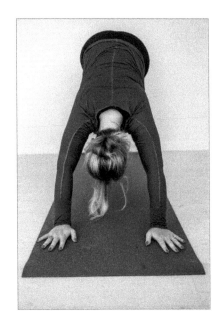

Downward Facing Dog: Adho Mukha Svanasana

1. Start in table position, with the hands firmly placed under the shoulders, and knees under the hips.

2. Press into the palms and fingers, especially the mound of the thumb and index finger.

3. Roll the armpits forward and the head of the arm bones back.

4. Make the belly flush to the spine.

5. Curl the toes under, breathe in, exhale and press into a downward V with hips raised.

6. Keep the hips lifted with bent knees.

7. Create a loop from the top of the tailbone down the back of the legs through the back heels, under the body to the heels of the hands and fingertips.

8. Continue to press firmly into the hands and lengthen the spine and the legs.

9. Release by bending the knees back into table pose.

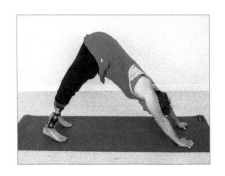
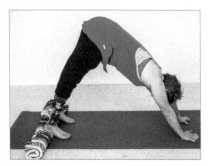
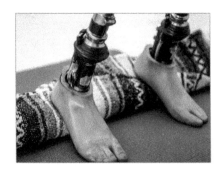

- Place a rolled yoga mat under the prosthetic leg.

- Bend the prosthetic leg to keep the hips even.

- Practice with the feet at the wall.

- Face the wall, press the palms into the wall and walk the palms down until parallel with the hips.

- Fold over a chair at the hips with the feet pressed into a wall.

- Place a yoga block under the prosthetic knee or thigh.

- Loop a strap around the upper arms for more stability.

- Fold forward, placing the hands at the edge of the seat of a chair.

UE amputees

- If strong enough, do the pose with one arm.

- If there is no pain rest the residual limb on a yoga block.

- Fold over a chair with the feet at the back of the wall.

- Place bolsters under the chest.

- Do the pose with one hand pressing at the wall as you fold in half, the hand parallel to the hips.

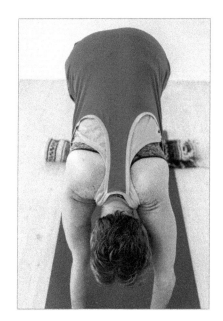

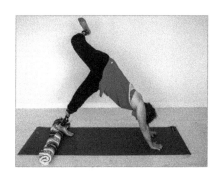

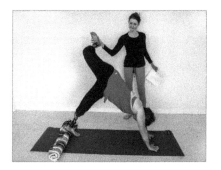

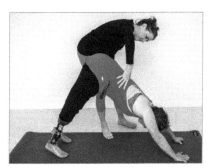

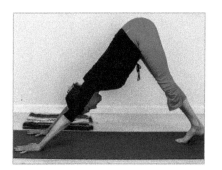

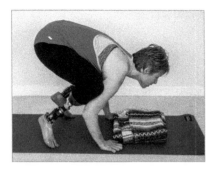

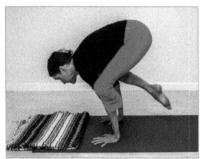

Crow: Bakasana

1. Stand in mountain pose.

2. Step the feet wider to allow for a full squat.

3. Begin to squat towards the floor, spine staying lifted.

4. Rock forward slightly, head staying lifted.

5. Press the palms flat into the mat.

6. Place the shins on top of the mid upper arms.

7. Draw the belly in.

8. Tiptoe onto the balls of the feet.

9. Lift one foot, or both off the floor a few inches.

10. Hug the limbs in towards the center.

11. Keep the head lifted.

12. Balance.

13. To release place the toes back on the floor and come into a standing forward bend.

BK and AK amputees

- Do this pose without a prosthesis.

- Be sure to safely bend the prosthetic leg to rest on the upper arm.

- Set a pile of blankets or a pillow in front of the head. That way, there is something soft to fall on if balance is lost.

- Place a yoga block or chair behind you to sit on when finished.

- Wear something long sleeved to avoid irritation from the prosthetic to the upper arm skin.

- Practice squatting to see how far a bend is possible while keeping the torso upright.

- Try side crow instead.

- Practice frog squats instead.

- Practice one handed push-ups and burpees.

Side Crow: Ardha Bakasana

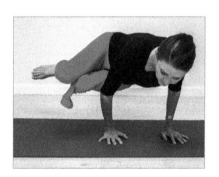

1. Come into a squat with the hands in prayer pose at the heart.

2. Twist the torso to the right.

3. Place the palms on the floor to the right, elbows bent, upper arms under the upper right thigh.

4. Look up.

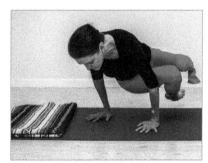

5. Draw the navel in to the spine and lift the feet off the floor.

6. Breathe deeply 3-5 times.

7. Gently come back to the squat.

8. Roll to standing.

9. Repeat on the left side.

- Do this pose without a prosthesis for an easier bend in the knee and lift off.

- Sit on a yoga block then place the palms to the right.

- Place folded blankets and pillows to the right before doing the pose on the right. Switch props to the left when ready to do the left side.

- Practice lifting the residual limb into the chest before attempting the pose.

- Place a blanket between the upper arms and upper thighs to avoid pain in the residual limb.

- Begin the pose on all fours if not wearing a prosthesis to avoid overuse of other leg. If a bilateral leg amputee, sit in an easy sitting pose. Place the palms on either side of the hips. Practice lifting the body off the floor before attempting side crow.

UE amputee

- Try a squat with a side twist, with or without sitting on a block, rather than full crow.

- Practice twisted lunge into twisted half-moon.

Boat: Navasana

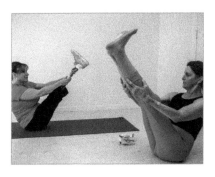

1. Sit on the floor with the legs outstretched.

2. Place the hands on both sides of the hips.

3. Tuck the tailbone, while extending the chest up.

4. Bend the knees, lifting the feet parallel to the knees.

5. Stay with the knees and feet parallel or extend the legs up so the body is in a V shape.

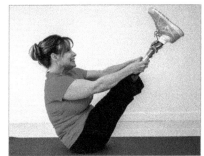

6. Continue to press the hands into the floor.

7. Lift the arms up parallel to the shoulders.

8. Hug the knees in and release.

BK and AK amputees

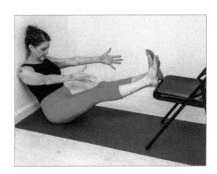

- If the prosthesis is too heavy to lift without injury, drape the back of the lower legs over the seat of a chair.

- Face a wall, lean back into the hands, and walk the feet up the wall.

- Sit against the wall in a slight diagonal, pressing just the mid back into the wall. Let the feet rest, with legs extended on the edge of a chair

- Keep the feet on the floor, knees bent and lean back into a V.

- Lift only one leg.

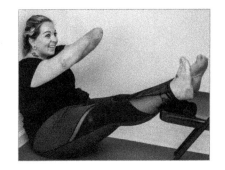

- Rest the legs on a bolster and folded blankets while leaning the mid back into a wall or immovable chair.

- Do this pose with the mid back to the wall, bolster or blanket between the lower back and the wall.

- Try lying on the back and rolling up 5-10 times until balancing on the buttocks in boat.

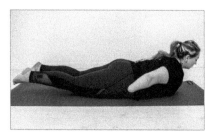

Locust: Shalabhasana

1. Lie on the belly with the feet close and arms, palms down, along the side of the torso.

2. The chin rests on the floor.

3. Drop the coccyx slightly to the pubic bone with a small tuck.

4. Inhale and lengthen from the navel to the crown and the navel to the toes.

5. Draw the thigh bones and shin bones up to the back of the legs. Exhale.

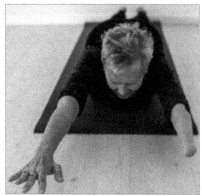

6. Press into the palms and pubic bone and extend through the toes, lifting the legs off the floor a few inches.

7. Exhale.

8. Release the legs to the floor, relax and receive the pose.

BK and AK amputees:

- Place a folded blanket or towel under the pubic bone to support the pubic area.

- Place a rolled blanket under the lower sternum.

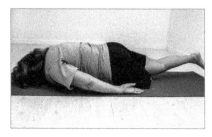

UE Amputees:

- Lift the lower and upper body away from the floor a few inches, maintaining length.

- Place the remaining forearm parallel to the chest, if available, leaning the forehead on the forearm.

MEET KELLY

"This is the life I was given. I'm not gonna change it. You can do it with a smile or you can be mad for the rest of your life."

Kelly is a shining example of embracing the body she has, living from her blissful nature daily. Kelly lost both her legs below the knees, as well as most of her fingers due to Meningococcemia, a bacterial form of Meningitis, as a one year old. She is a mother and full time internal auditor for an insurance company, who has an incredible network of support. She wears two vacuum system prosthetics daily and is extremely active, including teaching Zumba®! Fitness is extremely important to her, both as a woman but also as an amputee, to prevent injuries and weakness later in life. Kelly has done yoga off and on over the years.

For Kelly, wholeness means balance among work, family and personal time, which gives her peace of mind. She has gained so many life lessons she never would have gained if she wasn't an amputee. She shares her story almost daily, inspiring others to live with possibility. Her relationship with her limbs has changed over the years. She used to cover up her legs and hands often, but, depending on the person with whom she is speaking, she shows her limbs proudly

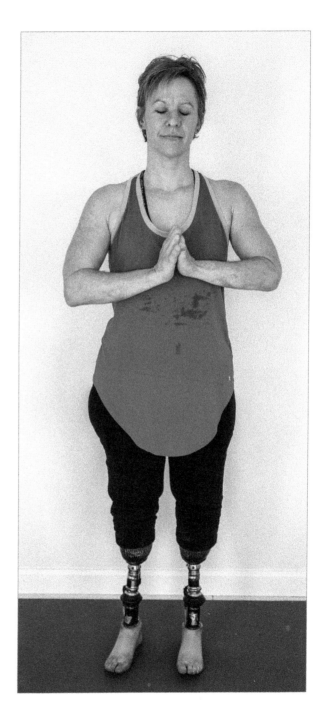

more often, reminding her how far she's come in her life. Kelly has met people who don't see her missing limbs or fingers at all, while others only see what is missing.

Kelly has endured a lot - at least two surgeries per year until the age of twenty and a revision on her residual limbs a few years ago. When she was around eight, Kelly had a moment that made her question whether God even cared about her, wondering why she had to endure her life as a quadruple amputee. She felt bad for asking, because at the time of her illness, her family was told she would be a vegetable if she ever woke up. She felt should have been more grateful.

Yet here she is today! Kelly has been able to reclaim her life and remember who she truly is; a joyful child of God. Kelly is proud to be who she is. So are we!

YOGA FOR BALANCE

We hear a lot of people talk about how they want more balance in life, but what does balance mean for an amputee? Amputation shakes a person to the core, with both his inner and outer world upset in challenging ways. Things we take for granted, like walking across a room, or washing the dishes, take on a whole new meaning after limb loss. Emotional and psychological balance can be off kilter, as can an amputee's physical reality. Yoga is a natural way to bring an amputee back to a sense of harmony, rebuilding one's self from the inside out. Balance requires finesse, as well as the skill to handle imbalances well. The poses below challenge amputees to find balance no matter what is happening .

Tree: Vrikshasana

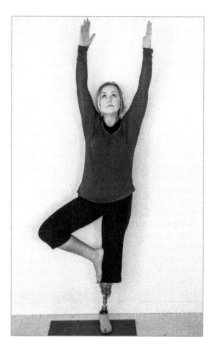

1. Stand in mountain

2. Bend the right knee, placing the right foot to inside of the inner left thigh or calf.

3. Root down through the left leg; lift the arms overhead, parallel to the shoulders or in a V.

4. Lower the right foot down.

5. Repeat on other side.

BK and AK amputees

- Stand sideways at a wall and press the hand closest to the wall into the wall.

- Keep the foot on the ground, turn out the knee and curl the toes near the opposite foot

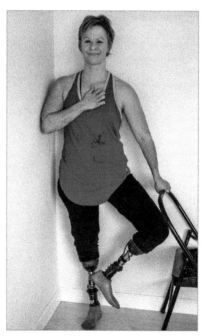

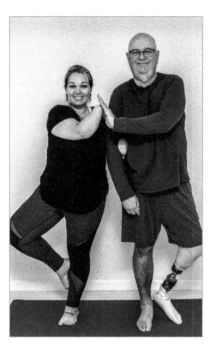

- Hold a strap around the shins.

- Place a yoga block under the prosthetic foot.

- Stand at the wall with a chair nearby for extra stability.

- Practice balancing on the prosthetic leg first.

UE amputees

- Lift through the armpits.

- Grab hold of the residual limb to form a square overhead.

- If the residual limb can lift, it may be more comfortable to extend the arms in front at shoulder level.

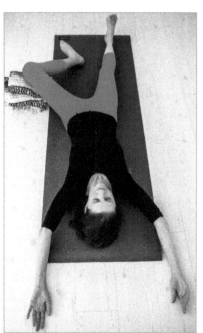

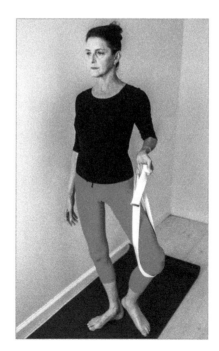

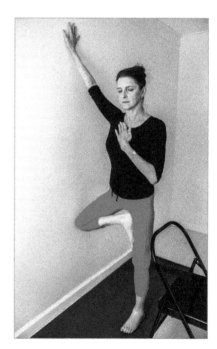

Warrior III: Virabhadrasana III

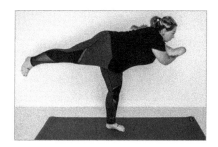

1. Stand in mountain pose.

2. Step the left foot back 3-4 feet, left foot turned in about 70 degrees towards the left front.

3. Pivot the hips square to the front, as in mountain pose.

4. Bend the right knee as you lengthen the tailbone down, draw the navel in to the spine, and lightly lift the left leg off the ground.

5. Lift the left leg fully off the ground.

6. Parallel the torso to the floor, as if the torso is the body of an airplane.

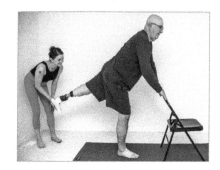

7. Firmly press into the standing leg.

8. Even the hips to be pointing towards the floor.

9. Place the arms in a 'T' position, close to the body, or interlocked and lengthened in front of the crown of the head.

10. Look to the floor to keep balance.

11. To come out of the pose, slowly land the left leg back into its starting position.

12. Step the left leg to meet the right.

13. Switch and repeat on the other side.

BK and AK amputees

* Do Warrior III against a wall or corner. Place the balancing leg closest to the wall, and lift the other leg as in the instructions above. If at a corner, press the foot of the lifted leg into the wall behind. Place hands to the floor, on a yoga block, leaning the shoulder and arm on the balancing side into the wall.

- Use a wall and a chair. Do as above, but place the back of a chair next to the non-balancing leg. Lean the arm on that side on the top of the chair.

- Try Warrior III on the hands and knees. Lift the left leg behind, parallel to the floor, foot flexed towards the floor, with hips even. For a more challenging pose, extend the opposite arm in front.

- Try Warrior III in a chair. Sit at the side edge of a chair, with the chair facing the wall vertically. Slide the front leg over the front of the chair, with the knee bent. Extend the back leg behind, leaning the top of leg or knee on yoga blocks, or pillows to support the back leg.

- Fold over the front bent knee, extending the leg and press the hands into the wall.

UE amputee

- From the balancing leg, work on tipping from the waist, forward and back to a place that feels challenging yet safe. Deeply hug the abdominal muscles in. Lift the chest slightly, which supports balance.

Firefly: Tittibhasana

1. Come into a squat, arms between the legs.

2. Wrap the upper thighs around the tops of the upper arms.

3. Spread the fingers and press the palms into the floor.

4. Lift the legs off the ground, facing the limbs forward in a wide 'V'.

5. Look forward.

6. To come out of the pose, bend the knees if available.

7. Place the feet on the ground, then gently slide the buttocks to the floor.

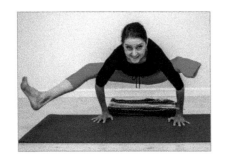

- Do this pose about 10-12" from the wall, with the back to the wall, for extra security.

- Place plenty of folded blankets behind and under the buttocks.

- Do the pose without a prosthetic for easier lift of the leg.

- Practice wide angle forward bend instead.

- Stay seated in a wide angle pose, and try to lift the legs off the floor into a wide 'V', any height from the floor.

UE amputee

- Come into wide angle forward bend or seated wide angle pose.

- Stay seated in a wide angle pose, and try to lift the legs off the floor into a wide 'V', any height from the floor.

Side Plank: Vasisthasana

1. Start in downward dog.

2. Revert to plank pose.

3. Place the feet together to the right.

4. Roll over to the right side, leaning into the right palm.

5. Keep hips lifted and in line with the right palm.

6. Extend the left arm up to the sky.

7. Look towards the top arm.

8. Come back to plank.

9. Repeat on the left.

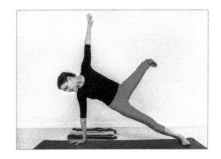

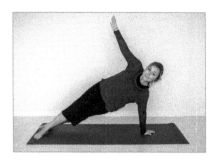

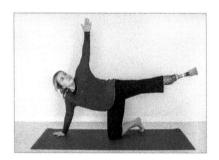

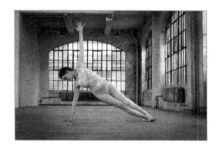

- Practice with the back to the wall.

- Practice with the feet leaning into the wall.

- Place the bottom knee on the floor, foot behind the knee.

- Place the top foot in front of the hip, knee bent.

- Do this pose sideways on the forearms.

- For the residual limb side, if practicing without the prosthesis, practice pressing the limb to the other leg.

- Do a push up or plank instead.

UE amputee

- If the forearm is available, practice on the forearm.

- Practice the pose standing, leaning slightly to the left and lift the right leg diagonally away. Repeat to the other side.

- Sit on the right edge of a chair leaning against a wall. Extend the legs out to the right side, pressing the feet into the wall. Flex the feet. Reach the top arm to the sky. The body will be in a diagonal.

King Dancer: Natarajasana

Be sure to have a yoga strap nearby.

1. Stand in mountain pose.

2. Lift the right leg behind, grabbing hold of the inside of the right foot with the right hand.

3. Draw the right knee parallel to the left standing knee.

4. Balance on the left foot.

5. Press the right foot into the right hand and the right hand into the right foot until an arch in the back begins to form. Use a strap around the right foot if the right hand does not reach the foot.

6. Extend the left arm overhead.

7. Keep pressing the foot into the hand as you bend at the hips, coming into a balance.

8. Your torso will be nearly parallel to the floor as the right leg extends up behind you towards the sky.

9. The chest lifts and the ribs expand.

10. Slowly come back to standing and release the right foot to meet the left.

11. Take a moment to feel the effects of the pose.

12. Repeat on the other side.

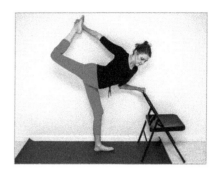

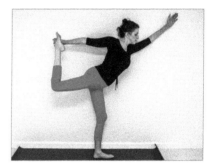

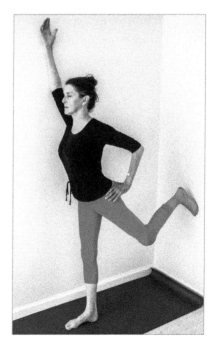

- Practice this pose against a wall. Lean the balancing leg against the wall and reach for the other leg.

- Practice the pose at a corner. Lean the balancing leg against one wall. Press the foot of the non-balancing leg into the bottom of the wall or if able, lift the leg with the knee bent and press the foot into the wall. Resist the foot into the wall for a greater backbend.

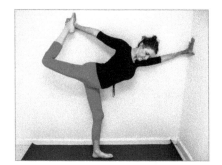

- Practice this pose in a chair with or without prosthetics. Come to the edge of the chair. Slide to the right and drop the right knee and right leg behind. Keep stretching the right leg back to get a quad stretch. Wrap a yoga strap around the left foot to create more backbend. If not wearing a prosthesis, support the residual limb on pillows or folded blankets and draw the navel into the spine, extending the sternum upward.

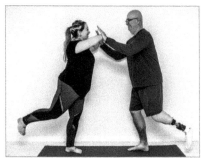

- Practice on the floor without prosthetics. Lie on the right side with legs lined up and extended. Bend the top right knee (when available) or the top of the right limb with the right hand. Press the hand into the limb and the limb into the hand as the back arches. A strap around the residual limb can also be used if the hand does not reach. Release and roll to the other side to repeat.

UE amputee

- When available, open the residual limbs into a T, drawing the shoulders together in a backbend. Lift the sternum up and arch the chest.

- Do the pose against a wall for better balance.

- Lift the back foot to a wall and press into the wall, expanding the chest.

- Practice the pose on the floor near the wall, lying to the side, with the back foot pressing into the wall.

- Stand at a corner. Place the chair behind you with the back legs of the chair pressing into the wall. Rest the top of the left foot on top of the chair as you stand on the right leg, the other wall to your right in case you need to lean in to the wall. Open the chest and expand the ribs like wings. Repeat on the other side.

Balancing Half Moon:
Ardha Chandrasana II

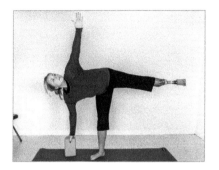

1. Stand in mountain pose.

2. Step the right foot back three feet, right foot turned in fifteen degrees, left foot at ninety degrees.

3. Open the arms into a T and lean the torso over the left leg, dropping the left hand towards the left shin, floor or ten inches to the left of the left foot.

4. Bend the left knee as you lift the right leg up, the right hip open, the right foot flexed to the side.

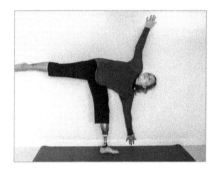

5. Press into the standing foot as you revolve your torso to the right.

6. Lean the left hand or fingertips into the floor diagonally to the left of the front foot.

7. Bend the left knee as you gently drop the right foot back to its original position.

8. Lift the torso up straight.

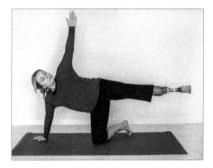

9. Step the feet together into mountain pose.

10. Repeat on the other side.

BK and AK amputees

* Do this pose against a wall. Place the balancing foot closest to the wall as you lift the other leg. Lean the balancing foot and buttocks into the wall. If unable to lift the other leg, keep it on the floor and have someone place the prosthetic leg on the seat or back of a chair. You can also put a strap around the upper thigh and lift the leg to place on a support such as a chair. It all depends on the weight of the prosthesis, the strength of the abdominals and the length of the residual limb.

THE FIVE 'B'S

135

- Stand against a corner, one leg's width from the edge of a wall. Press the lifted leg into the wall behind you. Lean the stabilizing leg into the side wall.

- Place a yoga block or chair in front of the balancing leg, leaning the hand on that side of the chair or yoga block.

- Do this pose on the floor. Lie on the back at a corner, leg's length from the wall. Open the right leg to the right wall. Roll over halfway towards the right buttocks as you press the left leg into the opposite wall. Open the arms, right arm reaching to the right foot, the left arm reaching above and behind the left shoulder, at an angle. Switch sides.

- If doing this without prosthetics, practice rolling the left thigh, hip or torso into the right and open the left arm out. Repeat to the left.

UE amputee

- Practice this pose against a wall with the back to the wall.

- If the amputee has an elbow, lean the elbow into a chair and lift the back leg.

- Have a spotter press the back hip open to avoid falling on the residual limb.

- Practice in increments, lifting the back leg up a few inches, developing balance.

- Practice standing triangle instead.

- Stand in mountain. Lift the left leg and swing it back and forth until the leg is behind. Try turning the torso to the left. Repeat to the right.

- Practice abdominal exercises to develop better core for balance and safety.

Eagle: Garudhasana

1. Stand in Mountain.

2. Wrap the left leg over the right thigh and wrap the left foot around the back of the right calf.

3. Open the arms wide as you inhale.

4. Exhale. Cross the left elbow under the right elbow.

5. Sink down as if about to sit in a chair.

6. Press in to the standing leg.

7. Slightly straighten, release the arms and stand upright.

8. Go to the other side.

BK and AK amputees

- Do this pose on the back.

- Sit at the edge of a wall with a chair in front to hold onto if balance is lost.

- Rather than cross the legs, hug the thighs into the midline.

- Do this seated in a chair.

- Place the crossed foot on a block.

UE amputee

- Cross the non-residual limb over to the opposite shoulder.

- Round the shoulders forward then back.

- Turn the inner arms up.

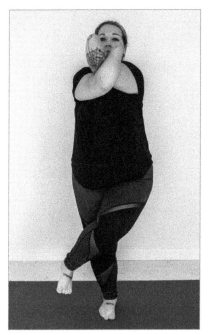

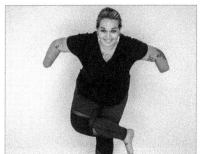

Warrior I: Virabhadrasana I

1. Stand in Tadasana.

2. Step the right foot forward about 3'.

3. Turn the left foot in about 15 degrees.

4. Square the hips forward.

5. Tuck the tailbone.

6. Lift the ribs up off the hips.

7. Draw the navel back to the spine.

8. Lift the arms up overhead.

9. Lift the heart.

10. Step the left foot to meet the right.

11. Step to the back of the mat.

12. Repeat on the other side.

Bk and AK amputees

- Place a rolled edge of a yoga mat under the prosthetic foot, heel or the ball of the foot, depending on alignment.

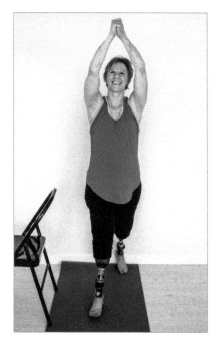

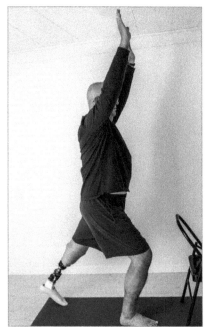

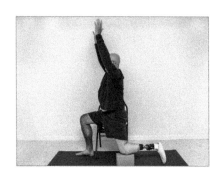

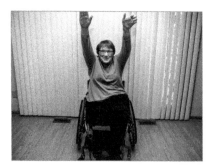

- Stand against a wall, leaning the extended back leg into the wall.

- Do this pose in a chair, the back leg extended, the front leg draped over a chair.

- Stay on the ball of the back foot.

- Do this pose between two chairs, placing the hands on the chair backs as needed.

- Place a chair at the wall, the seat facing you. Step forward, the front knee/shin pressing into the chair edge.

UE amputees

- Lift the armpits and expand the collarbone.

- Practice the cobra chest in this pose.

- Relax the shoulders.

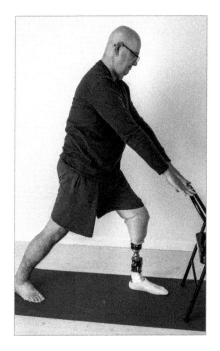

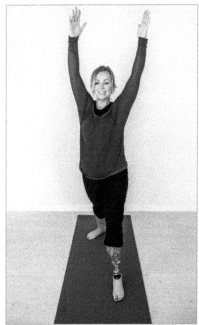

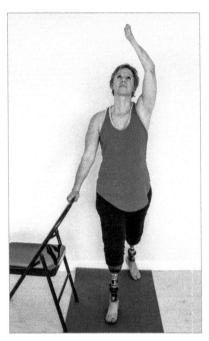

Crescent Lunge: Virabhdrasana I variation

1. Come to all fours.

2. Press back into downward facing dog pose.

3. Lift the right leg up behind you.

4. Deeply hug the abdominal muscles in toward the spine and bend the back right knee. Lift it toward the belly, then step it forward, the knee parallel to the ankle, placing the right foot on the floor.

5. The back toes will be curled under.

6. Lift the torso upright, hands interlocked overhead

7. Lift the chest.

8. Be sure the hips are facing forward.

9. Focus on a point 8-10 feet in front.

10. To come out of the pose, fold over the bent front knee, palms to the floor.

11. Step the right foot back to meet the left in downward facing dog.

12. Repeat the pose on the other side.

BK and AK amputees

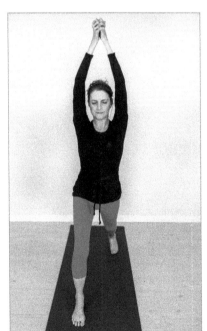

- Do the pose against the wall either horizontally, leaning the side of the body in the lunge against the wall or vertically, facing the wall with the front bent knee, elbows hugging into the ribs, palms pressing into the wall.

- Do the pose seated in a chair at a corner. Press the back leg into the wall, and the side of the front knee into the wall. Press the hand opposite the knee into the chair to align the hips square to the front and lift the chest.

- Wrap a yoga strap around the upper arms as you press the upper arms into the strap and expand the chest.

- Use yoga blocks, folded blankets and pillows underneath the extended back leg.

- Do the pose on the floor. Lie on the right side. Extend the left leg behind and back. Bend the bottom right knee parallel to the hip. Reach the arms overhead, the fingers interlocked.

UE amputee

- Do crescent lunge from a standing position. Come to the back of the mat. Step the right foot forward in a lunge. This can be done flush to the wall if more support is needed. Lift the torso from the belly button to the sternum, creating a backbend. To come out of the crescent lunge, round the spine, tuck the chin, draw the navel in and gently step the left foot to meet the right.

- Do the pose as above, in a chair, focusing on lifting the sternum and drawing the shoulder blades towards each other.

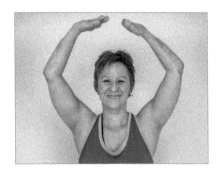

YOGA TO OPEN THE HEART

The heart is a powerful organ. Not only does it pump blood and oxygen throughout the body, the electromagnetic field of the heart has a resonance all its own, stronger than the mind, which profoundly influences our health, well-being and relationships. If you have ever been around a 'warm-hearted' person, you know what I mean! When the heart and mind work together, life feels clear, and congruent. Likewise, a resonant heart and mind build resilience, balance heart rate, increase brain function, improve relationships with others, and help us better cope with stress.

The heart's own system of intelligence guides all of us when we are willing to listen. Yoga is the perfect mix of body, mind and HEART which awakens our innate capacities to listen well. As amputees, we need to listen to all aspects of ourselves to be our own best advocates.

The word courage is derived from the Latin word 'Cor', or heart. Living with limb loss and limb difference requires tremendous heart, or courage, to thrive in life. From physical to emotional challenges, amputees know what courage really means.

This yoga practice is designed to build strength, resilience, courage and compassion in the heart of an amputee. Enjoy.

Extended Stretch: Parsvottanasana

1. Begin in Mountain with the feet hip distance apart.

2. Step the left foot behind, about 2 ½ feet.

3. Turn the left foot in 60 degrees. The right foot is at 90 degrees.

4. Press in to both feet and draw in from the groin, and up.

5. Take the hands behind in backwards Namaste, between the shoulder blades or, grab opposite elbows. Alternately, lengthen the spine behind the heart.

6. Inhale. Lift from the heart.

7. Exhale. Pour the heart over the front right knee, until the head rests toward the shin.

8. Inhale. Come up. Keep the hands in backwards Namaste.

9. Turn to the other side and repeat the pose.

BK and AK amputees

• Place the hands on a chair in front of you to open the hamstrings more.

• Place a chair with the back of the chair pressing into the wall. Fold over the chair, pressing the hands into the front seat of the chair.

• Sit in a chair facing a wall, with one leg outstretched, pressing that foot into the wall. The other leg is bent with the foot on the floor. Fold the torso over the extended leg, keeping the spine lengthened. If balanced, you can place the hands in backwards Namaste or interlock them as you fold over the extended leg. Switch sides.

• Sit on the floor with the legs extended. Practice seated forward bend.

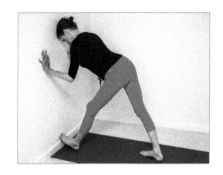

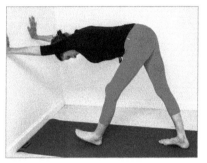

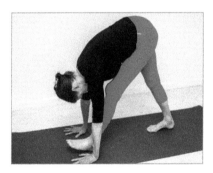

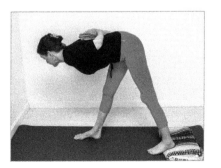

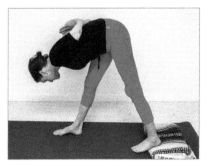

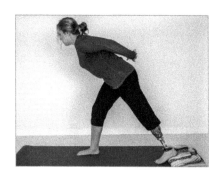
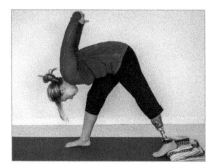

- Practice rolling the shoulder blades into each other.

- Lean against a wall with the front extended leg side of the body. Repeat to the other side.

- Lean against a wall with the back extended leg side of the body. Repeat to the other side

- Lean the chest on the back edge of a chair covered in a soft folded blanket. Avoid pressing directly into the Xyphoid process. Lengthen the heart and spine in opposite directions.

Triangle: Trikonasana

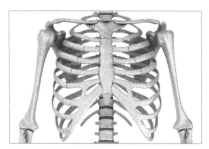

1. Come to the left side of the mat in Mountain pose, arms overhead or sides of the torso lengthened.

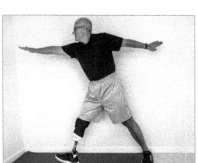

2. Step feet 3 - 4' apart and spread the arms or collarbone into a T.

3. Rotate the right hip inwards towards the pubic bone, the right foot facing in about 15 degrees.

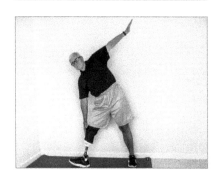

4. Turn the left hip out, the left foot facing straight ahead.

5. The left heel lines up with the center of the right arch.

6. Reach the right hip out to the right.

7. Fold the torso sideways over the crease of your left hip.

8. Elongate through the torso and keep reaching.

9. When reached far enough, pivot the torso so the left arm reaches to the inner left leg, calf or floor.

10. The right arm lifts to the sky, the inner arm facing forward, fingers spread.

11. Extend from the heart out to your fingertips.

12. To turn the head up, roll the chest around and turn the head to look to the sky.

13. Press into the feet to come up.

14. Reverse to the other side.

BK and AK amputees

- Do this pose with the back to a wall.

- Place the rolled edge of a yoga mat under the prosthetic heel or ball of the foot depending on alignment.

- Bend the front knee.

- Press the back heel into a wall.

- Reach the hand into a chair placed near the extended leg.

- Loop a yoga strap around both shins and resist into the shins.

- Bend the extended arm, placing the hand on the shoulder rather than pointing to the sky.

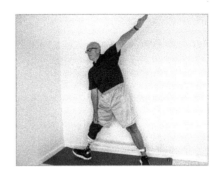

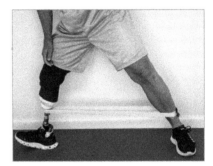

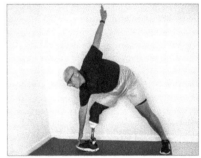

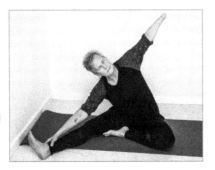

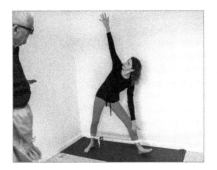

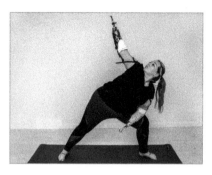

- Lean the side of the torso over the back of a chair.

- Practice the pose with the back against a wall.

- Expand through the center of the chest.

Side Angle: Utthita Parsvokonasana

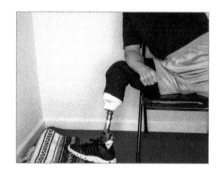

1. Stand wide on the yoga mat.

2. Turn the right foot straight ahead 90 degrees, the left foot turning in 15 degrees.

3. Bend the right knee, so the knee is over but not beyond the right toes.

4. Come into Warrior II arms.

5. Reach over the bent right knee with the arm still extended, then rest the right forearm on the upper right thigh, to the outside of the bent knee, pressing the palm into a block or the floor.

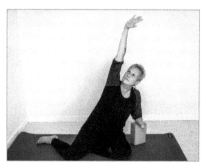

6. Press into the left foot, especially the inner and outer heel.

7. Reach the left arm over the left ear towards the right.

8. Roll the ribs up towards the ceiling.

9. Reach into the feet to come back to standing and switch to the other side.

BK and AK amputees

- Do the pose sideways against a corner wall, with the back heel pressing into the back wall.

- Practice this pose at the edge of a chair.

- Loop a strap around the lower shins for stability.
- Face a wall with the chair at the wall. Press the bent knee into the seat edge.

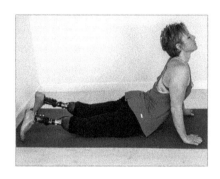

UE amputees

- Focus on revolving the ribs open.
- Do the pose with the back to a wall.
- Place rolled blankets or a soft yoga block between the mid-ribs and mid-thigh of the bent knee.

Cobra: Bhujangasana

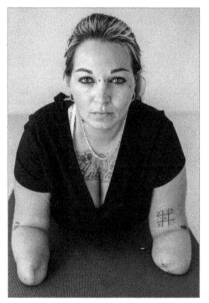

1. Lie on the belly with the legs outstretched.
2. Zip up the legs as if there were a zipper between them.
3. Place the palms under the shoulders, hugging the ribs with the upper arms.
4. Spread the fingers, then isometrically slide the hands back to the toes.
5. Lift your heart forward.
6. Roll the thighs in toward the pubic bone.
7. Spread the toes and press into them.
8. Lift the thigh bones and lengthen the legs.
9. Push into the palms and slide the chest through, lifting it up.
10. Let the throat open and reach the head up high.

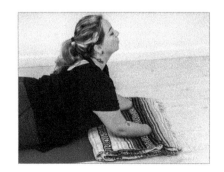

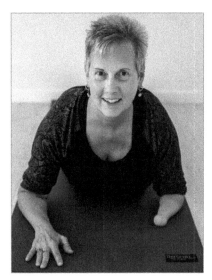

- Place a folded blanket under the pelvis to even out the hips and thighs.

- Roll a towel under the lower belly to support the back.

- Place a folded blanket under the thighs to even out the legs.

- Press the toes to a wall to create a lift in the chest.

- Place a rolled towel or yoga mat under the prosthetic foot.

- Wrap a strap around the upper arms for stabilization.

UE amputees:

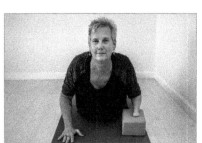

- Place the forehead on a yoga block.

- Place weighted bags on the backs of the upper thighs.

- Place a rolled blanket under the lower belly.

Sphinx

A variation of Cobra, place the forearms on the floor, elbows beneath the shoulders.

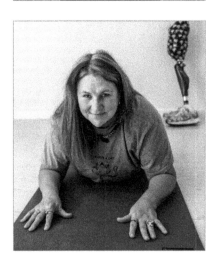

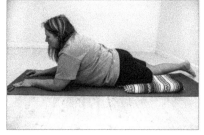
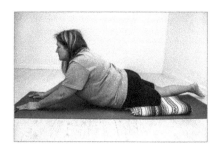

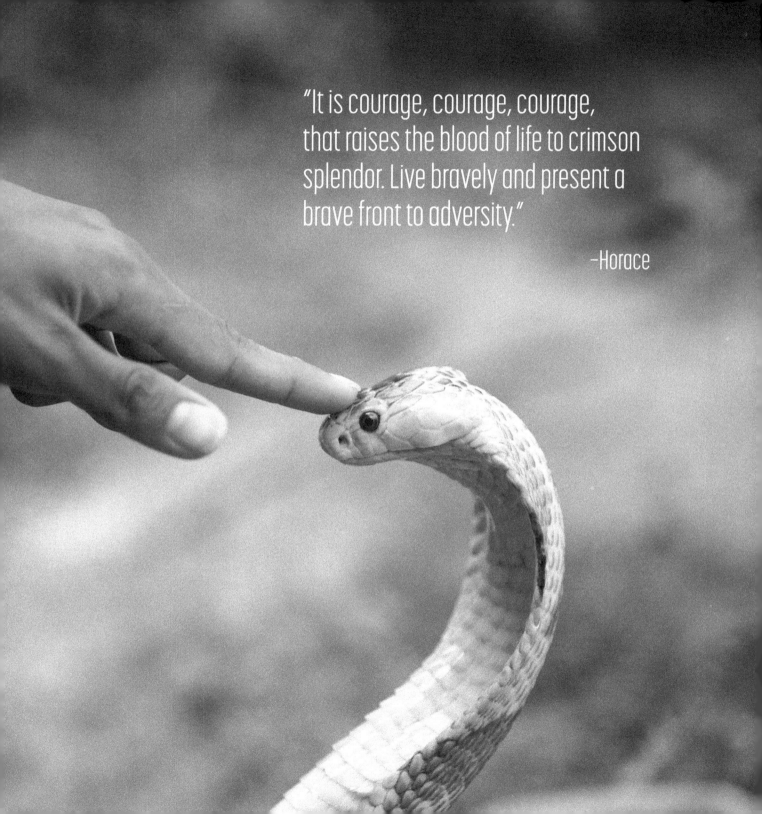

"It is courage, courage, courage, that raises the blood of life to crimson splendor. Live bravely and present a brave front to adversity."

–Horace

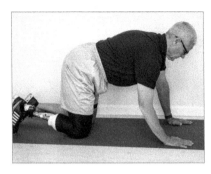

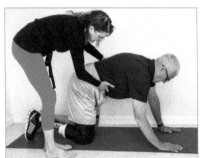

Cat/Cow :Bidalasana

1. Start in table pose with all four limbs on the floor.

2. Draw the tailbone under.

3. Reach the hands into the floor.

4. Draw the belly in.

5. Spread the sacrum.

6. Round the spine.

7. Draw the chin in to the chest, dropping the head.

8. Exhale.

9. Reverse direction, lifting the tailbone up to the sky.

10. Extend the belly forward and up as the head lifts to the sky.

11. Repeat three to five times.

BK and AK amputees

•   With a prosthesis, place a folded blanket under the knee or hip that may be lower than the other.

•   Do the sequence in a chair if scar tissue does not allow pressure on the knee.

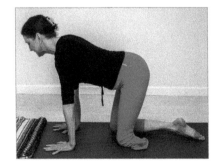

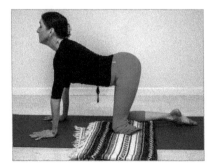

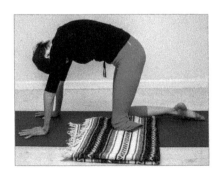

- Come to a wall, pressing the prosthetic foot into the wall for more stability.

- Place many folded blankets under the residual limb to even the shoulders.

- Lean into the wall with the side of the body to get extra support.

Camel: Ustrasana

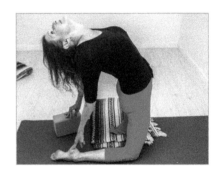

1. Kneel on the ground with the knees parallel to the hips.

2. Spread the toes and drop the tail bone slightly.

3. Draw the lower belly in and up towards the belly button.

4. Roll the inner thighs in and hug the hips in.

5. Drop the pubic bone then slightly lift the lower belly up.

6. Lengthen the front of the pubic bone.

7. Lift and lengthen the torso.

8. Place the hands and fingers pointing up on the top of the buttocks, near the tip of the hips.

9. Draw the flesh down and continue to tone the lower belly in and up.

10. Reach the top of the thigh and hip forward.

11. Hug the shoulder blades towards each other.

12. Lift the heart.

13. Place the hands to the back of the thighs, the heels , yoga blocks on either side of the feet or a wall behind you.

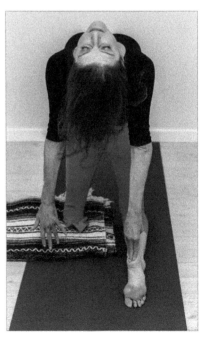

THE FIVE 'B'S

151

14. If the hands reach the heels, firmly grip the heel edge and press down into the hands.

15. Allow the head to tilt back, lining it up with the neck.

16. To come out of the pose, place the hands on the buttocks, twist to the right slightly and roll up.

17. Transition from camel pose with a twist to the right and left thigh.

18. Fold back into Childs pose.

BK and AK amputees

- Place yoga blocks on either side of the feet.

- Face the wall, reaching the pubic bone and fingers into the wall.

- Place a folded blanket underneath the knees.

- Kneel with the back to the bottom of a chair. Reach for the chair with the hands.

- For some amputees, kneeling is off limits. Instead, sit at the edge of a chair and grab the back edge of the chair to experience the backbend. Alternately, if able to stand, stand to the back of a chair, reaching the arms behind to the top of the chair. Lift the chest in a backbend.

- Lie on the back with a rolled yoga mat or yoga blanket lengthwise. Sit at the edge of the blanket, then lie back on the blanket, allowing the arms to relax to the sides.

UE amputee

- Focus on lifting the back of the heart up to the sky.

- If unable to transition to the knees, practice camel pose in a chair or standing, drawing the navel in, dropping the shoulders down and opening the throat.

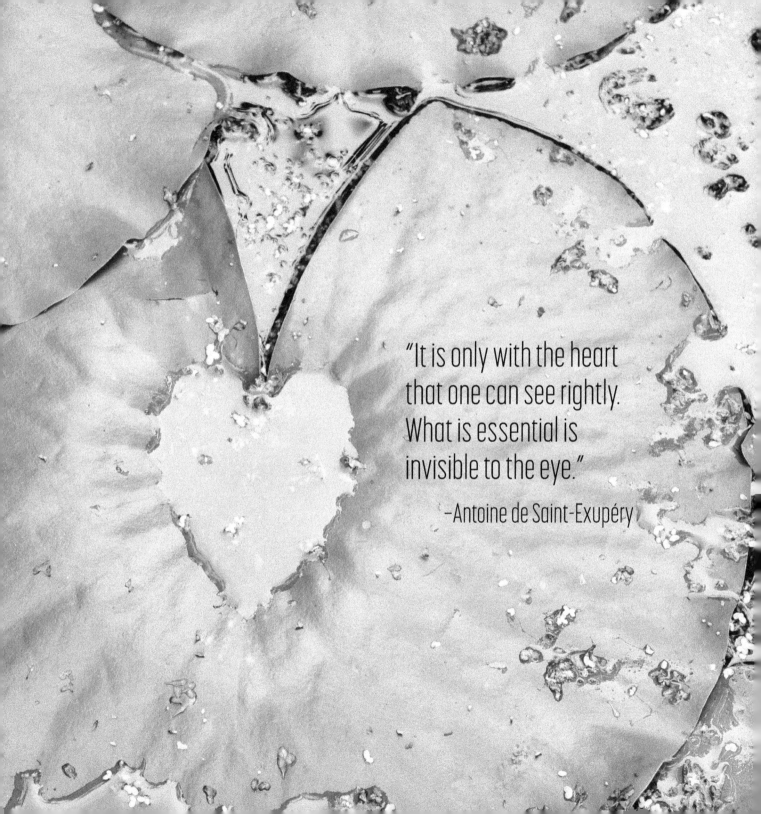

"It is only with the heart
that one can see rightly.
What is essential is
invisible to the eye."

–Antoine de Saint-Exupéry

Bridge: Setu Bandhasana

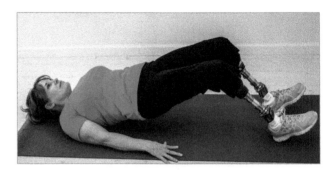

1. Lie on the back with the knees bent, ankles underneath the knees, knees in line with the hips.

2. Relax the shoulders to the ground, turning the palms down.

3. Lift the tailbone under and press into all four corners of the feet.

4. Take a deep breath in.

5. Lift the hips up to the sky.

6. Push into the feet as if trying to reach back to the shoulders.

7. At the same time, take the arms underneath or the palms down to the side.

8. Lift the heart towards the throat.

9. Come down slowly from the top of the spine to the bottom.

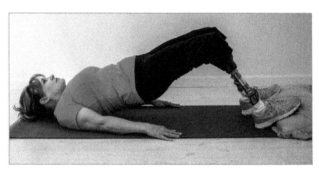

BK and AK amputees

- Practice with the feet to the wall, reaching the knees towards the wall.

- Do this pose with the legs draped over bolsters and blankets.

- Loop a strap around the thighs, then lift up into the pose.

- Place a yoga block under the lower back.

- Fold a yoga mat under the heels or toes for greater evenness of the hips.

- Place a folded blanket crosswise under the upper back.

- Press the feet into the wall.

- Add a folded blanket under the residual limb for better balance in the shoulders.

- Place a rolled towel lengthwise at the lowest height under the top center of the spine.

Fish: Matsyasana

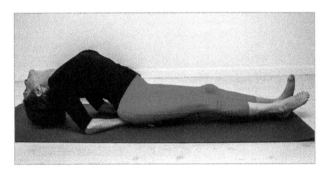

1. Lie on the back with the legs outstretched and the hands, palms down, under the body, near the buttocks, elbows close.

2. Flex the heels and press out through the midline of the heel.

3. Exhale, lifting the waist off the floor, reaching the hip bones forward, pressing down into the sitz bones, pushing firmly into the floor with the elbows and forearms.

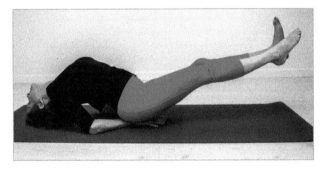

4. The buttocks stay on the floor.

5. Lift up through the chest and gently place the top of the head on the floor.

6. Zip the legs together like a fish tail.

7. Inhale and exhale, relaxing into the pose.

8. Release.

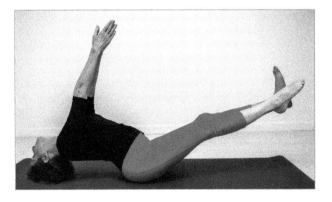

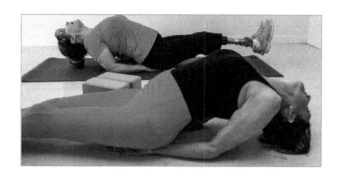

- Place the hands to the sides of the body or grab the thighs.

- Place the back of the head rather than the crown on the floor.

- Roll a blanket under the chest and do a restorative fish pose with the head and shoulders resting on the floor.

- If doing this pose without a prosthesis, place a folded blanket under the residual limb, especially the thigh, to balance the pelvis.

- Do this pose with the feet (whether prosthetic or not) pressed to the wall.

- Do this pose in a chair. Sit at the edge of a chair. Reach the hands to the back of the chair. Lift the sternum up, bend back and open the chest. Allow the head to reach back without collapsing the neck.

UE amputee

- If the arm is not available, come to the floor. Have a rolled blanket or yoga mat placed lengthwise on the floor. Slide the center of the spine to the top of the rolled blanket or mat so the shoulders drape down towards the floor. The head rests on top of the blanket, mat, or yoga block.

- Practice the pose seated in a chair. Draw the shoulder blades together and lengthen the sternum.

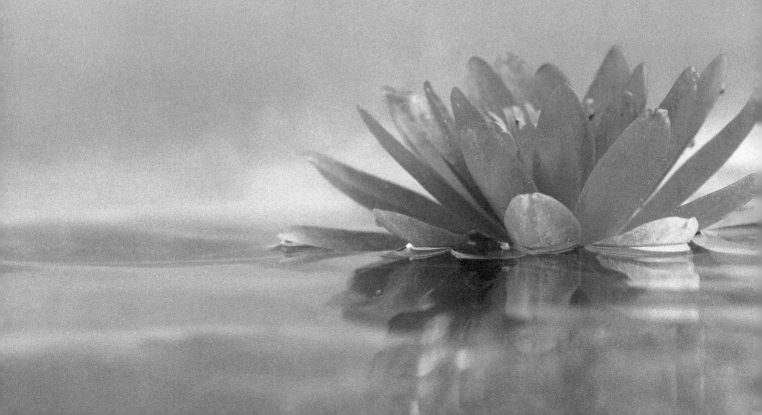

"I am blooming from the wound where I once bled."

-Rune Lazuli

Great Seal: Maha Mudra

1. Sit in staff pose, with the legs out in front, feet flexed.

2. Press down in to the sitz bones and lengthen out of the crown.

3. Draw the right knee back parallel to the hip.

4. Bring the right foot in to the left thigh.

5. Press the thigh into the foot, foot in to the thigh.

6. Inhale. Raise the arms overhead.

7. Lengthen out of the spine.

8. Keeping that length, exhale and bend forward from the hips over the extended leg.

9. Keep the shoulders relaxed.

10. To come out, press firmly in to the legs, inhale and raise the arms and torso back to the original position.

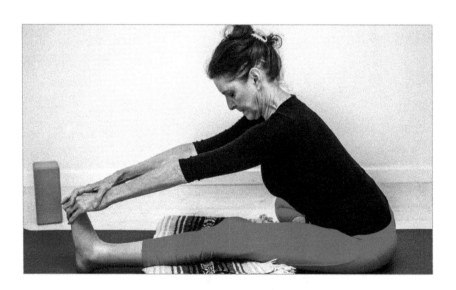

11. Exhale the hands to the side.

12. Repeat on the other side.

- Lean the back against a wall and fold forward.

- Wrap a yoga strap around the front extended foot.

- Place a chair in front of the body. Lean forward, resting the forearms and forehead on the chair.

- Place a folded blanket or yoga block under the bent knee if the prosthesis or leg does not open to the side

- Do the pose pressing the extended leg into the wall.

- Place a pillow or folded blankets over the extended leg and fold the torso over.

- Lean the top of the chest on the edge of a chair that is placed in front.

Lotus: Padmasana

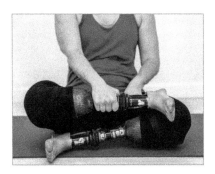

1. Sit on the floor in staff pose.

2. Grab the right foot with the left hand, the right knee with the right hand.

3. Flex the right foot.

4. Roll the right thigh and right shin out as you place the outside of the right ankle to the top of the left thigh or crease of the left hip.

5. Repeat with the left leg.

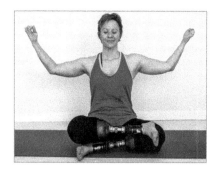

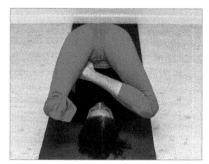

6. If the knees are too high off the floor, sit on the flat edge of a yoga block or a folded blanket.

7. Lengthen the spine, close the eyes, and concentrate on the breath.

8. Come out of the pose very slowly, leaning to one side, unfurling the opposite leg.

9. Repeat on the other side.

This pose can only be done if you are able to sit erect in half lotus with no strain on the knee.

BK and AK amputees

- Do this pose one leg at a time, keeping the other leg extended.

- Do this pose in a chair with one leg at a time, focusing on opening the piriformis.

- Lie on the back with the knees bent, feet flat on the ground. Place the right ankle on top of the left thigh.

- Do the pose without a prosthesis, focusing on turning out the inner thigh, when available, then rolling the outer thigh in. This releases the glutes.

- Sit in a chair or on the floor. Place a yoga strap around the outside of the upper leg. Lift the leg with the strap, and then tug at the outside edge of the strap to stretch the outer hip.

UE amputees

- Practice sitting on the floor, crossing and uncrossing the legs to see if able to do so comfortably. If so, practice as above, if at least one arm is available. If no arms are available, avoid this pose if hips have limited flexibility. Instead, try a seated twist.

Half Bound Lotus Intense Stretch: Ardha Baddha Padma Paschimottanasana

As above with **lotus**, follow the steps with the following changes.

1. Keep one leg extended with the foot flexed.

2. The arm on the same side as the extended leg wraps around the back to grab hold of the toe now resting in the hip crease of the opposite leg.

BK and AK amputees

- As with **lotus** pose, practice with a strap or on the back.

UE amputee

- As with **lotus** pose, focus on drawing the shoulder blades (when available) together.

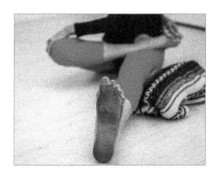
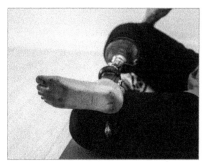
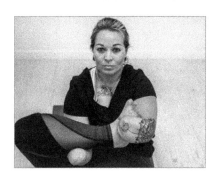

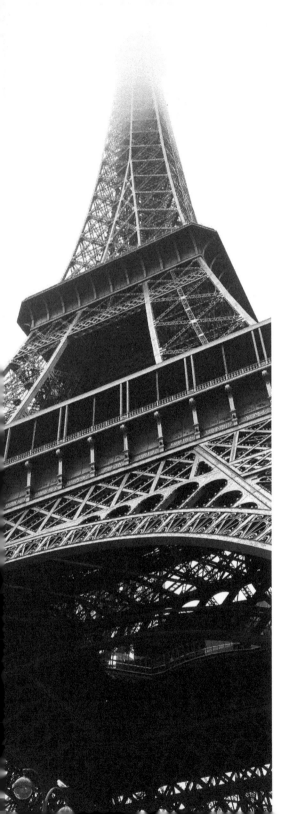

BUILD

When a builder begins a new project, the first thing she does is create a foundation that can support the weight of the building, keep the foundation dry, properly insulate the building, and endure the test of time. The architect, on the other hand, designs the building based on its function and aesthetic. Together, they hope to create a substantial building that is structurally sound and visually appealing.

Our bodies are similar. By strengthening our core, we are both the builder and the architect of our bodies. Our core, the center of our body that sustains us, guides our health, well-being, alignment, structure and overall demeanor. Even without limbs, our core matters, and indeed directs all our actions. This is no small thing. Proper breath, digestion, spinal health, emotional harmony, nerve strength, circulation, and hormonal balance all reside in the CORE.

For an amputee, a strong, supple core, is essential to our sense of self. We get our ground from our core. We also get our physical freedom and inspiration. The practices below teach amputees how to access their core and build their inner strength.

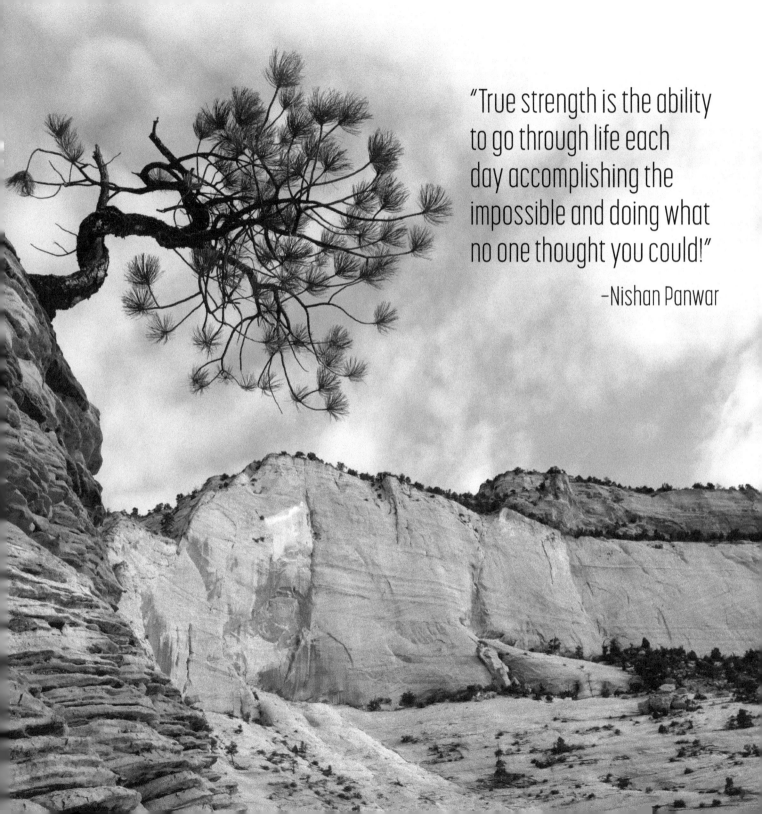

"True strength is the ability to go through life each day accomplishing the impossible and doing what no one thought you could!"

–Nishan Panwar

CORE BUILDING PRACTICE

Ujjayi breath

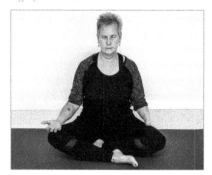

Seated Twist

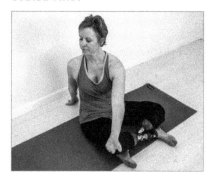

Breath of fire

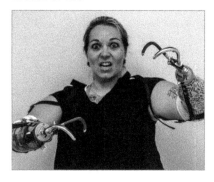

Cobra

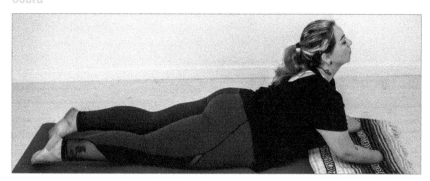

Butterfly pose

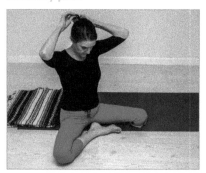

Locust

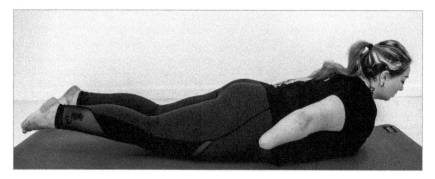

Plank

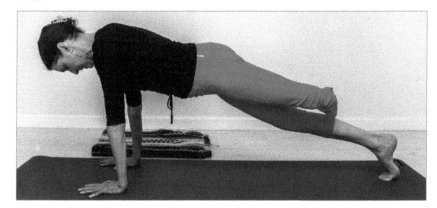

Four Limbed pose

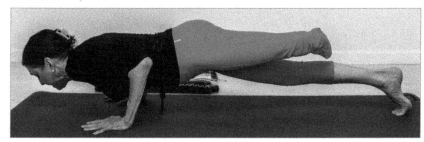

Upward Dog

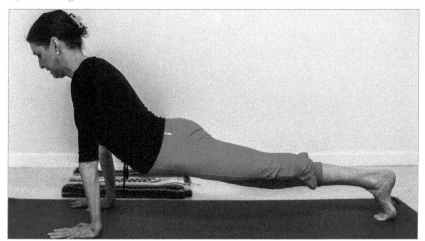

Downward Dog

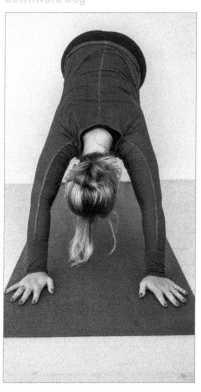

Childs

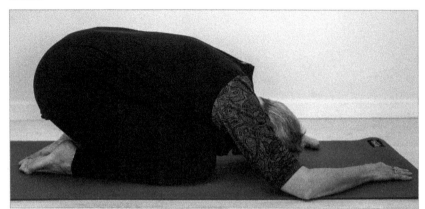

Abdominal crunches

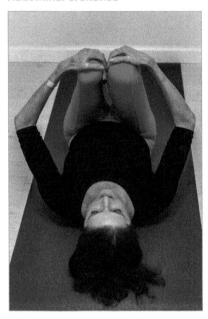

Supine Twist

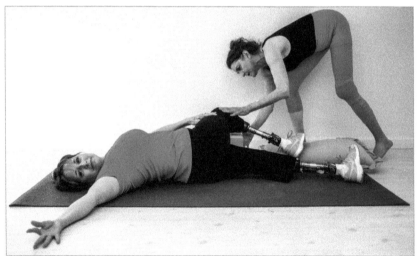

Relaxation

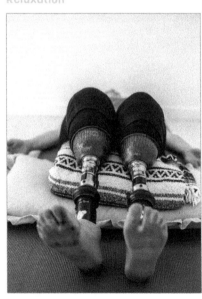

The core is located just above the pubic bone, spreading up and out to the solar plexus. It is the center of movement and strength in the physical, spiritual and emotional body. All actions result, ultimately, from this core, such as the physical action of lifting an arm wearing a prosthesis, or the emotional action of standing up for yourself.

In practices like Qigong and Tai Chi, the core is known as the Dantian, or sea of treasures. In yoga, the core is the combination of three energy centers, or chakras; the root, the lower belly and the upper belly. Amputees need a strong, balanced core to keep upright, with good spinal alignment. A healthy core means excellent digestion, elimination, and proper self-esteem. Practice these yoga and abdominal exercises to build your core and feel your best.

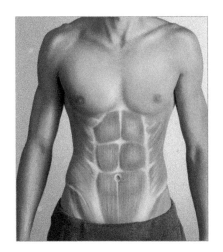

ABDOMINAL TONING EXERCISES

Abdominal toning teaches amputees to use energy efficiently, keeping the back protected, the breath steady and the spine aligned. Digestion improves, physical stamina increases and most importantly, balance is strengthened. The following are some abdominal exercises which tone the deeper muscles of the abdomen.

Abdominals in a chair

1. Sit up, pressing the torso to the back of the chair.

2. Draw the belly button back toward the spine.

3. Pump the belly button in and out 10 times.

4. Place the hands behind the neck, with the elbows spread wide.

5. Repeat step 2.

6. Draw the belly button in to the spine.

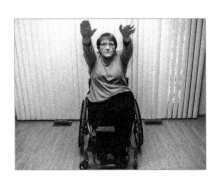

7. Crunch the elbows forward, tucking the chin in slightly, exhaling.

8. Inhale as you lift back up.

9. Repeat ten times.

Belly pump

1. Lift the arms at a diagonal from the shoulders.

2. Inhale.

3. Exhale.

4. Pump the belly button into the spine for ten counts with the breath suspended.

5. Release.

6. Repeat three to five times.

Abdominals on the floor

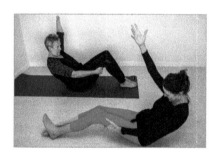

1. Laying on the back, draw the pelvic floor in and under, pressing the entire back into the floor.

2. Press the belly button deeply toward the floor as you exhale.

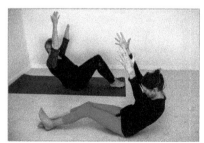

3. Inhale and release with an exhale.

4. Do this ten times.

5. Keeping the spine and belly button position, wrap the hands behind the head, elbows wide.

6. Tuck the chin slightly as you crunch up ten times.

Leg Lifts

1. Laying on the back, draw the pelvic floor in and under.

2. Press the lower back into the floor.

3. Reach the hands towards the feet as you lift the arms off the floor.

4. Tuck the chin and lift the head off the floor as you lift the legs off the floor to a 45-degree angle.

5. If comfortable, lift one leg towards the forehead, then the other.

6. Keep the tailbone tucked as you lower the legs, arms and head to the floor.

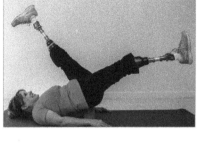

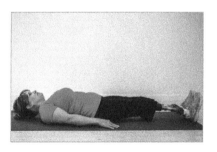

Life nerve stretch

1. Draw the pelvic floor in and under, then soften the lower back to the floor as you extend the lower legs.

2. Keep your arms by your side, palms facing the hips.

3. Take a deep breath in.

4. On the exhale, lift the legs, shoulders and head off the floor a few inches, eyes gazing towards the toes.

5. Take three to five deep breaths.

6. As your stamina increases, increase your number of breaths, until you can sustain the position for ten minutes.

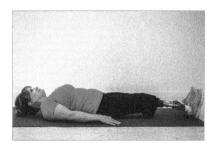

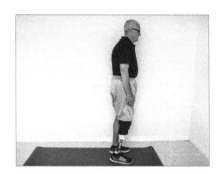

Abdominal pumping standing

1. Draw the navel into the spine.

2. Hug the ribs around the navel.

3. Take a deep breath in.

4. Before exhaling, pump the lower belly, lifting back and up towards the spine.

5. Exhale when the need to exhale is strong.

6. Take a deep breath in, suspend the breath, and repeat the belly pumping.

7. Exhale.

8. You will feel energized, clear headed and more alert.

Boat: Navasana

(See page 123).

Practice abdominal exercises regularly to become comfortable with your body's movements and abilities. Coordinating your breath with your movements teaches you how to listen to your body and cooperate with it in a mindful, compassionate way. Abdominal exercises prepare your body, mind and spirit for your complete yoga practice.

*Tucking your tailbone

The tailbone tuck is a common phrase used in yoga. To properly 'tuck', lift the pelvic groin area, take the inner thighs back, draw the hips towards each other and draw the lower belly and the pubic bone towards each other. If you are dealing with **lordosis***, or sway back, a slight tuck of the tailbone works well. For yogis who have* **kyphosis***, or rounded lower*

back, the tailbone tuck is counterproductive. Instead focus on lifting the inner pelvic muscles upward, without squeezing the buttocks.

BANDHAS

One way to build the core in yoga is to use something called the **bandhas**. Bandhas are internal body 'locks', or holds, which lift up the torso and tone the abdomen. Think of the bandhas like locks in a canal. Before a barge can move forward, a lock must open and another close. Within each of us we have energy (**prana**) that moves upward from the root to chin and energy that moves downward from the chin to root (**apana**). Apana and prana meet at the belly in what is known as **samana**, where the prana and apana are processed into the body systems through digestion, absorption, elimination and circulation.

For amputees, bandhas provide internal support and spinal alignment. Bandhas also help amputees move from the center, rather than overuse peripheral muscles, joints and tendons. Over time, bandhas help amputees gain even more control of their movements, breath and mind, providing them with more confidence to master their inner and outer terrain.

There are three main bandhas in the body, with a fourth bandha that unites the first three together. The **Mulabandha** is the root lock. The Mulabhanda draws muscular energy into the perineum and pelvic bowl, including the pelvis, tailbone, pubic bone and sitz bones. Mulabhandha provides foundational strength. It also stimulates the parasympathetic nervous system which then calms and restores equilibrium and resilience. *This internal lift in the lowest portion of the torso is greatly beneficial to the stability and range of motion for all levels of amputation*, even when the pelvis is missing. **Mulabhanda, or root lock**, coordinated with pranayama, or yogic breathing, greatly helps amputees maintain strength, flexibility and grounding.

Those who are rooted in the depths that are eternal and unchangeable and who rely on unshakeable principles, face change full of courage, courage based on faith.
—Emily Greene Balch

Steps to mulabandha

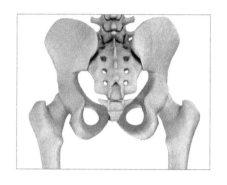

1. Sit cross legged if possible, or in a chair.

2. Roll the outer flesh of the thighs inward allowing the sitz bones to move apart.

3. Drop the pubic bone down and wrap the hip bones inward, opening the sacrum.

4. Exhale until the breath reaches its natural end.

5. Feel pressure in the lower abdomen.

6. Inhale from 3 inches below your navel as you drop the tailbone to the earth.

7. With each inhale feel the tailbone magnetizing towards the pubic bone, growing heavy.

8. Allow space in front of the sacrum.

9. Tilt the sacrum slightly forward into the body.

10. Draw the pubic bone towards the sacrum.

11. Draw the pelvic floor in and up.

12. Notice how muscles engage in the conversation between the pubic bone and tailbone.

For women, Kegel lifts are similar to mulabandha technique. With mulabandha, the inner core becomes firm, like an energetic pillar drawing you up from roots to crown. This creates a feeling of being lifted up.

The next internal lock, the **uddiyana bandha**, is the abdominal lock. When we practice uddiyana bandha, energy flies upward from the lower belly into the chest. Uddiyana Bandha also pulls energy from the root into the lower belly, just under the ribs about three inches below the navel. Uddiyana Bandha creates space in the diaphragm and lower belly for breath retention practices, as well as energizing the heart, which helps support full breath rather than strained, upper chest breathing. For amputees, uddiyana bandha stabilizes the deeper muscles of the core so that movement can emanate from the center rather than from the periphery of the body. Energy gets used more efficiently with less wear and tear on residual limbs, spine and joints. Uddiyana Bandha stimulates the pancreas, adrenals, liver, ovaries and pancreas. Uddiyana bandha progresses from mulabandha.

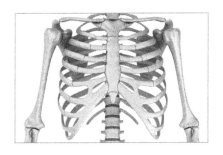

Steps to uddiyana bandha

1. Continue to sit as in Mulabhanda.

2. Take a deep inhale.

3. Press the navel back to the spine as you exhale.

4. Feel the solar plexus soften as the back body expands.

5. Feel the sides of the mid-chest and upper chest expand.

6. Breathe in and out naturally while maintaining the lift in the belly.

The third bandha, the chin lock, is known as **Jalandhara Bandha**. Jalandhara bandha 'locks' the net of nerve plexes at the neck to better circulate life force, or prana, throughout the body. Jalandhara tones the thyroid and parathyroid glands. In addition, jalandhara bandha is said to stimulate the pineal gland which has a direct positive effect on mood. Jalandhara bandha opens the vocal diaphragm which is involved in better breathing and personal confidence.

Steps to jalandhara bandha

1. Begin as before with mulabandha, adding uddiyana bandha.

2. Align the shoulders.

3. Open the collarbone, taking the head of the arm bones back.

4. Externally rotate the shoulders so the palms face forward.

5. Bring the elbows in close to the body and relax the hands to the sides. Alternately hug the ribs into the center of the body.

6. Take the top of the throat back by guiding the chin toward the back of the head.

7. Feel the back of the neck lengthen.

8. Soften the head toward the heart as the heart lifts.

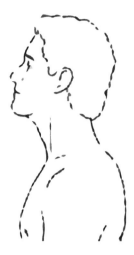

When all three bandhas are combined: **mulabandha, uddiyana bandha** and **jalandhara bandha**, a master bandha is attained, known as **Maha**, or **Great Bandha**. Mulabandha and uddiyana bandha are intelligent support for amputees. Jalandhara bandha is a more advanced technique refined over time through consistent yoga practice. Often Maha Bandha is practiced separately toward the end of a yoga sequence, before meditation and relaxation, to seal in the energy of the practice. A common yoga pose called **Maha Mudra** is used to achieve **Maha Bandha**. For us as amputees, maha bandha shows us our own capacity for healing and our ability to control our life force for our benefit.

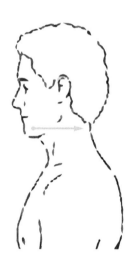

MEET RAY

"Healing is not the same as curing. Healing does not take us back to what was before. Rather, healing brings us closer to our true Self."—Ram Dass

Ray is an IT specialist for a major insurance company. He lost his leg in 1998 from a blood clot due to Peripheral Arterial Disease. He wears a Willow Wood elevated vacuum system. He practices yoga with and without props.

Before Ray lost his leg, he wasn't very active. After amputation, that changed. Yoga is his number one activity to exercise his body and mind. He enjoys getting in tune with his body through yoga poses, breath and relaxation. He feels better than ever adding yoga to his life.

To Ray, feeling comfortable with himself makes him feel whole.

His world has expanded after limb loss. He has met so many people from around the world, traveled to conferences and taken more risks outside his comfort zone then he ever did. He would never have considered yoga before amputation or attending a support group. Now, he is a regular at both. This has boosted his confidence and given him a whole new lease on life.

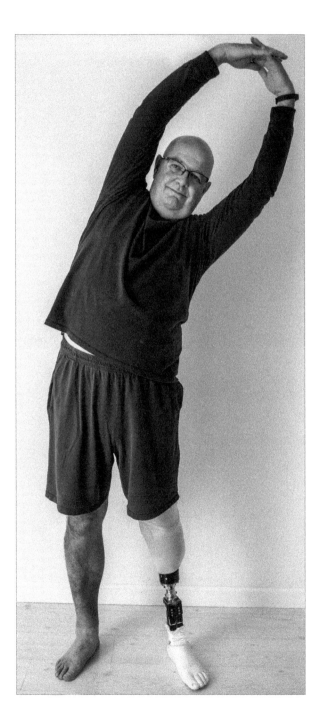

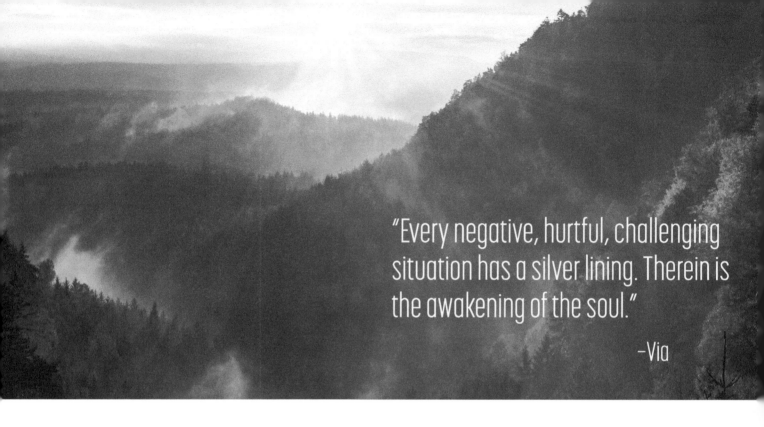

"Every negative, hurtful, challenging situation has a silver lining. Therein is the awakening of the soul."

–Via

Ray believes that once an amputee gets over feelings of shyness and vulnerability, he recommends being proud of who you are now. After all, the limb is not going to grow back. Getting on with life is a decision that **can** be made. There is always a silver lining.

BE

MEDITATE

What is meditation?

Meditation is a practice of redirecting our minds to a calm state, stilling its fluctuations so that we have higher levels of consciousness. The gift of meditation is the ability to be present, totally in the magnificent now, with no demands on ourselves other than to Be. Centering paves the way. Meditation can take many forms: movement meditation such as walking a labyrinth, contemplative prayer, Vipassana meditation, mantra (a repeatable phrase) meditation, Buddhist meditation, and focus on a single object. All are means to the same end: inner peace.

When a person meditates, amazing things happen. Harmful behaviors, habits, beliefs and stress reactions become less prominent in a person's life. Peace of mind, a broader perspective, heightened creativity, healthy habits, and compassion become more commonplace.

Moment by moment self-awareness can appear counterproductive or "a waste of time" in our driven-to-success, fix-it-now society. In fact, with meditation, the very opposite occurs. A relaxed mind and body *accomplish more* when devoid of the burdens of overthinking or stress.

Research has shown that meditation reduces symptoms of PTSD, pain and anxiety, all of which amputees can have. Amputees can enjoy physical and psychological relief through the simple practice of meditation!

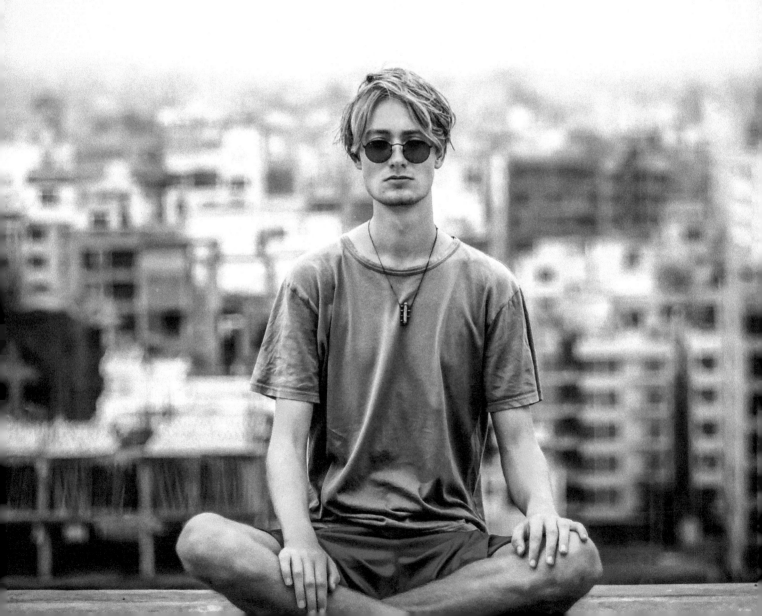

"Meditation is not a means to an end.
It is both the means and the end."

–Jiddu Krishnamurti

What are the benefits of meditation for amputees?

There is much study being done on the benefits of meditation. Meditation is a win-win for amputees. Because meditation is self-directed and self-controlled, the practitioner actively participates in his/her own health and wellness. When a person meditates, the brain literally changes. The hippocampus, the part of the brain associated with retaining information, gets larger. This means that for an amputee, more peaceful mental energy is available for the rest of life.

Meditation has been found to positively affect a person's sense of self in the world, after a traumatic experience, such as an amputation. This means that meditation has the potential to aid amputees find their space and place in the world and feel whole again.

Amputees are living with unique mental and emotional challenges. As amputees age, or for those who are new older amputees, additional challenges related to secondary health conditions, such as diabetes and heart disease, can cause a greater risk of breakdown in the residual limb, greater risk of falling, and lowered mental acuity. Meditation can play an active role in reversing those secondary conditions, both in the aging amputee population and with any age. According to one recent study *"Our initial results suggest that meditation may be associated with structural changes in areas of the brain that are important for sensory, cognitive and emotional processing. The data further suggest that meditation may impact age related declines in cortical structure."*

For new amputees the stressors are more immediate. Pain, anxiety, fear, and worry are palpable. As amputees adjust to their new life, there are many changes that happen, adding extra layers of stress, such as new prosthetics, changes in health, change of prosthetist, or sports injuries. For all amputees, certain everyday stressors become a fact of life. Worries like "There is no parking. How far will I have to walk? "And "I have a blister and can't wear my prosthesis. How will I work today? "are common. These can affect an amputee's mood and outlook. Meditation turns that around.

Anxiety and stress are significantly reduced by practicing meditation. Many amputees suffer from sleep deprivation due to mental agitation, phantom pain and discomfort. Meditation has been found to reduce insomnia and improve sleep.

Immune response increases with meditation, which has incredible health benefits for many amputees, especially those who are recovering or dealing with chronic disease. The insula, the "intuitive" part of the brain, grows with regular meditation. The insula serves as a cushion for stress. A strong insula means more resilience and less stress for an amputee when facing these multiple challenges.

Meditation has the capacity to reduce reactivity such as anger and increase thoughtful responsiveness. This is especially helpful for amputees dealing with pain, depression or overwhelm.

A foundational practice of meditation does not have to be difficult. Regular meditation gives an amputee a sense of belonging in the world. For amputees who have felt isolated by their limb loss, meditation builds empathy, compassion, and a sense of unity with the world. For all these reasons, meditation is a vital practice for an amputee, to be done on its own or in conjunction with a traditional yoga practice.

Special needs of amputees in meditation

There are special considerations for amputees wanting to practice meditation, which are different from the public. *Comfort is paramount.* Comfort includes elevated hips, relaxed thighs (if the amputee has them), a place to rest residual limbs, support for the belly, support for the neck, and the ability to elongate and hold up the spine. Some amputees have grown accustomed to dangling residual limbs over pillows or edges of chairs, so extra support may or may not enhance their experience. Options are always good.

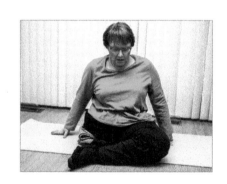

Pillows and low yoga bolsters underneath the buttocks and residual limbs can really help elevate the spine. Pillows, rolled towels and rolled blankets placed behind the spine and/or head, or underneath the residual limbs can be excellent as well. An amputee's hips should be in alignment as much as possible, hence the extra props and support.

Part of yoga practice is the ability to become more comfortable with the discomfort of rambling thoughts, by using the tools of mindful meditation. The ability to respond to life with greater peace of mind is enhanced with meditation. Amputees need added strength daily to handle all the ups and downs of limb loss.

Meditation for amputees is a way to welcome more wholeness into life.

Here are the steps to a basic meditation practice

1. Sit in a chair or on the ground.

2. Keep the spine erect.

3. The hips should be in line with the knees (if you have them) or slightly above the knees.

4. For AK amputees and UE amputees, sit on a yoga block, soft pillow or folded blanket so the hips are above the thighs if the hips are not flexible.

5. For those with balance issues, sit at the back of a chair or sit on the floor leaning against a wall. Some amputees need two sturdy chairs on either side to lean on for added security.

6. If in a wheelchair, be sure the wheels are in locked position.

7. Relax the upper body by rolling the shoulder blades down the back.

8. If the arms or hands are available, let them rest in the lap.

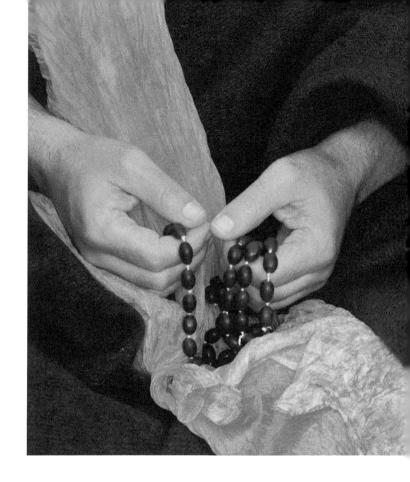

9. Begin taking easy breaths in and out.

10. Lengthen these breaths.

11. Close the eyes.

12. Continue with easy breaths in and out.

13. When the mind begins to "chat", causing you to be distracted, simply notice the mind distracting you, make a mental note, such as "my mind is speaking right now", then return to easy breaths. You do not need to engage in the thoughts or judge them in any way. Let them float away like soft clouds.

14. When the body begins to "chat" with discomfort, itchiness, or fidgeting, make a mental note, such as "my body is fidgeting right now", then return to easy breaths.

15. When emotions pop up, make a mental note such as "I have an emotion right now". Do not label the emotion or analyze it.

16. Start with 5 minutes of meditation.

17. As your body and mind become accustomed to the practice, increase the length of time, up to one hour, once or twice a day.

You will know that your meditation is making a difference, even if you do only five minutes per day, when you can tune out distractions and tune in to you. You will feel more relaxed during the day and look forward to taking time to meditate. You will have less desire to criticize yourself or judge your experience. Eventually, you will be able to easily access your "meditation mind". Challenge yourself to sit in stillness for 5 minutes every day. Note any positive changes in your daily life, or personal behavior throughout the day.

Below are some simple meditation techniques to awaken your inner wholeness.

Meditation Techniques

Meditation One	Meditation Two	Meditation Three	Meditation Four
Meditate on an uplifting word or phrase.	Repeat a mantra. Examples include: So hum, Om namo bhagavate vasudevaya, Om, Hallelujah.	Focus on the in and out breath to get grounded.	Meditate on the phrase "I am whole"
Meditation Five	**Meditation Six**	**Meditation Seven**	**Meditation Eight**
Bring your attention to your heart. Imagine opening your heart to connect with your Higher Self and with others.	Meditate on the brow point (the space between the eyebrows) for wisdom and clarity.	Sit and witness yourself as you are, with no preconceived notions.	Meditate on the breath going in and going out, rising up and falling down, with a mantra- "Breathing in I am breathing in, breathing out I am breathing out."
Meditation Nine	**Meditation Ten**	**Meditation Eleven**	**Meditation Twelve**
Meditate on a single repetitive prayer, using mala beads or a rosary.	Meditate on an inspirational color, then allow the color to infuse your whole being.	Sit in a comfortable position while listening to sacred music, inviting the music to fill your cells with vibrant sound.	Meditate on the phrase "I am complete".
Meditation Thirteen	**Meditation Fourteen**	**Meditation Fifteen**	**Meditation Sixteen**
Take a mindful walk in nature or in a labyrinth. With each step, take a breath.	Practice Vipassana meditation. Vipassana, translated as "seeing things in their true nature", encourages you to observe your breath, then body sensations, then exterior sounds. Continue to stay present with yourself.	Meditate on a body part. Notice how it feels. Remain neutral.	Sit silently for a period.
Meditation Seventeen	**Meditation Eighteen**	**Meditation Nineteen**	**Meditation Twenty**
Nada meditation: Focus on a sound.	Listen to a soothing piece of music, practicing stillness and mindfulness.	Mindfully move and breathe, dancing to music.	Softly gaze at the light of a candle or other object for five or more minutes. Notice how your breath slows down and your body relaxes.

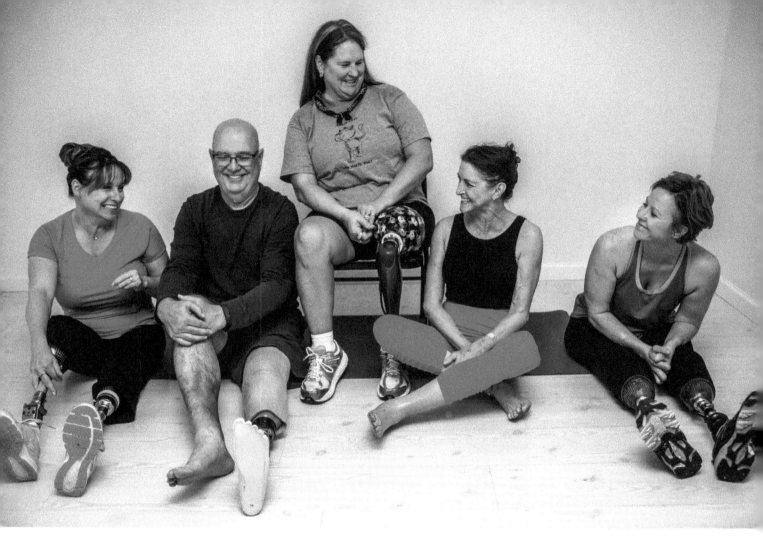

CREATIVE VISUALIZATION

What is creative visualization?

Many years ago, a story was told of an American prisoner of war captured and kept in solitary confinement. His daily ordeal of abuse, deplorable conditions and extreme isolation were combatted by his brave decision to use his mind to think of something hopeful. He envisioned himself playing piano perfectly; reading the music, turning

"You must live in the present, launch yourself on every wave, find your eternity in each moment. Fools stand on their island of opportunities and look toward another land. There is no other land; there is no other life but this."

—Emily Greene Balch

the pages, and moving his hands easily across the piano keys. When he was finally released and returned to the United States, he was able to play with expert precision. He not only used his mind to endure his hardship, he was able to make the physiological connection to his body solely through his thoughts. This is the power of creative visualization.

By visualizing a task or feeling as if it is already happening, we can create a new reality. Like daydreaming, creative visualization is NOT mind over matter. It is mind and matter co-creating a desired outcome, a walk through our imagination toward a pleasurable or healing experience. For amputees, envisioning any activity they want to accomplish as already happening, teaches their mind and muscles to work together to complete events that haven't yet occurred, but can. Amputees enduring pain, anxiety, stress and suffering can use creative visualization to not only positively affect the body's physiological responses to these challenges, but also to change the brain's reactions. The more an amputee practices creative visualization, the easier it is to access a new, more hopeful reality.

Can creative visualization work for amputees?

Yes! A mind forcing a body to "believe the impossible" through affirmations alone constricts the body and stresses it out. If the result doesn't occur then the person my feel they have failed, the body is their enemy, or the world is stacked up against them. However, when the body feels and trusts that the action is possible, the mind relaxes. In fact, research is being done with amputees and veterans, using virtual reality, a form of creative visualization, to help amputees visualize walking, running and feeling pain free, with promising results.

For example, the scent of cinnamon has an instant response in the body and mind. It can bring up a positive sensation, such as the taste of homemade apple pie at a family gathering or can remind the body and mind of a time when homemade apple pie caused illness.

A creative visualization has the same effect on an amputee. Envisioning a good feeling as already existing in the body will ease pain in the body. Similarly fearing that the pain will never go away (also a form of creative visualization) can induce more pain and stress. This does not mean we dishonor or diminish real experiences of pain. On the contrary, creative visualization allows the body and mind moments of respite from pain and suffering. The more moments of relief we have, the more we can trust that our bodies and minds DO work together to restore our wholeness. Creative visualization enhances the brain's ability to produce more theta

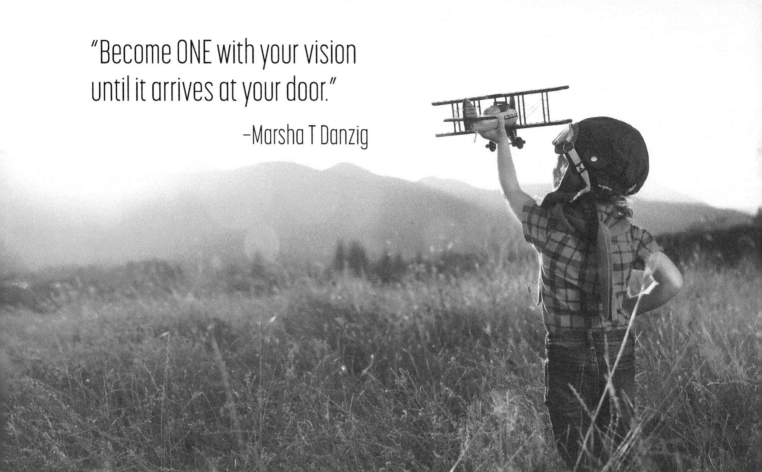

"Become ONE with your vision
until it arrives at your door."

–Marsha T Danzig

waves, which expand spiritual insight and connection to all of life. Letting the mind reside in this pleasurable state more often offers an amputee real hope and a powerful connection to the mind and body.

What happens in a creative visualization practice?

To begin, the amputee is guided to feel a positive feeling such as better range of motion in the shoulder, or the ability to walk with a perfect gait. Once he/she has a sense that the positive feeling is a reality, it is easier for the body to make it so.

Steps to creative visualization

1. Sit or lie down comfortably.

2. Close your eyes.

3. Envision a goal or feeling you would like to have.

4. Create a visual image, story, or event in which you will participate.

5. Focus on that happening right now.

6. Allow yourself to feel the reality of your vision.

7. Anchor that reality in your body.

8. Notice your body and mind sensations as you do this.

9. When you are ready, open your eyes.

10. Come back to the room you are in. Look around. Feel yourself sitting or lying down.

11. Note how you feel.

12. Remind yourself that the feeling you created is available any time you want.

13. Repeat your creative visualization as many times throughout the day as you'd like.

14. The more positive energy you put into a desired outcome, the more likely it is to happen.

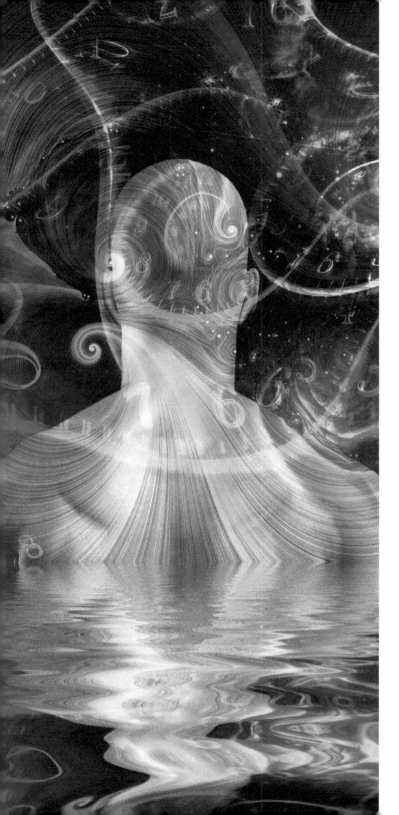

Creative visualizations for amputees

Universal connection for infinite possibility

Accept the reality that we are all connected. There is no part of you that is separate from the universe, and there is no part of the universe that is separate from you. You and the universe are composed of the same material. An interdependence between you and the vastness of the universe always exists. Within this infinite universe, anything is possible. Imagine yourself walking through this endless universe. Everywhere you go, you are welcomed. Strings of light connect you to the universe. You can put anything you want in this universe, for it is the field of infinite possibility. In this universe there is only love, acceptance and hope. Come to this universe often. What does it look like? What are you doing? How do you feel being as free as the universe? Create the reality you desire in the universe, and feel it manifesting in your life through all your senses: touch, smell, taste, sound, and sight. Notice how you feel. Bring that feeling into your present reality. And so it is.

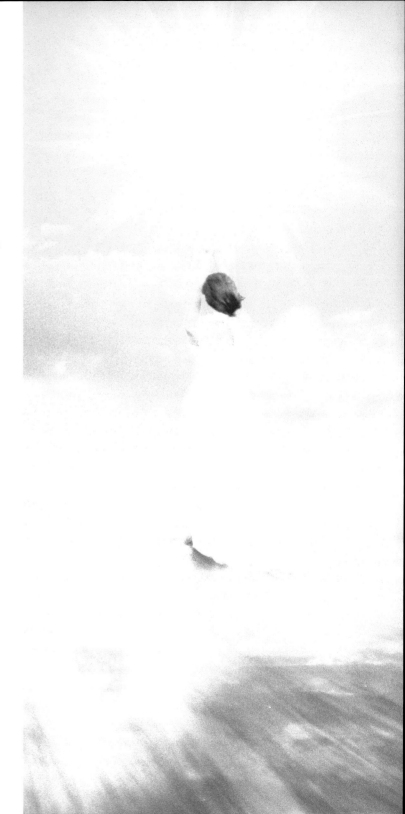

Pillar of light for security and safety

Sit erect with your spine elongated. Rock on your bottom until you feel secure and stable. Roll your shoulder blades down your back. Open your heart and relax your throat. Imagine a tall pillar of light that descends from the crown of your head through the center of your spine into the center of the earth. Feel how connected you are to the earth as the earth reaches up to meet and support you from its center. Notice how anchored you are, how secure, how rooted. Now imagine the pillar of light ascending from the center of the earth up through your body into your spine, out the top of the head, reaching up into the heavens. The light flows through the center of your spine and spreads out to your whole body. You are filled with the power of this light that comes to you from the center of the earth and the heavens. The light intersects at your heart. You are safe, and full of the power of heaven and earth. You can do anything.

Body scan releasing pain and discomfort

Scan your body for any area of pain or discomfort. Once you find this area of the body, bring all your attention there. Imagine this area is like a rock. As you breathe in and out, watch the rock disintegrate before your eyes. Stay with your visualization until the rock is completely dissolved. Replace the rock with a calm stream of clean running water. Notice how you feel in this area of your body after your visualization. You can also do this visualization for an unhealthy or painful feeling.

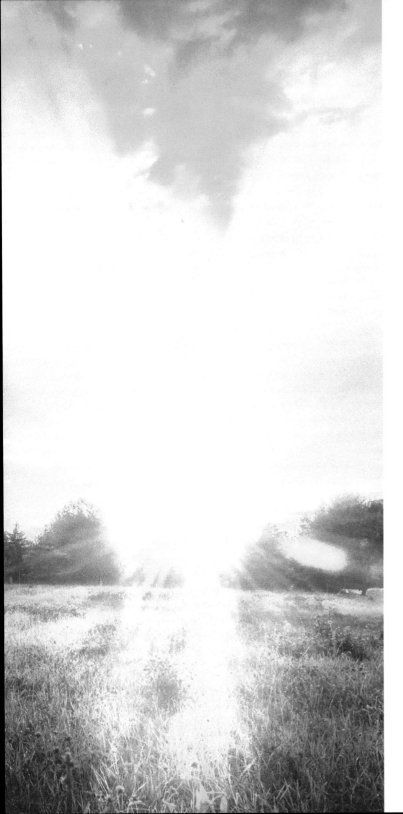

Imagine sitting on the beach. The waves are calm, the breeze soft, the sun shining, and the sand warm. As you enjoy this peaceful scene, you see a person coming towards you. You look over, thinking the person looks familiar. Eventually, the person is by your side. You realize that person is you, as your Highest Self, the wisest, kindest, and truest part of you. You smile at each other. Your Highest Self embraces you and asks if there is anything you would like to know. You may ask a question, like "How can I be happier in my life?" or, "Why did I lose my leg/arm? What purpose is there for me in this?" Remain curious and open to the guidance of your Highest Self. When you feel complete, thank your Highest Self. Know that your Highest Self is available to you all the time.

Creative visualization can add a whole new dimension of healing and possibility thinking to your life. It is a process that encourages you to remember your innate wholeness, with or without limbs, through the amazing power of the mind and body connection. After all, thoughts become things. Choose your thoughts with care.

Relax-Release

The word relax comes from the root 'to loosen' or 'widen'. Loosening tension in the body and mind through yoga loosens stress, anxiety, and tension. Certainly, amputees can be under a lot of stress, which affects the body and mind. Too much stress causes disease, but we do need some short gushes of stress to make the body and mind function at maximum capacity. When a yogi practices yoga asana, there are certain natural stressors on muscles, joints and willpower, that help the yogi to grow more proficient in their practice. These necessary stressors, followed by relaxation, become extra sweet.

The following yoga sequence is designed to create small doses of stress to tear and heal the muscles, building focus and strength. At the end of each challenging pose, a restorative pose is added to receive the benefits of the challenging pose.

Crane: Krounchasana

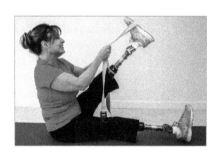

Steps to Krounchasana

1. Sit on the floor in staff pose.

2. Lean over to the left. Bend the right knee, placing the right foot to the outside of the right hip.

3. Realign the hips so they are even.

4. Bend the left knee.

5. Lean back slightly.

6. Grab hold of the left foot with both hands, or a yoga strap.

7. Extend the left leg up in a 'V".

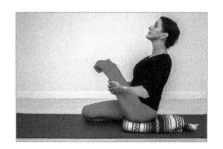

8. Lift and lighten the spine, keeping the collarbone open.

9. Gently release the extended leg when ready.

10. Repeat on the other side.

BK and AK amputees

- Hold the ankle, calf, or thigh instead, with hands or a strap.

- Lean the extended leg on the edge of a chair.

- Lean the upper back into a wall and let the extended leg rest on the edge of a chair in front of you.

- For most amputees wearing a prosthesis, the knee will not bend deeply. Instead, place the inside foot of the prosthetic leg to the thigh or calf of the extended leg.

- The extended leg, if it won't lift, can stay on the ground. Provide support with pillows and folded blankets underneath the buttocks as needed.

UE amputee

- If able, place a yoga strap behind the extended leg and hold on with one hand.

- If unable to grab hold of the extended leg, practice lifting the leg up and down slowly with the knee slightly bent and lean against a wall to build abdominal strength.

- Lean the chest into a folded pillow between the extended leg and torso, then lean back into the wall.

- Wrap a looped strap or two around the entire body, from around the back, under the armpits and around the extended leg. Lean back into the strap, like a hammock, and lift the leg.

Head to Knee Pose: Janu Sirsasana

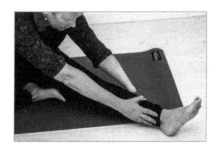

1. Sit with the legs outstretched.

2. Flex the feet.

3. Bend the left knee, placing the left foot in towards the right inner thigh or calf.

4. Lengthen the spine and press the sitz bones down.

5. Lift the arms to the sky, palms facing each other.

6. Inhale.

7. Exhale. Bend at the hips and reach the heart over the legs towards the toes with the hands resting on either side of the extended right leg or grab the right toes.

8. Keep the sternum lifted while the chin tucks in slightly.

9. Walk the hands up the right leg until sitting upright.

10. Switch legs and repeat.

BK and AK amputees

- Place a yoga block or folded blanket under the bent knee with or without the prosthesis.

- Wrap a strap around the extended leg.

- Place a folded towel or blanket under the extended knee.

- Sit in a chair, extending the chest forward over one extended leg. Repeat on the other side.

- Lean against a wall with a supportive blanket or pillow lining the spine.

- Face the wall, pressing the extended foot into the wall.

- Place the hands on blocks at mid-thigh level.

- Place a yoga block between the knees or thighs and lean the forehead on the yoga block. Drape blankets over the block for added neck support if needed.

UE amputees

- Tuck the chin under while folding forward.

- Press the extended foot into a wall.

- Fold the torso over a blanket or bolster.

- Place a yoga block between the knees or thighs and lean forehead on the yoga block. Drape blankets over the block for neck support.

Eight Angle Pose: Astavkrasana

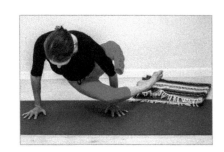

1. Sit on the floor with the legs extended into staff pose.

2. Lift the legs to the right with the feet flexed and crossed at the ankles.

3. Place the right hand between the thighs, right palm to the floor.

4. Place the left hand behind the left hip.

5. Lift the hips off the floor and bend the arms, sliding the right elbow closer to the right knee.

6. Swivel the hips towards the right.

7. Legs lift off the floor and extend.

8. Bend the knees to gently come back to the floor.

9. Repeat on the other side.

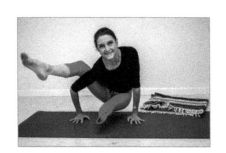

- Do this pose without a prosthesis.

- Place folded blankets underneath the hips and residual limb in case of a fall.

- Practice push-ups to be sure this pose is an option.

- Place the extended bottom leg on a yoga block.

- Do boat pose instead.

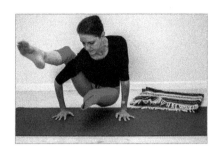

UE amputee

- Lie fully on the side. Place the right foot in front of the left thigh. Lift the left leg up. Roll to the other side and repeat. Have soft folded blankets under the residual limb if needed.

Childs: Garbhasana

1. Come to all fours with the hands directly beneath the shoulders.

2. Take a breath in.

3. Sit back on the heels.

4. Exhale.

5. Bend at the hips and fold the torso over the thighs, chest to the knees.

6. Rest the forehead to the ground.

7. Place the hands towards the feet, palms up. Breathe.

8. To release, slide the hands under the shoulders and press up into a seated position.

9. Rock the hips to one side and stretch the legs out in front.

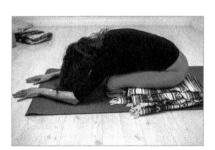

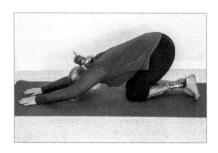

- With a prosthesis, keep the hips off the feet unless the prosthesis can bend completely at the knee. Extend the arms in front (puppy pose).

- Sit on the remaining leg, extending the prosthetic leg back with props underneath as needed.

- Lie on the back and hug the knees into the chest.

- Without a prosthesis, place a folded blanket under the thighs lengthwise at the calves.

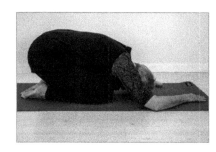

- Elevate the residual limb under folded blankets.

- Place a bolster lengthwise under the chest and fold forward.

- Lie on the side, curling the legs into the chest.

UE amputees

- Straddle the legs in a V and fold the torso over a bolster.

- Place folded blankets under the residual limb.

- Place a yoga block under the forehead.

Boat: Navasana

(See page *123*).

Knee to Chest Pose: Pavana Muktasana

1. Lie on your back.

2. Hug your right knee into your chest, drawing it towards your right shoulder.

3. Keep the left leg extended, with the left foot flexed.

4. Switch legs.

5. Hug both knees into the chest.

6. Release the feet, when available, to the floor in easy resting pose.

BK and AK Amputees

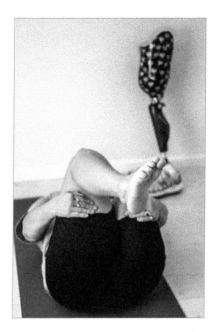

- Wrap a strap around the residual limb as you bring it in towards your chest.

- Sit in a chair and draw the knee into the chest with the hands or a strap.

- Press the extended leg into a wall.

- Bring both knees into the chest.

- Place a pillow under the prosthetic limbs to avoid hitting your face.

- Place the back edge of a chair into the wall. Lean the top of the prosthetic foot of the bent knee into the front edge of the chair.

- Place a folded blanket under the extended leg for support and evenness.

- Place a folded blanket under one or both buttocks to even the hips.

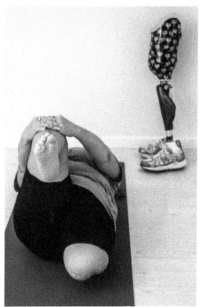

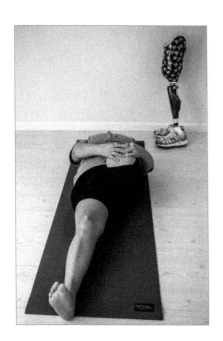

- Roll to the side and draw the knees into the chest.

- Do child's pose instead.

- Rest the knees on the back of a chair and try to bring the knees in to the chest from there.

Easy Resting Pose

1. Lie on the back.

2. Knees are bent, feet flat on the floor.

3. Soften the sacrum into the floor.

4. Allow the arms to rest by the side, palms down.

5. Melt into the floor.

6. Close the eyes and take at least five deep breaths.

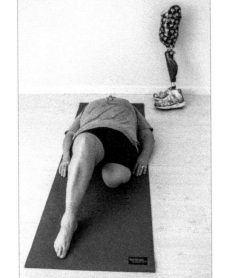

BK and AK amputees

- Do this pose at the wall, with the prosthetic foot/feet pressing into the wall.

- Place pillows and folded blankets under the knees.

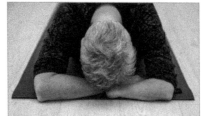

UE amputee

- Rest the arms on folded blankets.

- Do this pose on the belly, resting arms under the head when able, or to the side.

MEET MOLLY

Being an amputee is a mind game, much more than the physical sometimes. Trusting your prosthetics, the space around you and your own body's wisdom to be able to walk again means trusting YOU.

Molly lost both her legs below the knee, as well as two fingers, in 2008, from a strep throat infection that turned into sepsis. At the time, she was an elementary school teacher who adored her job. After her limb loss, over two years of rehabilitation and the dissolution of her marriage, she felt sad and lost. She could no longer teach (her passion) because her immune system was compromised. Eventually, she found her way to a job at a new prosthetics company as a patient liaison, where she feels truly blessed. "I work for a prosthetist and I work with new patients. That feeds me in ways that no amount of money could ever do. This job happened because of what happened to me. I've been placed in this incredible position to go in and talk to someone who just lost a limb and tell them there is life. It's not easy. But you can live your life missing a part or two."

She has two pairs of prosthetics, one set with adjustable heels that are more cosmetic, and one uncovered set with more energy storing feet. She wears her prosthetics twelve hours per day.

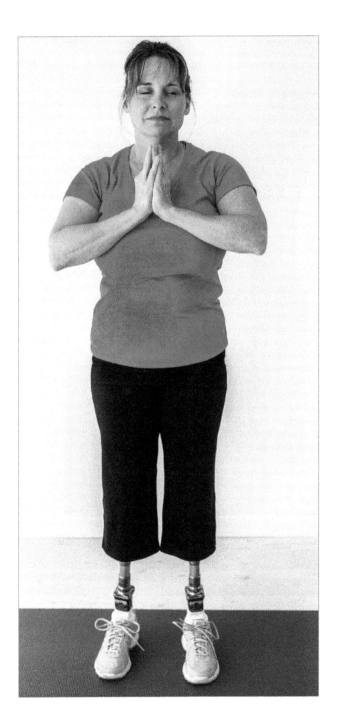

Molly believes wholeness is internal, being able to still be you, with or without limbs. Even though Molly had a lot of support, the decision to feel whole as an amputee came from within herself. Molly explains "Being an amputee is a mind game, much more than the physical sometimes. Trusting your prosthetics, the space around you and your own body's wisdom to be able to walk again means trusting YOU. "

Molly has always had a lot of drive, which she knows contributed to her recovery, but it was the circle of other amputees that got her back into life. She has learned patience with herself as she lives each day, knowing that some days there will be temporary setbacks, but they will pass. After losing her legs, Molly saw how strong she truly was to overcome so many hardships. She remarks "Wow, I didn't realize I could do the things I've done."

Molly started doing yoga after she lost her legs. She found that it strengthened her core, so she could walk better, which made her feel more secure. Molly is a bright star in our lives. She has coped with her major life transitions with incredible grace. She is a blessing to anyone who meets her.

Learning to rest

Rest is a necessary part of life. Depending on the culture in which you live, rest may or may not take precedent. Certainly, in the United States, rest is often limited to a fitful sleep after a hard day, or a two-week vacation. In American culture, stillness is often seen as unproductive. If an amputee has been still for too long due to rehabilitation or a sedentary lifestyle, rest seems redundant. Conscious mindful stillness and relaxation, though, are different. When we finally get still, we come face to face with how we are really feeling, what we may be avoiding in our day to day life, and what needs to be transformed or healed. The body is a storage center for every experience, good and bad. A conscious practice of stillness gently allows those experiences to fill us with pleasant sensations, or help us release pain, anxiety, stress and suffering.

Many people find relaxation in yoga to be challenging. Their mind moves a million miles a minute, they can't get comfortable, or they feel anxious, like they should be doing something more productive. The reality is: choosing conscious rest makes you the master of your thoughts, restores balance in your body, mind and spirit and heals those broken parts begging for relief. I encourage and challenge you to give yourself the luxury of constructive rest in **Savasana or Relaxation** pose. Your entire being will thank you.

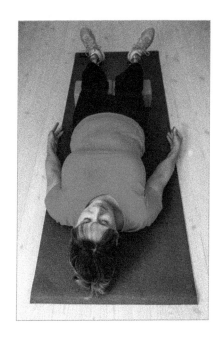

Savasana

Savasana, or relaxation pose, is usually practiced at the culmination of a yoga practice. From the outside, it may look like a nap. On the inside, there is a whole different series of events taking place. While some people do fall asleep during savasana, savasana is meant to be done fully awake and alert, but in an altered brain wave state. When we fall asleep and rest well, our brain follows a pattern of different waves.

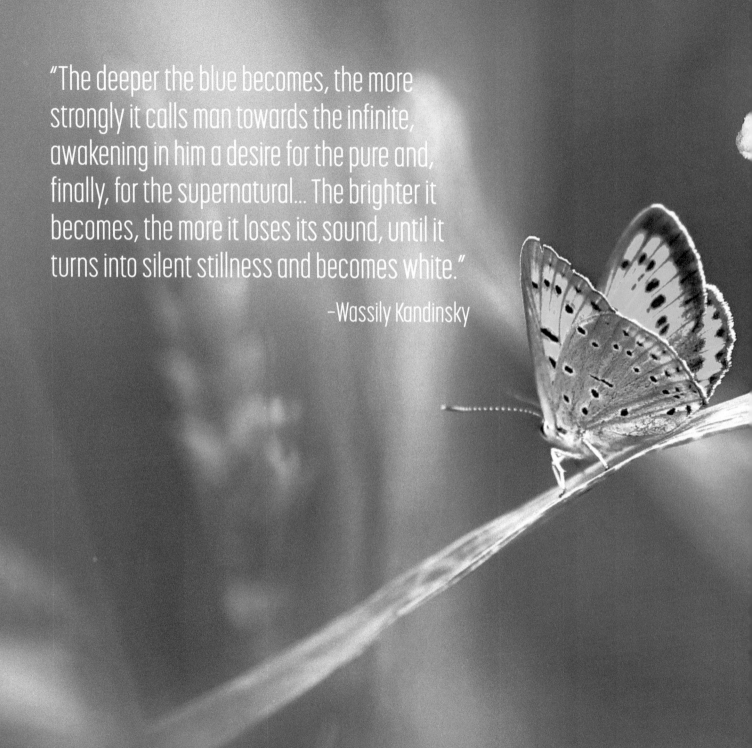

"The deeper the blue becomes, the more strongly it calls man towards the infinite, awakening in him a desire for the pure and, finally, for the supernatural... The brighter it becomes, the more it loses its sound, until it turns into silent stillness and becomes white."

–Wassily Kandinsky

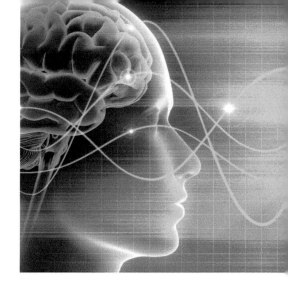

In savasana, keeping alert without falling asleep activates the important healing functions of the body and mind in a more relaxed state. Savasana significantly affects the peace of the body and mind, which means better sleep, better metabolism, and a generally more relaxed state throughout the day.

Brain waves on savasana

We live in a high stress, high productivity culture. Our brain, for the most part, stays in beta waves, or high activity waves, most of the day, and then we crash into bed exhausted, diving right into deep sleep, or *delta* waves. We often miss out on the benefits of *alpha* and *theta* waves. During our delta deep sleep state, the body and brain get to work, cleaning out the systems and restoring balance.

Alpha waves are our 'chill pill' waves, where we begin to connect with the subconscious. They provide us with fresh insight, inspiration and creative vision. They keep us "in the bliss zone". Time has no bearing. This is the state where pain diminishes, blood pressure lowers, and creative visualization occurs. These waves cushion our ability to handle stress better. Like delta waves they increase our immunity *and* our serotonin, the 'feel good' hormone. Savasana, because it is a heightened state of deep meditation and relaxation for the mind and body, strengthens and lengthens the *alpha* waves.

Theta waves are even longer than *alpha* waves but still allow a person to be conscious and present yet connected to a larger part of themselves and the universe. Orgasm produces excess *theta* waves, as does any activity that causes a person to experience bliss. In deep relaxation, *theta* waves help heal anxiety, reduce fatigue, restore deep peace and heal the tissues of the body. Through active yoga techniques, many yoga practitioners can experience these *theta* states regularly. Not a bad way to live!

Delta waves, our slowest waves, bring us into deep meditation, sleep and healing. Many hormonal changes occur in the *delta* wave state, which affect our waking state. Some yoga practitioners can obtain this delta state, which is a waking dream state, without falling asleep. For example, there are some yogis with intensive yoga practices (six to eight hours per day) who need only a couple of hours of sleep to feel restored. Most amputees won't be living the ascetic yogi's life, but a thirty-minute daily savasana practice is certainly doable.

The benefits of savasana for amputees

Yoga students often report feelings of profound calm, renewed energy and clarity as if they had taken a nap. Memories from their past are released for some after savasana. But, some students are uncomfortable in savasana. The idea of lying down and resting, even for five minutes, causes anxiety. Their minds go all over the place. They can't get comfortable. They go into high alert. These reactions shine a light on what is really happening. A restless mind is a mind that is "on" all the time, taking a heavy toll on a person's health and mental state. Awareness of this restlessness is the first step to changing that behavior to a calmer, more centered self that heals the body and mind.

Strong emotions which have been pushed away may come to the surface during relaxation. They will keep knocking more loudly until they are dealt with.

A person with PTSD may find it dangerous to close his eyes, or completely surrender into savasana, which is fine. They can keep their eyes open, sit against a wall, and position themselves so they can see the entire space, including the exit, and still receive some benefits from savasana.

Some people fall asleep right away, indicating that they are far more exhausted than they realize, or they are not ready to handle difficult emotions that may show up when the mind has time to rest.

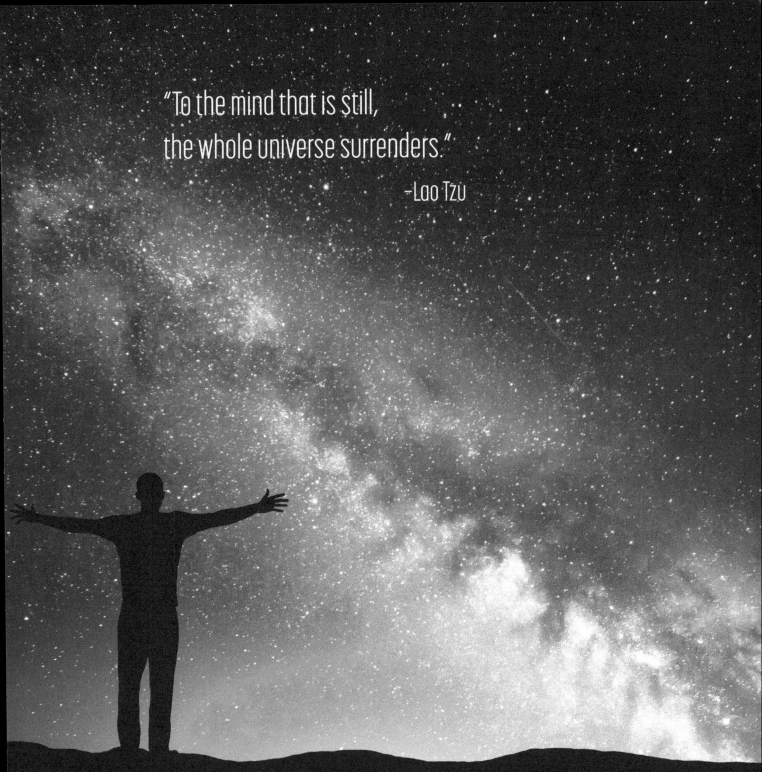

Savasana is of such great benefit to the body, mind and soul. Stressed out people get less stressed. Muscles get a chance to relax. The body systems have time to recuperate and repair. The echoes of yoga practice, especially the increase in prana, or life force, have time to absorb into the body and mind. The chatter of the mind diminishes as the nervous system heals. The mind gets clearer as does the body, gently removing toxic buildup naturally and efficiently. Tension unwinds. A sense of all things working together, or balancing for good, is achieved.

For amputees who practice savasana often, savasana transforms. So often we try to get through life, but we aren't actually in it. Savasana is that rare opportunity in yoga practice to see your life as it truly is, not what you expect or demand it to be. While it can be challenging to feel certain emotions such as grief, anger or even happiness, the physical practice of conscious rest allows the body to better handle life, to know what it's like to feel content and relaxed. Many people in savasana shed tears, laugh, reduce their pain, resolve problems, become aware of how uncomfortable they are in their own skin, or have an old memory pop into their minds that they are gratefully able to release. Some even report visions, and spontaneous healing. The point is: deep relaxation is a natural equalizer for the body, mind and spirit which restores us to wholeness.

Being whole means feeling complete as you are. Savasana, in its truest form, is just that. 'Sava' means corpse. Savasana, then is "sitting in the consciousness of a dead corpse." While it sounds macabre, the significance is quite meaningful. A person practicing savasana is saying, "In this moment I am so complete within myself that if, in this moment, I die, I am whole, fulfilled and clear within my spirit." Yoga's purpose is to remove all that keeps us from our highest best selves so that we remember our divine nature and our wholeness. Savasana takes us there.

How to practice Savasana

Below we will explore the practices of savasana and yoga nidra, a deeper relaxation technique. For some amputees, getting down to the floor is challenging. They do better practicing savasana in a chair. Some amputees can get to the floor, but may need to lie on their belly, or side, to avoid discomfort. For those amputees who keep their prosthetics on during yoga, they will continue to do so in savasana with the aid of yoga props such as a bolster under the knees. Other amputees may decide to take their prosthetics off during relaxation.

Savasana

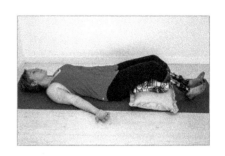

1. Stand in easy mountain pose.

2. Take a deep breath in, breathe out, and find your way to the ground

3. Bend your knees, feet flat on the floor and sit up tall.

4. Hold your hands beneath your thighs, if available, then slowly roll back, stretching your legs out as you lie on your back.

5. Alternately roll to one side and slide onto your back.

6. Bend your elbows, and then push the upper arms into the ground as you draw the shoulder blades towards each other to open the chest.

7. Place your hands by your hips, palms open and relaxed.

8. Let your hips fall out to the side.

9. Close your eyes.

10. Relax your jaw.

11. Relax your body completely, bringing all your attention softly to your breath at first.

12. Eventually let even that focus go.

13. Let your thoughts float away like little clouds.

14. Surrender to the pose.

15. Stay in the pose if you'd like. A minimum of ten minutes is recommended.

16. When your savasana is complete, follow the instructions below to transition to a seated position.

Savasana can be practiced on the belly as well for those who need to feel more connected to the earth or need to settle their bellies.

- Place a folded blanket or bolster under the knees of the residual limb or prosthetic. If the feet hang over the blanket, add another folded blanket or yoga block under the feet.

- Do the pose leaning back in a chair, with legs extended or resting on the seat of another chair.

- Do a forward fold in a chair if unable to get to the floor.

- Sit in meditation with the eyes closed if unable to get to the floor.

- Lie on the side with supportive props under the residual limb or prosthetic.

- Lie on the side with a yoga block or folded blanket between the thighs, if available.

- Place a chair upside down at a diagonal on the floor, a blanket folded over it, and place the legs over the chair, folding at the knees.

- Place legs, at the knees, over the seat of a chair, while resting the back on the floor.

- Put weighted bags over the lower belly.

- Lay in supine bound angle for a variation.

- Place a yoga block under each knee.

- Rest the feet against the wall.

UE amputees

- Place a folded blanket under the shoulders and back of the head.

- Place a yoga block underneath a bolster laying lengthwise. Sit at the edge of the bolster and roll onto your back.

- Place a folded blanket under the residual limb.

- Place a weighted bag lengthwise over the center of the chest and horizontally over the lower belly. Be careful not to put too much pressure on the sternum.

How to come out of Savasana

1. Keep your eyes closed.

2. Take some deep breaths.

3. Place one hand on your heart and one hand on your belly.

4. Focus on your breath.

5. Become more aware of the sounds around you.

6. Rub your palms together, and then cup your eyes with your palms, eyes still closed.

7. Open your eyes as you pull your hands away.

8. Circle your wrists and ankles (or hips and ribs if ankles, knees, wrists, elbows or shoulders are not available).

9. Roll your head side to side.

10. Rock your knees and hips side to side.

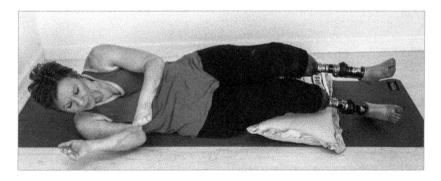

11. Stretch your entire body.

12. Roll to your right side.

13. Press into your left hand and roll up to sit comfortably, using any props necessary.

14. Notice how you feel.

Savasana techniques

- Scan your body from head to toe, mentally telling each part to relax.

- Tighten all your muscles as you inhale, then release as you exhale.

- Place a bolster under your knees.

- Cover yourself with a blanket.

- Bend your knees, placing your feet on the floor.

- Listen to a guided visualization.

- Imagine there is a screen underneath you. As you relax, all that you don't need sifts through the screen. What remains is all that you need to feel whole.

- Be aware of how and where your body touches your surroundings, like the floor, or your clothes.

- Visualize yourself becoming calm and relaxed.

- Imagine becoming a gentle wave by the shore, pulsing with breath.

- Feel your body getting heavy, settling deeply into the floor.

Yoga Nidra

A deeper layer of savasana is a practice called **yoga nidra**, or yogic sleep. Yoga nidra can be beneficial for some amputees, but not all. To enter a deep state of relaxation and stay there for an extended period can be traumatizing for some individuals who are unaccustomed to deeper states of meditation. These states can arouse emotions around limb loss and pain that are better served with movement or psychotherapy. For example, a beginner amputee yoga practitioner may become uncomfortable with the descriptive language of yoga nidra which mentions body parts. In that case, a guided relaxation or creative visualization will do.

Yoga props can be wonderful during savasana but upsetting during yoga **nidra** for some amputees dealing with PTSD, such as veterans. Blankets may feel like traps; weighted bags may seem like war trenches and eye bags too vulnerable. For any amputees who are dealing with PTSD, sitting upright in a chair, or on the back with the eyes open, may suffice.

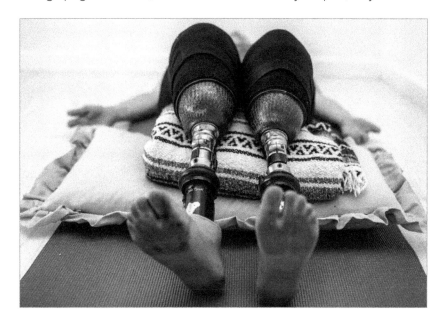

While it is not always possible to know if an amputee is going to react negatively to yoga nidra, it is possible to clue in to whether the practice would be a good fit for them. Watch how they move in the space around them. Watch their eyes, their body language and the words they use. Watch to see if they are present or far away. For amputees, if you feel that the practice is beneficial to you but feel afraid to try it, ask to have a yoga teacher present with you. Do not attempt yoga nidra alone if you are living with ongoing PTSD.

Yoga nidra offers the opportunity to witness and therefore heal the body on many levels. In yoga, the body is seen as multi-dimensional. Each layer, or **kosha**, is affected by the other layers. A hopeful mental state will give the body better blood flow, more energy and clear thinking. A distracted mental state will cause the body tension, lack of focus and low energy. All five koshas of the body: the physical, the emotional, the mental, the intellectual and the spiritual layers, are activated and explored in yoga nidra. Therefore, an amputee needs to be properly prepared with yoga practice before moving into yoga nidra. Familiarity is safety in this case.

Yoga nidra is done on the back with supportive props when necessary. Please follow the instructions for savasana to come into yoga nidra. Like savasana, yoga nidra restores the body and mind. Because yoga nidra addresses the layers of the body more directly, there are additional benefits as well. The pineal gland, a master gland of the body which is involved in melatonin production, is stimulated during yoga nidra. Blood pressure, for many amputees dealing with circulatory issues, can be lowered. Aging slows down, and immune function speeds up. Old patterns of mind and body are upgraded or eliminated to make way for healthier, happier patterns. Yoga nidra creates a sense of overall well-being in the body and mind, a quality of restfulness, and inner peace for amputees on their path to wholeness.

Standard yoga nidra script adapted for amputees

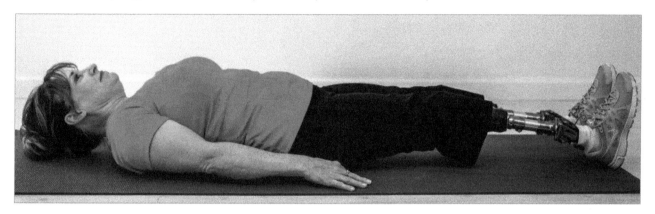

1. Set up all necessary props so that you can go deeply into the practice with no disturbances.

2. Get comfortable.

3. Lie down.

4. Close your eyes if you feel okay to do so. Otherwise keep them open with a soft gaze.

5. Allow your body to feel heavy.

6. Feel the room around you.

7. Become aware of your breath but do not control it in any way.

8. Create a *Sankalpa, or intention*, for your practice of yoga nidra if one comes to you.

9. Tell yourself the following: *"I am aware that I am about to practice Yoga Nidra. I will remain alert and awake during the practice."*

10. Become aware of your whole body. Breathe in. Breathe out.

11. Feel the floor. Breathe in. Breathe out.

12. Feel your skin. Breathe in. Breathe out.

13. Become aware of your bones. Breathe in. Breathe out.

14. Become aware of your muscles. Breathe in. Breathe out.

15. Become aware of the systems of your body. Breathe in. Breathe out.

16. Become aware of your navel to your lowest portion of your body. Breathe in. Breathe out.

17. Become aware of your navel to the crown of your head. Breathe in. Breathe out.

18. From the navel, become aware of your right side lower torso all the way down to the lowest portion of your body. *(Amputees who feel okay and have been practicing yoga for some time may be able to focus directly on individual body parts such as right hip, right femur, right knee, right shin, right ankle, right foot, right toes, and each individual toe, whether the limb is there or not)* Breathe in. Breathe out.

19. From the navel, become aware of your left side lower torso all the way down to the lowest portion of your body. Breathe in. Breathe out.

20. From the navel to the right become aware of the upper right side of the body, to the highest portion of the torso on the right. *(Amputees who feel okay and have been practicing yoga for some time may be able to focus directly on individual body parts such as right hip, right ribs, right upper chest, right collarbone, right shoulder, right upper arm, right elbow, right forearm, right wrist, right hand, and each individual right finger, whether the limb is there or not)* Breathe in. Breathe out.

21. From the navel to the left become aware of the upper left side of the body, to the highest portion of the torso on the left. Breathe in. Breathe out.

22. Become aware of your whole right side. Breathe in. Breathe out.

23. Become aware of your whole left side. Breathe in. Breathe out.

24. Become aware of your whole right arm as it is. Breathe in. Breathe out.

25. Become aware of your whole right leg as it is. Breathe in. Breathe out.

26. Become aware of your whole left arm as it is. Breathe in. Breathe out.

27. Become aware of your whole left leg as it is. Breathe in. Breathe out.

28. Become aware of your whole lower body. Breathe in. Breathe out.

29. Become aware of your whole upper body. Breathe in. Breathe out.

30. Become aware of your whole right side of the back. Breathe in. Breathe out.

31. Become aware of your whole left side of the back. Breathe in. Breathe out.

32. Become aware of your whole back. Breathe in. Breathe out.

33. Become aware of your whole right side of the front.

34. Become aware of your whole left side of the front. Breathe in. Breathe out.

35. Become aware of your whole front. Breathe in. Breathe out.

36. Become aware of your whole back. Breathe in. Breathe out.

37. Become aware of your whole body. Breathe in. Breathe out.

38. Become aware of your whole body. Breathe in. Breathe out.

39. Become aware of your whole body. Breathe in. Breathe out.

40. Become aware of your natural breath. Breathe in. Breathe out.

41. Feel the breath BREATHING the Body. Don't regulate the breath. Begin to count the breath. Inhale 27, Exhale 27. Inhale 26, Exhale 26. Continue counting backwards to 1.

42. Allow the counting to fall away. Just BE.

43. Repeat this sentence. "I am aware that I am practicing yoga nidra. I will remain alert and awake during the practice."

44. Feel heavy in your entire body, as if you were a large boulder. Breathe in. Breathe out.

45. Feel light in your entire body, like a feather floating. Breathe in. Breathe out.

46. Feel hot in your entire body. Breathe in. Breathe out.

47. Feel cold in your entire body. Breathe in. Breathe out.

48. Feel pleasure your entire body. Breathe in. Breathe out.

49. Feel pain in your entire body. Breathe in. Breathe out.

50. Feel sadness in your entire body. Breathe in. Breathe out.

51. Feel happiness in your entire body. Breathe in. Breathe out.

52. Feel centered and open-hearted in your entire body. Breathe in. Breathe out.

53. Feel irritated in your entire body. Breathe in. Breathe out.

54. Feel hate in your entire body. Breathe in. Breathe out.

55. Feel love in your entire body. Breathe in. Breathe out.

56. Repeat this sentence. *"I am aware that I am practicing yoga nidra. I will remain alert and awake during the practice."*

57. Imagine the color red infusing your entire body. Breathe in. Breathe out.

58. Imagine the color orange infusing your entire body. Breathe in. Breathe out.

59. Imagine the color yellow infusing your entire body. Breathe in. Breathe out.

60. Imagine the color green infusing your entire body. Breathe in. Breathe out.

61. Imagine the color turquoise infusing your entire body. Breathe in. Breathe out.

62. Imagine the color purple infusing your entire body. Breathe in. Breathe out.

63. Imagine the color indigo infusing your entire body. Breathe in. Breathe out.

64. Imagine the color white infusing your entire body. Breathe in. Breathe out.

65. Imagine your favorite smell. Sense how you feel as you imagine this smell. Breathe in. Breathe out.

66. Imagine a bright light in the center of your heart. Breathe in. Breathe out.

67. Watch this bright light become smaller and smaller, until it is a flicker of light within your heart. Observe how this flicker of light can light up your entire being. Breathe in. Breathe out.

68. Ask yourself 'Who am I?". Breathe in. Breathe out.

69. Repeat your affirmation from the beginning of your practice.

70. Resist the need to move.

71. Stay in yoga nidra.

72. Feel your breath breathing your body.

73. Feel your tongue resting in the mouth.

74. Move your tongue.

75. Feel your skull.

76. Feel your breath.

77. Feel your body resting on the floor.

78. Feel your lower body.

79. Feel your upper body.

80. Feel your back body.

81. Feel your front body.

82. Feel your whole body.

83. Deepen your breath.

84. Open your eyes.

85. Look around.

86. Breathe.

87. Move your body.

88. Notice if there is any place where the body needs loving touch.

89. Place your hands there, if able. Alternately, place your thoughts there. Breathe in. Breathe out.

90. Move slowly out of yoga nidra just as you would savasana.

91. Your practice of yoga nidra is complete.

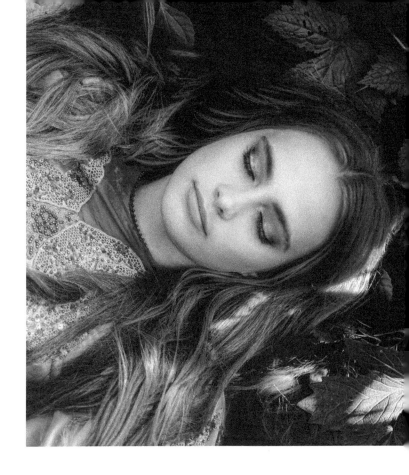

Spend time after yoga nidra in quiet contemplation. Allow yourself to receive the full benefits of yoga nidra before moving on to your next task. **Yoga nidra** deeply heals the body and mind. It is highly beneficial to an amputee's sense of wholeness and personal fulfillment. Enjoy its benefits.

OM

At the beginning and end of yoga practice, practitioners and instructors often chant the sound of **"Om."** **Om** is a combination of three sounds: A, U and M. Each sound is pronounced in the chant, followed by the sound of silence at the end of the 'M'. 'A' 'U' 'M' represent the divine aspects of creation, sustaining, and completion.

Om has great physical, mental and spiritual significance, especially for an amputee. The sound of **Om** has an omnipresent quality to it, as if it were the vibration pervading all living things. It is like an electric current, one seen from its end results rather than from the form of the current itself. When an amputee chants **Om** that quality of an all-encompassing universal connection restores any feeling of separation from one's self or the world. Chanting **Om** positively affects the nervous system, helping amputees learn to redirect strong sensations such as phantom pain, or tense scar tissue, away from pain and toward the healing sound of **Om**.

There are many reasons to chant 'Om'. The main reason is that chanting 'Om' feels good! Since a human being is like a microcosm of the larger universe, chanting **Om** reminds an amputee that her life is part of the cycle of life itself, always creating, sustaining and completing. For example, an amputee practicing a yoga posture creates the posture by beginning the posture. She then sustains the posture with breath and completes the posture by coming out of the posture, feeling the effects of the posture in a moment of silence.

While 'Om' is not for everyone, either because it seems weird, or their religion does not allow the chanting of 'Om', for most of us, 'Om' is a great comfort to the body, mind and spirit. It feels eternal, and familiar. As amputees, our sense of wholeness needs that dose of heaven to remind us we are so much more than our amputation. We are limitless.

How to chant Om

1. Close the eyes.

2. Place the palms, if available, in a prayer position in front of the heart. Alternately, reverently focus your attention on the heart.

3. Bow the head slightly toward the heart.

4. Take a deep inhale.

5. Exhale.

6. Take another deep inhale.

7. As you exhale, chant Om, beginning in the belly with an 'Aaaah' sound.

8. Sustain the chant with 'Uuuuu', feeling it in the mid –torso.

9. Complete the chant with 'Mmmm', letting the sound rise to the throat.

10. Repeat the Om three times.

11. End with a few minutes of silent meditation.

To be or not to be. That is the question. All the yoga practices in this chapter offer opportunities to simply BE. Try being for a while. You may be surprised by how magical life really is, with or without limbs. Choose to BE.

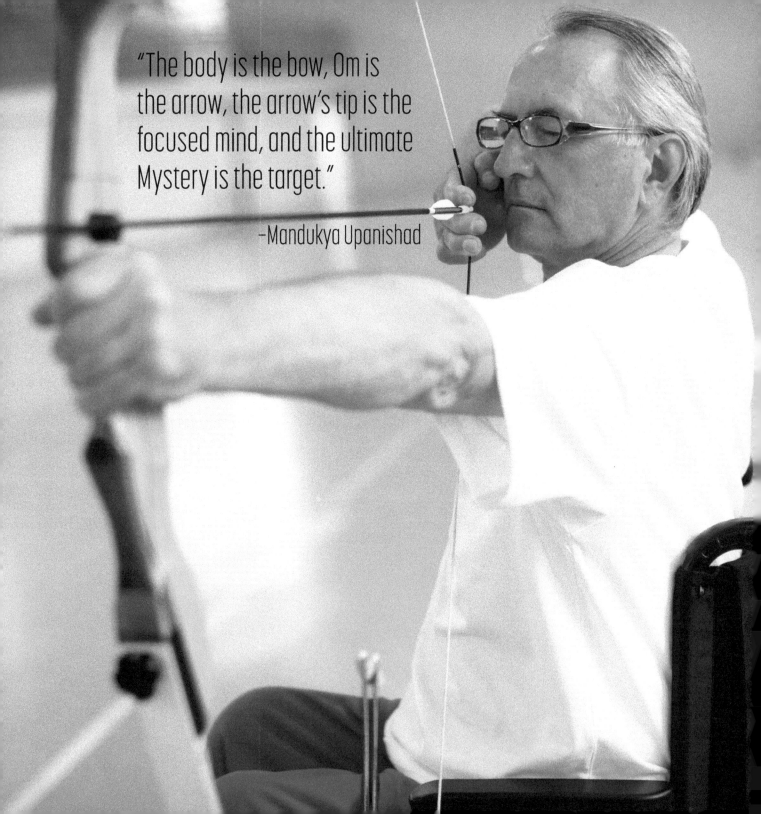

"The body is the bow, Om is the arrow, the arrow's tip is the focused mind, and the ultimate Mystery is the target."

–Mandukya Upanishad

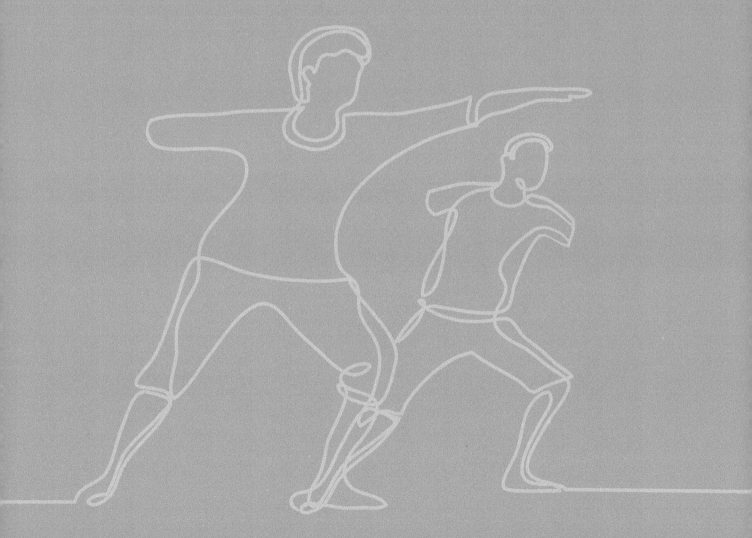

The day I received my kidney transplant, I was reminded once again that life flows when we let it. I waited desperately for over 11 years for relief from dialysis. After a few transplant misses, I finally received my kidney at the right time. There were many days, in my years facing life threatening illness, when I fought tooth and nail for every breath, every freedom and every passion. Yoga helped me find the flow within my battles, and before I knew it, I was loosening my grip, a little at a time, until I could trust the process of life more fully. I still have my moments, but going with the flow, I believe, creates *more* flow in your life. The following yoga practices remind us to flow through life with more ease.

ALIVE

Greet the Sun

Surya Namaskar, or sun salutation, a flow of yoga postures moving one to another(vinyasa), is a prayer, a devotional thank you(Namaskar) to the creative force of the sun(Surya) that illuminates everything and brings life to all of us. A reverent attitude for the sun and the gift of life enlightens an amputee, elevating her beyond the mundane to see the sacred in everything. The twelve poses, both bowing down and lifting in gratitude, form a complete cycle, representing 12 months, the 12 Sanskrit names for the sun, and the balance of the feminine and masculine aspects of nature. Sun Salutation is both a warm-up and a yoga practice. Traditionally, 12 rounds of sun salutation are done, but for amputees, do what is available. For some amputees, vinyasa flows are easier to manage because there is less chance of falling due to dynamic sequencing. Other amputees need to transition in poses very slowly when practicing vinyasa or feel better with a static yoga practice. As you explore each vinyasa, which means 'to place in a certain way', let your heart, mind and body be placed in a new experience of wholeness.

"... let me repeat that no asana practice is complete without sun worship. Without its focusing of mental energies, yoga practice amounts to little more than gymnastics and, as such, loses meaning and proves fruitless. Indeed, the Surya Namaskara should never be mistaken for mere physical exercise –for something incidental, that is, that simply precedes the asanas of yoga. Therefore, it is necessary, before beginning the sun salutations, to pray to Surya [...] to bestow upon us the good fortune of having only good thoughts, of hearing and speaking only good words, and of attaining a sound and strong body, so that we may have a long life and, one day, achieve oneness with God." — Sri K. Pattabhi Jois

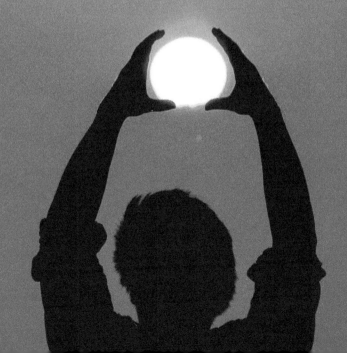

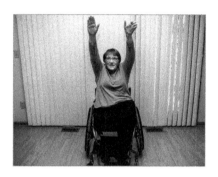

Sun breath

1. Place the hands, when available, next to your side.

2. As you inhale, raise your arms up overhead until you are at your maximum level of inhale.

3. Exhale float the arms back down to the side.

4. Repeat this breath three times.

UE amputees: If one arm is available use that arm. If no arms are available, lift the sternum and draw the lower shoulder blades towards each other. Then return to your original position. If shoulders/one shoulder are available, roll them back on inhale then return to the original position on exhale.

Sun Salutation: Surya Namaskar

1. Stand in mountain pose.

2. Inhale. Lift the arms overhead.

3. Exhale. Fold into a forward bend.

4. Step the right foot back into a lunge.

5. Step the left foot back to meet the right in plank pose.

6. Bend the elbows into the ribs as you hover towards the floor in chaturanga, four limbed pose.

7. Push up the chest into a cobra pose, lifting the collarbone up to the sky.

8. Fold forward into a downward dog, or upside down 'V'.

9. Step the right foot forward into a lunge.

10. Step the left foot forward to meet the right in a forward bend.

11. Circle the arms over head as you come back to stand in mountain pose.

BK and AK amputees

Follow the instructions for each of these individual poses first. Once you feel comfortable, make necessary adjustments to put the flow together.

Sun salutation can be done seated in a chair, pressing against a wall, or on hands and knees, with or without a prosthesis.

UE amputee

Follow the instructions for each of these individual poses first. Once you feel comfortable, make necessary adjustments and put the flow together.

Sun Salutation in a chair

- Sun breath

- Seated mountain

- Seated forward bend

- Hug abdominals into the core for plank pose

- Seated cobra with or without arms

- Seated forward bend

- Seated mountain

- Sun breath

Sun Salutation with a prosthesis

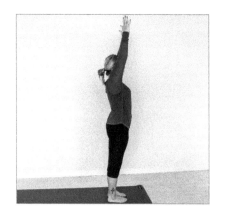
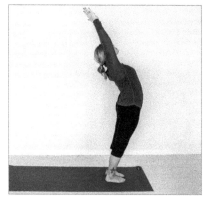
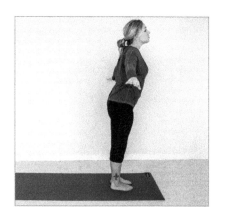
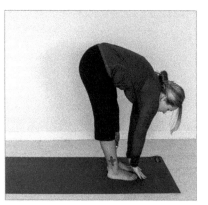
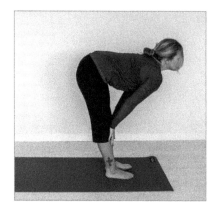
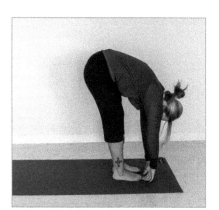
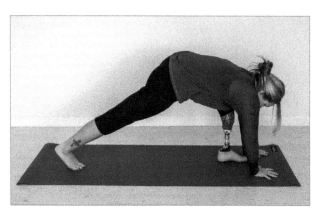
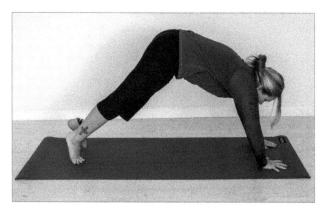

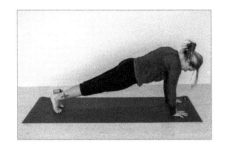 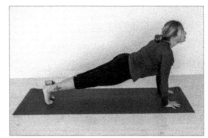 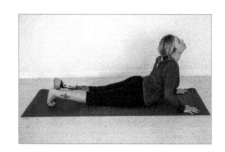

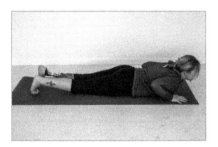 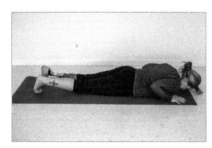 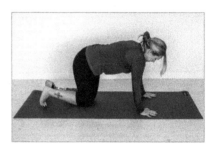

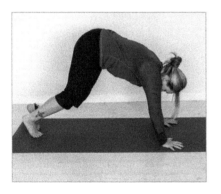 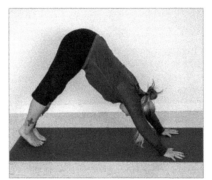 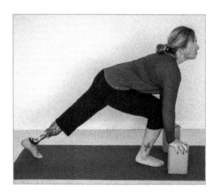

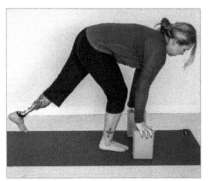 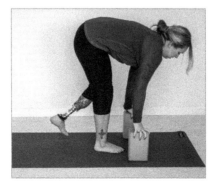 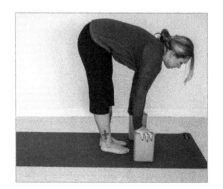

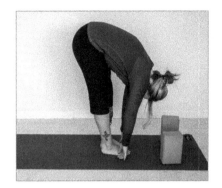

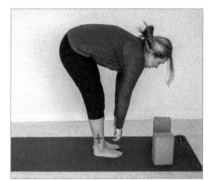

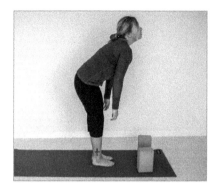

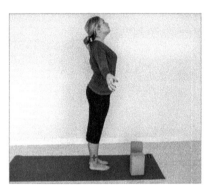

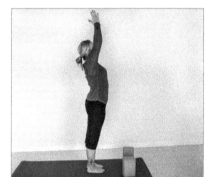

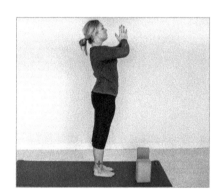

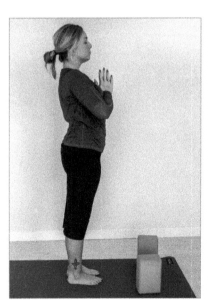

Sun Salutation without a prosthesis

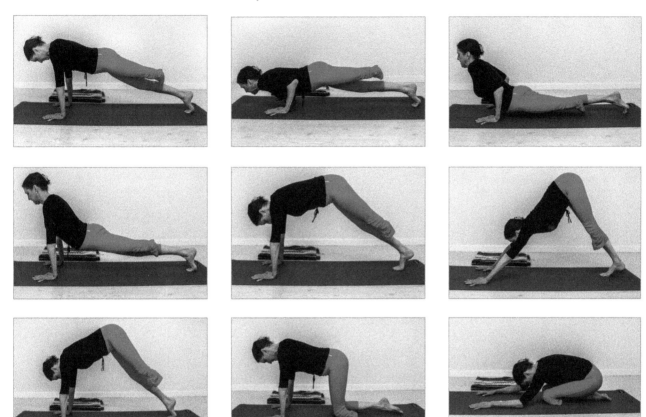

Done daily, sun salutation (Surya **Namaskar**) benefits all major systems of the body, stimulates creativity and restores balance in the body, mind and spirit.

Practice Surya Namaskar!

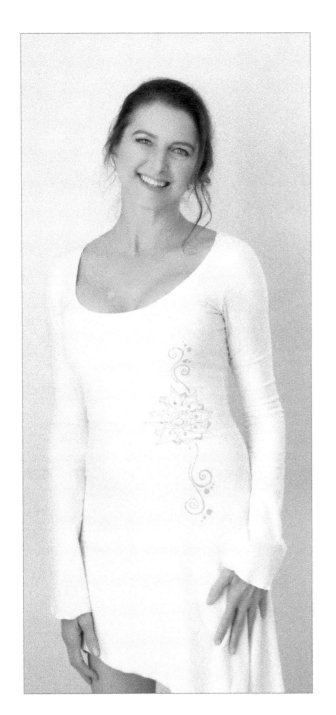

MEET MARSHA

On my yoga mat, as I practiced yoga in a physical, tangible way, I came to accept myself fully after all these years of thinking I already had!

Like many amputees, I have gone through periods of grief, discouragement, pain and trauma. The process of recovering from limb loss and learning how to live as an amputee, has changed over the years. Dancing and movement are who I am. Losing my left leg as a thirteen-year old girl was devastating. There was almost no support network set up for amputees back then. Naturally, everywhere I went, I stood out as the "girl who was sick and handicapped." The bald head didn't help! Disability had a stigma back then that still exists, but thanks to the activism of people within the disability community and beyond, attitudes have improved. The process of emotional and psychological recovery was gradual. As I got better at walking with my prosthesis, I was able to pursue, at least awkwardly, some of my passions, such as working out and dancing.

*When I first encountered yoga as a young girl, before I lost my leg, I was under the impression that it was a practice to bring people into altered states of consciousness. I saw pictures of yogis in very awkward positions, and I was intrigued to try them myself. Little did I know that my own yoga journey would lead me not only into altered states of consciousness, but also into **more consciousness about my own body,** my breath, my feelings, my intuition and the spiritual universe.*

That is the true practice of yoga, a seamless interplay of everyday mindfulness and profound spiritual awareness. All and everything is included. Harmony is simply an acceptance and acknowledgement of all that is. There is nothing to achieve in yoga. There is only greater and greater awareness /consciousness of what IS. When we are constantly living in the future, in what needs to be done and what comes next, we may be awake, but we won't be aware.

I started doing yoga again in my mid-twenties, mostly because a friend convinced me to give it a try. The friend is gone but the yoga stayed. I'll be honest. Before I found yoga, I thought I had gotten over my amputation. I'd done talk therapy and prayer groups as a young woman. I had volunteered at hospitals, working with sick children. I owned my own design business, traveled regularly, and lived my life the way I wanted to. All along, I had been hiding how alone, vulnerable and 'ugly' I still felt. Yoga changed all that.

From the moment I found yoga as an adult, I took a deep spiritual dive into what wholeness meant to me. After about ten years of yoga practice, I became a yoga teacher. Almost immediately in to my yoga training, I was brutally aware of all the sore spots in my body and soul. My body was telling me the truth not only about my hamstrings, but also about my held emotions of sadness and anger, old hurts, both medical and personal, and unconscious beliefs that had shrouded my light. I listened to my body, mind and spirit. I breathed compassion into the broken parts. I rocked my thirteen-year old girl to sleep at night. I released years of tears. I relaxed into my life. On my yoga mat, as I practiced yoga in a physical, tangible way, I came to accept myself fully after all these years of thinking I already had!

Yoga taught me to be aware of how I behaved when things got tough, boring, tiring, sad, or hostile. It is no coincidence that my inner habitual voice would tell me "Go on, push through. Ignore your feelings. You can deal with them later." as I plowed through a challenging yoga flow, only to see the same voice show up later in the day. "Go on; Clench that jaw, Stiff upper lip. Stop complaining, ignore your feelings. You can deal with them later." I saw how judgmental I had been towards myself for so long and how lacking in compassion for myself I was. Wow. What an awakening!

Slowly, over thousands of days on and off the yoga mat, I have reclaimed the me that had been missing for so long. Now I understand. Yoga, this ancient healing practice, makes it safe for me to get right down in to the very thick of it, to be fully alive in my body, and to see things as they really are, not as I wish them to be. This makes each moment full of possibility, new and unique. There will never ever be a breath like the one I am breathing right now. There will never be another life like the one I am living now. I choose to live that life knowing I am whole. This is my lifelong yoga practice.

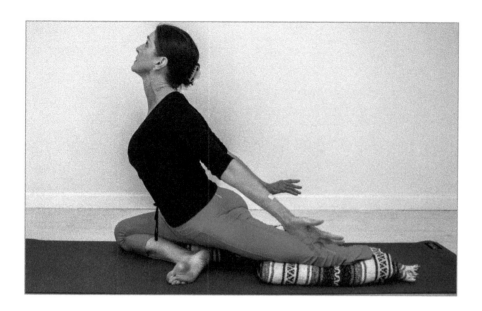

Adapt

Each amputee I meet has an amazing, and often heartbreaking story to tell. Losing a limb or limbs is very difficult, but the human spirit has a built-in mechanism to face incredible odds, quite evident in the joy and strength of the amputees in this book. Amputees must adapt to their lives in every possible way. And for the most part, they do it with incredible finesse. We just don't see all the effort that goes into it.

The same is true for yoga. Yoga is not simply stretching. It is a mental and emotional challenge that offers amputees tremendous opportunities for personal growth and happiness. Yes, some amputees will need more props than others. And yes, some amputees will not be able to practice the yoga pose the way "the yogis do it". So, what? The truth is that yoga is a grand personal experiment. We are the creators and the recipients of its benefits. Life as an amputee brings with it countless situations that demand we go with the flow, trust our body and learn to love ourselves even more. Love yourself well by practicing the yoga poses with curiosity and a welcome smile. You'll be so glad you did.

ADAPTIVE FLOW

Seated Twist: Ardha Matsyendrasana

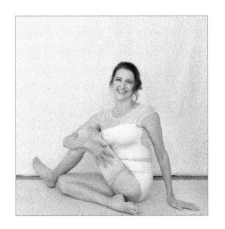

1. Sit with the legs outstretched, spine long, head reaching up to the sky and the bottom pressing down into the earth. Flex the feet.

2. Bend the right knee, then place the right foot on the outside left thigh.

3. Wrap the left elbow around the right knee, and then twist from the lower torso to the right, placing the right hand behind on the floor.

4. Allow the head and eyes to twist last.

5. Release from the pose by drawing the belly into the spine and unwind the spine back to center.

6. Repeat on the other side.

BK and AK amputees

- With a prosthesis, bend the knee as much as able, with the option to place the prosthetic foot to the inside of the extended leg.

- Elevate the hips on a yoga block or bolster.

- Sit lengthwise at the wall. Keep the bent knee to the inside of the extended leg, twist to the wall, and press the hands to the wall.

- Sit at the wall with the extended leg pressing into the wall.

- Place the hand that is outside the hip on a block.

- Without a prosthesis, wrap the strap around the residual limb including the bent knee (when possible) to twist.

- Rest the residual limb on the opposite thigh, then twist.

- Keep the residual limb forward (or the prosthetic limb when needed), rest on a folded blanket to remain even with the extended leg. Place the fingertips or hands on the outside of the extended leg and twist.

UE amputees

- Sit with the back against the wall. Draw the navel to the spine and twist the torso to one side then the other.

- If able to bend the knee and place on the outside of the extended leg, focus on lifting the sternum and twist.

- If unable to lift the bent knee, slide the foot flat on the floor until parallel with the calf or thigh of the extended leg, then twist the torso.

- Place a folded blanket on top of the thigh of the bent knee and lean into the thigh with the torso as you twist.

Cow: Gomukhasana

1. Sit in seated staff pose.

2. Place the left foot underneath the right hip.

3. Place the right knee on top of the left, resting the right foot to the outside of the left hip.

4. Rest the knees on top of each other.

5. Lift the left arm up.

6. Bend the left elbow, placing the left palm between the shoulders.

7. Reach the right hand behind the back, between the shoulder blades, until it can grab the left hand or a yoga strap.

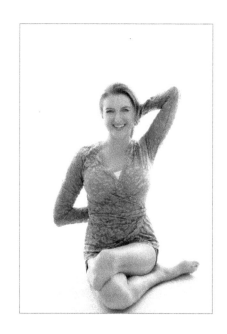

8. Breathe deeply 2-5 breaths.

9. Release the arms slowly.

10. Place the hands behind the buttocks, lean back and uncross the legs back into staff pose.

11. Repeat on the other side..

BK and AK amputees

- Do this pose without a prosthesis to get better range of motion in the hips and ankles.

- Do this pose one leg at a time, keeping the other leg extended in half-staff pose.

- Do a variation of this pose, focusing on the outer hip opening, by coming into a seated pose on the floor, with or without a prosthesis, crossing one leg over the other.

UE amputee

- Lift what you can of your residual arm to the sky. Roll the opposite shoulder down and back, drawing the shoulder blades towards each other.

- Practice crossing and uncrossing your legs to learn your level of hip flexibility.

- Sit at the wall. To feel extension in the spine and head, gently press the head into the wall with or without a yoga blanket behind, drawing the shoulder blades towards the wall.

Flow between cow-faced pose and seated half twist two to three times.

End your practice in Childs pose. (See page *195*).

"The cows have come and have brought us good fortune. In our stalls, contented, may they stay! May they bring forth calves for us, many-colored, giving milk for Indra each day. You make, O cows, the thin man sleek; to the unlovely you bring beauty. Rejoice our homestead with pleasant lowing. In our assemblies we laud your vigor." — Rig Veda (4.28.1;6)

AWARE

What does it mean to be aware? Awareness is a state of mind that keeps us present and connected to life. Have you ever talked to someone who makes you feel like every word you say is of great value? You feel like you matter, don't you? Or maybe you have talked with someone who said all the right words, but clearly wasn't listening to you. It doesn't feel very good, does it? Give your mind, body and spirit the courtesy of listening to them in this yoga flow. Be surprised by how much they can tell you. Allow yourself to trust them. They always tell the truth.

For each pose, follow this simple awareness formula. Be aware of:

*   The space around you

*   The space beneath you

*   The space above you

*   The space within you

AWARENESS FLOW

Five-Pointed Star

1. Step out wide with the feet.

2. Spread the arms wide in a 'T' formation.

3. Lengthen through the spine.

4. Focus the eyes straight ahead.

BK and AK amputees

*   Do this pose with the back to the wall.

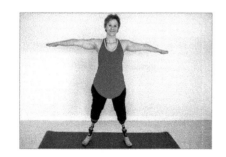

- Step sideways and lean the prosthetic foot into the wall.

- Sit in a chair. Open the legs into a wide V at the edges of the chair. Open the arms into a 'T'.

- Lie on the floor. Spread the body into a starfish shape, with or without prosthetics.

UE amputees

- Open the collarbone.

- Do the pose against the wall, leaning the back of the prosthetic arm into the wall.

- Imagine lengthening through the center of the spine.

- Radiate energy in all directions from the navel.

Gate: Parighasana

1. Come onto your hands and knees.

2. Rise up to a kneeling position.

3. Extend the right leg out to the side, flexing the right foot.

4. Lift the left arm up to the sky.

5. Lengthen the left side of the waist.

6. Lean the torso over to the right as you reach the right arm to the right leg or grab the right foot.

7. Arch the left arm toward the right foot.

8. Keep your body in one plane.

9. Lift the left arm back to center as you realign your torso.

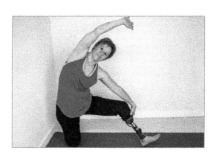

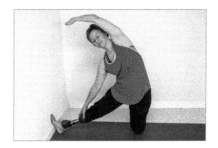

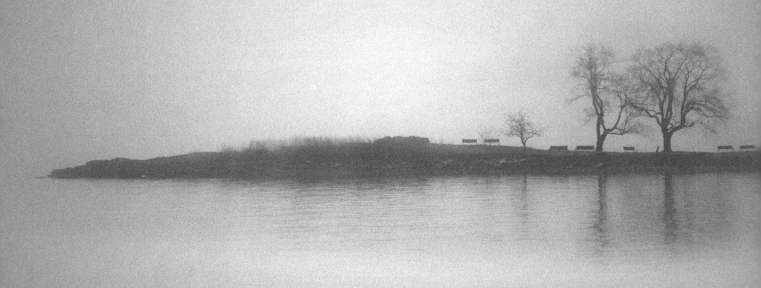

"Just for now, without asking how, let yourself sink into stillness."

-Danna Faulds

10. Come back to a kneeling position with the right leg.

11. Repeat the pose on the other side.

BK and AK amputees

- Lean your prosthetic foot into a wall.

- Bend your prosthetic leg, placing the prosthetic foot flat on the floor.

- Do the pose at a corner with the back to a wall and the extended leg pressing into the other wall.

- Place a chair to the right of the wall. Kneel with the left side to the wall. Arch over to the right in gate pose. Press the right hand on top of the chair or grab the edge of the chair.

- Sit in a chair. Extend the right leg out at the edge of the chair. Lift the left arm and arch over to the right leg. Switch legs and repeat on the other side.

UE amputees

- Do the pose at a corner with the back to a wall and the extended leg pressing into the other wall. Lean the ribs into the wall for support.

- When leaning to the right, lean the torso into the seat of a chair as you extend the right leg beneath the chair.

- Wrap two looped straps around the body. Place one end of the loop at the extended right foot, the other into the mid ribs of the left side. Tighten the loops as needed for added stability.

- If feeling wobbly, do triangle pose with the back to the wall instead.

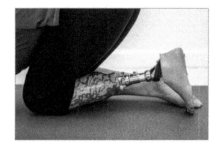

Puppy: Uttana Shishasana

1. Come onto the hands and knees.

2. Extend the arms forward as you stretch the spine.

3. Press the palms into the floor.

4. Slightly lengthen the arms at the front of the chest.

5. Walk the hands back underneath your shoulders.

6. Roll to one side to sit on the floor when complete.

BK and AK amputees

- Do this pose standing, pressing the palms into the wall as you stretch the spine.

- If unable to come to hands and knees, sit instead. Interlock the fingers, flip the palms and press the palms to the sky with lengthened arms.

- Place a bolster or yoga block under the chest.

- Place folded blankets under the buttocks.

- Do this pose with the feet to the wall. Press the feet into the wall for added spinal stretch.

UE amputees

- If one arm is available, extend that arm while supporting the residual limb with a folded blanket.

- Fold the torso over a bolster.

- Place the forehead on a yoga block against the wall. Put folded blankets under the chest to avoid collapse.

- Lie on the back draped over a bolster to open the chest.

Vishnu's Couch: Anantanasana

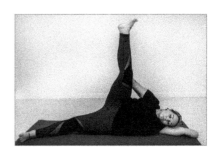

1. Lie sideways on the right, legs forward 45 degrees.

2. Lengthen the right arm underneath the right side of the head.

3. Flex both feet.

4. Draw the navel into the spine.

5. Lift the left leg up to the ceiling.

6. If available, grab hold of the left foot or a strap, and extend the leg.

7. Release the left leg to meet the right.

8. Roll to the other side and repeat.

BK and AK amputees

*   Use a strap to lift the leg up and down.

*   Lean the back of the body into a wall for extra support.

*   Press the lower foot into a wall.

*   Lean the extended leg on a chair which straddles the body.

*   Do the pose with or without a prosthesis.

*   Do the pose with bent knees.

UE amputees

*   Rest the head on a low pillow or folded blanket.

*   Lean the back of the body into a wall.

*   Place a bolster or yoga block between your midback and the wall. Lean into the prop.

"I flow into the whirlwind of God when
I am lost at sea, knowing I will find my way
back home."

– Marsha Therese Danzig

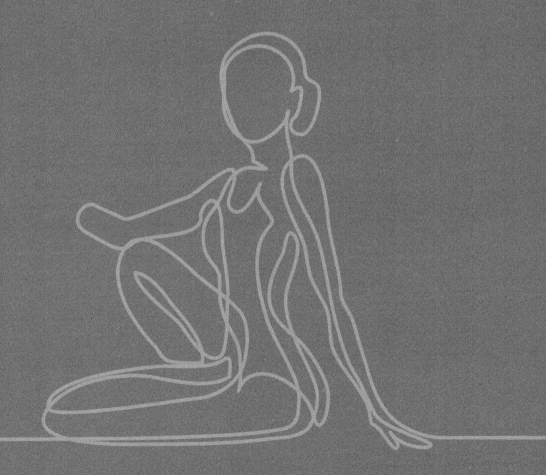

CHAPTER
SEVEN | HEAL

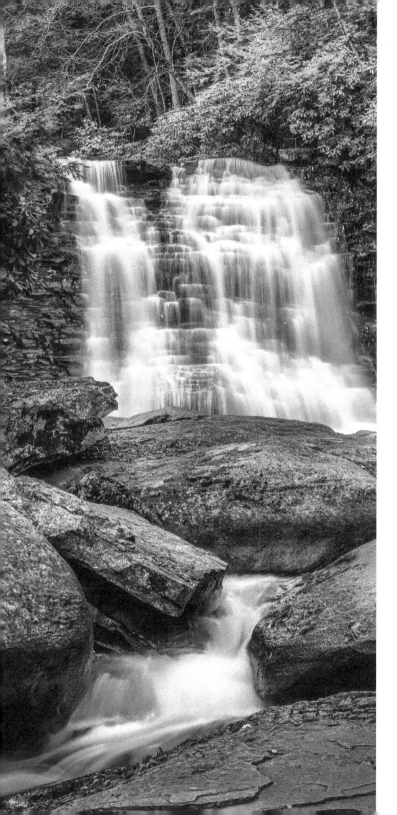

OVERCOME PAIN

The mere thought of amputation, for most of us, evokes feelings of extreme pain and suffering. Amputation is violent, whether a person is prepared for it, or not. The recovery for some is quick and relatively uneventful but for some amputees, pain is not just an acute sensation which happens from time to time, but an ongoing battle to live a normal life despite the pain.

According to *Miriam Webster online dictionary*, the very definition of pain carries with it the notion of punishment. Pain is a penalty for causing suffering in oneself or others, inflicted by an angry god. Pain, in practical terms, is the way the brain interprets messages that a sensation in the body isn't pleasant and is interfering with daily life. Many amputees experience pain, related not only to the residual limb, but referred pain due to an uncomfortable prosthetic fit, phantom pain or pain in another overused part of the body.

When pain takes over daily life, the mental and emotional energy to rise above the pain, handle daily tasks, and function normally drains an amputee's sense of well-being, many times to the point of desperation. Most humans have experienced pain at some point in life, but amputation hurts, a lot.

Phantom pain, a unique pain for amputees, is the brain's way of interpreting messages that a sensation in a part of the body that is now missing isn't feeling good and is interfering with daily life. The challenge, of course, is that the pain cannot be soothed using normal means, because the limb is not there. According to Keith Cornell, former president of the AOPA (American Orthotics and Prosthetics Association), phantom pain is a result of the brain's misinterpretation of signals it can't make sense of. Phantom pain occurs more often with new amputees, but long-term amputees also deal with phantom pain, often induced by stress or illness. Many amputees take analgesics initially to handle the pain, but can become dependent or addicted, prolonging recovery and complicating recovery. Usually, phantom pains do subside over time, but they can be frightening and debilitating when they occur.

Yoga reduces mental stress aggravated by limb loss, increasing the body's capacity to regulate and manage pain effectively. Through the practice of yoga and mindfulness, phantom pain can be lessened.

Some prosthetists and orthopedic surgeons maintain that phantom pain does not exist; that the mere mention of phantom pain can set an amputee up to experience its symptoms. The power of suggestion is the problem. The more research that can be done in this area, the better. Until then, phantom pain needs to be addressed for those who do feel its effects.

Phantom Pain vs. chronic pain

Phantom pain is most prevalent at the beginning of the limb loss journey, and normally subsides over time. However, certain stressors, such as health issues, job problems, insomnia, the onset of illness, visiting a hospital, and physical intimacy, can bring on phantom pain. The length of the pain, while acute, can be seconds, or days. Since phantom pain's origin is not localized in the limb, but in the brain and spinal cord, phantom pain treatments focus on the sources of the pain. Acupuncture, bio-feedback, nerve stimulation, brain stimulation, mirror therapy, virtual reality, meditation, exercise and psychotherapy are alternatives to pain medication.

Yoga reduces mental stress aggravated by limb loss, increasing the body's capacity to regulate and manage pain effectively.

HEAL

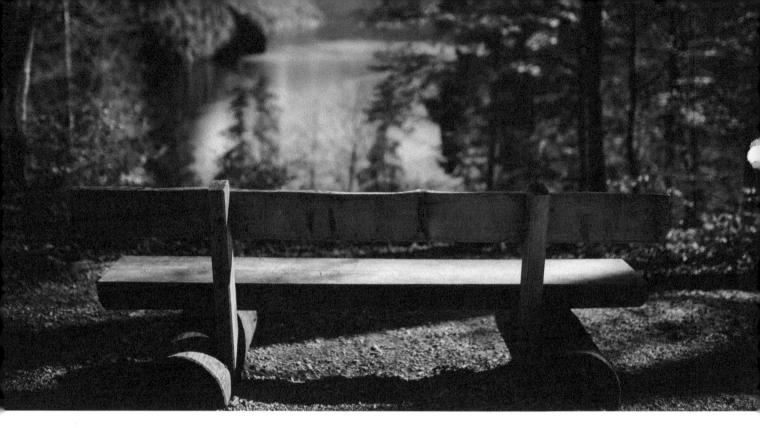

So is yoga.

Research is showing that the practice of yoga enlarges the gray matter of the brain. This is important for cognitive functioning and executive control, both of which are needed to avoid addiction to pain killers. Grey matter is also linked to the insula, the center of the brain associated with managing chronic pain. Yoga, rather than killing pain, invites positive feelings while awakening consciousness and helping an amputee control and indeed master their pain until it dissipates or ends.

Below are some practices to help an amputee cope more effectively with pain.

The **three-step meditation process** is an excellent way to cope better with pain.

1. First, practice sitting in stillness.

2. Second, be with the stillness exactly as it is.

3. Third, watch the stillness.

4. Notice how you feel.

5. Repeat throughout the day.

This **basic breath practice** to reduce pain works for all levels of pain.

1. Breathe in and out through the nostrils three times.

2. Extend the spine as you inhale.

3. Round the spine as you exhale.

4. Repeat steps 2 & 3 three times.

5. Practice this sequence any time you feel anxious or tense.

This **simple yoga sequence** invites feelings of calm, peace and trust. Repeat the sequence twice, daily, until you see changes.

1. Set an intention to care for yourself throughout this practice.

2. Do two rounds of sun salutation.

3. Do Kurmasana, or turtle pose. (see steps to the pose below)

4. Do Garbhasana, or childs pose, rolling side to side on the forehead to stimulate the pineal gland.

5. Do Jathara Paravritti, or knee down twist. (see steps to the pose below)

6. Focus on the action of each pose, then the sensations and feelings. Build stamina first.

7. Rest in Savasana, or relaxation pose.

8. Roll to the side and sit up.

9. Meditate on the space between the brow points.

10. End your practice with 5-10 rounds of alternate nostril breathing.

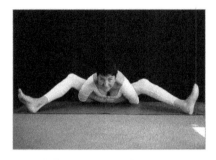

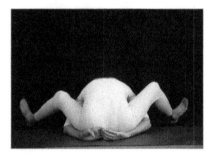

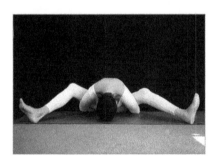

Turtle Pose: Kurmasana

1. Sit on the floor with the legs wide open, knees bent, feet flexed, arms inside the inner legs.

2. Walk the arms forward with the spine long.

3. Slide the arms underneath the thighs as the legs begin to extend fully or stay bent

4. If available, wrap the arms behind the back.

5. Settle the chin on the ground, as the torso rests fully on the ground.

6. To come out of the pose, bend the knees deeply. Slide the arms out from under the thighs

BK and AK amputees

- Press the feet against a wall.

- Keep the knees bent if wearing a prosthesis, and place a strap around each foot, pulling forward with the strap.

- Walk the arms forward rather than slide them under the thighs.

- Place the torso over a bolster resting on a yoga block, or multiple folded blankets.

- Do this pose in a chair, with the legs wide open. Lean the body forward, resting the head on a chair or table in front.

- Open the hips, roll the inner thighs inward when available, and lengthen the spine.

UE amputees

- Rest the torso on a bolster pressing against a wall or resting on a yoga block.

- Do this pose with the back to the wall. Lean forward over multiple folded blankets or a bolster.

- If elbows are available, fold forward and rest the elbows on yoga blocks.

Childs: Garbhasana

*Please refer to Chapter 5 for complete instructions.

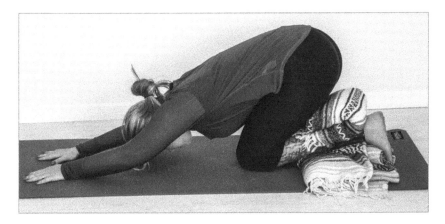

Knee Down Twist: Jathara Paravritti

1. Lie on the back. Bring the knees into the chest, or extend the legs straight up to the sky,

2. Place the arms in a T position.

3. Pull the navel in and feel the core activated as you inhale.

4. Exhale, sway the bent or straight legs to the right, towards the right elbow.

5. Turn the head to the left.

6. Rest in this position for a few breaths.

7. Bring everything back to center.

8. Repeat to the left.

BK and AK amputees

- Keep the feet on the ground and sway the knees to the right then left if wearing a prosthesis.

- Place a yoga block or bolster underneath the bent knees or residual limb on the right side then the left, when twisting.

- Lie on the left side. Roll the right arm to the right in a T position. Repeat on the other side.

UE amputees

- Place a single folded blanket under the shoulders and spread the space between the shoulder blades as you twist the legs in one direction then the other.

- For more stabilization, press the knees into a wall to feel the spine elongated.

- Place a folded blanket under the residual limb.

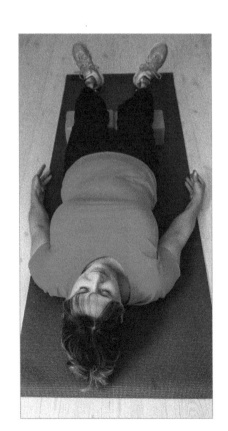

Relaxation: Savasana

*Please refer to Chapter 5 for complete instructions.

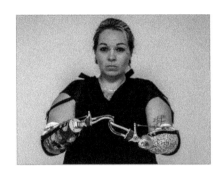

Our sorrows and wounds are healed only when we touch them with compassion.
—Buddha

PAIN AND YOGA

In yoga there are three qualities of nature which inform all of life. These qualities are called the **Gunas.** Understanding these gunas, or qualities, can provide a pathway through pain. The gunas are: **tamas/**inertia; **rajas/**fire; and **sattva/**harmony. For an amputee living with pain, staying stuck in **tamas** (or inertia) can increase pain, while being in constant movement (rajas) can aggravate pain and injury. A balanced state (**sattva**) flows from inertia (**tamas**) through movement (**rajas**) to restful harmony. These qualities of nature possess both 'positive' and 'negative' aspects, all a part of the nature of the universe. The negative aspects of **tamas** include inactivity, depression, and rigidity of mind and body. The positive aspects are potential, restoration, and inner reflection. The negative aspects of **rajas** are aggression, chaos, and selfishness while the positive aspects are movement, passion and generosity. **Sattva's** negative aspects are complacency, false virtue, and spiritual austerity. The positive aspects of sattva are contentment, pleasure and balance.

Gunas	Qualities of Nature	Positive	Negative
Tamas	Inertia	Potential, reflection, restoration	Depression, inactivity, rigidity
Rajas	Fire	Movement, passion, generosity	Aggression, chaos, selfishness
Sattva	Harmony	Contentment, pleasure, balance	Complacency, false virtue, spiritual austerity

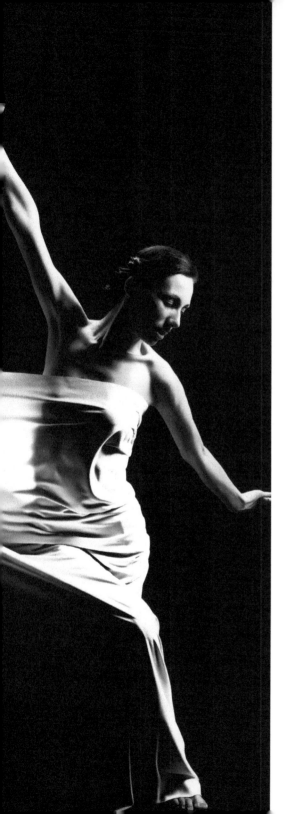

Movement is usually the best course of action to address pain naturally. No matter how miniscule, movement uplifts and heals. According to the Mayo clinic, exercise manages weight, controls medical conditions such as high blood pressure and diabetes, boosts endorphins and increases energy. Many amputees are dealing with excess weight, cardiovascular issues, diabetes, low energy and depression. Yoga, movement for body, mind and spirit, changes these problems into opportunities for better health and well-being.

Too much aggressive movement, however, which some amputees attempt after limb loss, to reclaim their sense of normalcy, can set an amputee back, causing injury and more discouragement. Staying stuck in a state of inertia does us no favors either, but at times, our bodies and mind need to restore first before we can become more active. Because yoga shows amputees how to listen well to their bodies, their relationship with their pain can change. They can learn to gain control over their lives, their bodies and their outlook when they notice and adjust the body/mind state.

Phantom pain is best addressed by a steady balance of movement and rest, mirroring these three aspects of nature (**gunas**). The physical and mental benefits of yoga can be felt immediately. This is **sattva**. These benefits then build up a healthy antidote to pain.

In addition to the gunas, yoga has a system called the **koshas** which offer a unique perspective on how to address pain. The koshas are layers of the body, from the physical to the spiritual. Each influence the other, and each is influenced by the gunas, or the states of nature. For example, a person who exercises regularly is activating rajas, or the natural state of movement and energy. This will shape her **pranamaya kosha,** or breath layer with more life force, her **manomaya kosha,** or mental state layer with an uplifted mood, her **annamaya kosha,** or physical body layer with better fitness, her **vignamaya kosha,** or intellectual layer with more clarity, and her **anandamaya kosha,** or

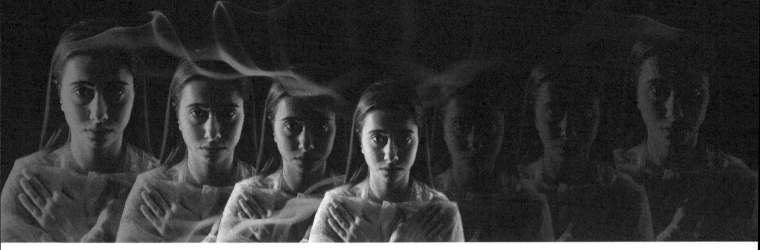

spiritual body, with greater connection to her essence. This high energy input affects all five layers of the body: her physical life, breath, emotional, mental and spiritual aspects.

Koshas	Physical, psychological, psychic and etheric
Annamaya kosha	Food, shelter, rest, exercise, asana
Pranamaya Kosha	Prana awareness; our essence or spirit
Manamaya Kosha	Based on beliefs and what the body tells it
Vijnanamaya	Wisdom and intellect: Pure self-wisdom
Anandamaya Kosha	Pure rest and relax in bliss and connection

Behind these layers is the **Atman,** or Highest SELF; the timeless Self that is never subject to death, life or rebirth. The depth of who we are as divine lights in the world can counteract the immediate noise of pain in the body. Through yoga we can see all things, even pain, as stemming from the same source and having the same divine Atman. Although this may be difficult to accept, there is a truth to seeing and feeling beyond our circumstances, that can restore hope and diminish suffering.

Below are some healing meditations to help the amputee reduce layers of pain, naturally.

Meditation One:

What color is your Atman?

1. Close your eyes to tune out the outer world.

2. Imagine that you are sitting in the center of your heart, as if it were a beautiful temple.

3. Become aware of a spark of light in the center of your heart.

4. As you breathe, the spark grows bigger and fuller, until it seeps into your entire being and beyond.

5. What color is this spark? Let this color fill you up completely. (You may be filled with multiple colors).

6. How does this color affect you?

7. Allow these positive effects to soak through your entire being.

8. You may notice that your pain has subsided.

9. This is the color of your Highest Self, the one that is beyond time and space.

10. Practice this meditation any time you are feeling the onset of pain.

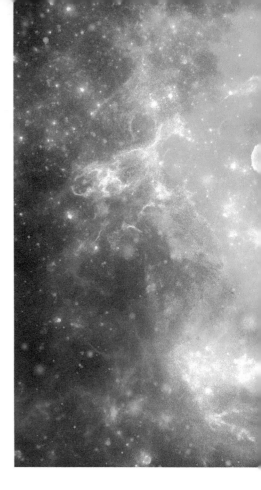

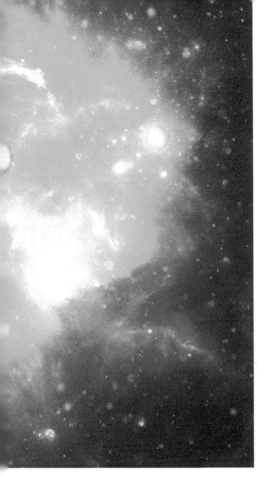

Meditation Two

Embracing Love

1. Close your eyes.

2. Imagine that your right hand right hand, or alternately right side of the torso, represents pain.

3. Your left hand represents love.

4. Take deep slow breaths as you feel sensations in your hands and notice how those sensations carry into your body.

5. Place your hands in a prayer position.

6. Blow breath into your prayer hands.

7. Invite your right hand to welcome love.

8. Invite your left hand to welcome pain.

9. The POSSIBILITY that emerges between the two is the relationship.

10. If we place any connotation/expectation on either hand, then neither can work together.

11. Open the palms. Breathe into the open palms, stoking the fire of possibility.

12. Follow the prana created in your hands with natural movement, for 1-2 minutes. See where the prana takes you.

13. Rest for few moments.

14. Practice one minute of deep reflexive breath.

(If arms or hands are unavailable, focus on the left and right side of the body individually, then draw the energy of both sides together at the heart.)

Ways to address the pain body through the koshas

Annamaya, or physical layer	Movement, yoga postures
Pranamaya, or breath layer	Yogic breathing
Manomaya, or mental layer	Meditation and creative visualization
Vignamaya , or intellect layer	Inspirational books and yoga scriptures
Anandamaya , or spiritual layer	Yoga nidra, relaxation pose, or any of the above practices

Beautiful people don't need coats. They've got their auras keeping them warm."
— Jennifer Donnelly

Using yoga to address pain takes commitment and discipline, both mental and physical. Unlike pain medication, which addresses immediate pains temporarily, masking the root causes of the pain, yoga sifts out those route causes, offering amputees a more long-term solution. It can be discouraging to take the slow route to pain free living, but the results endure, without negative side effects.

Below are two yoga practices that, when done consistently, can help an amputee reduce the need for excess pain medication.

Chronic Pain management practice I

BE: Close the eyes or softly focus on a spot in front of you. Lengthen the spine, establishing the seat. Find your inner calm. Open the eyes.

BREATHE: Breathe in through the nose for a count of 3, feeling the breath rise from the lower belly to the ribs to the chest. Breathe out through the nose down through the chest through the ribs to the lower belly for a count of 4. Do this 5-10 times.

BEND: Flex and extend the spine. Stretch laterally on each side. Twist the spine left and right.

BUILD: Breathe in. Draw the navel into the spine and pump the navel 7 times. Exhale.

BE: Close the eyes. Inhale. Tighten up the body. Exhale. Relax. Remain relaxed with the eyes closed.

BEINGNESS: Practice Meditation One above-'**What color is your Atman?'**

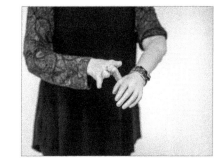

Chronic Pain management practice II

Support the cerebral spinal fluid (CSF).

CSF is the 'membranous fluid 'that moves through the brain, spinal cord and spinal nerves. CSF creates a sense of spaciousness, which counteracts the contracted state when dealing with pain.

1. Sit.

a. Breathe: Imagine, on the inhale, breath filling up the channels of the CSF and moving from the bottom to the top. On exhale the breath expands through the narrow pathways of the spinal nerves and moves down.

b. Add movement at the exhale from any part of the body that feels compelled to move.

c. Become aware of the nervous system by fanning out the tailbone, showing the body the concepts of receptivity and expression (rather than contraction and release).

2. Sit. Wait for movement. Notice if there are any blocks somewhere in the body.

a. Move fluidly around the block OR rest within the blocks.

3. Lie on the back if able.

a. Feel the head as if filled with sand (the brain).

b. Roll the head from side to side.

4. Extend that feeling to the body, shifting the head and body to one side then the other.

5. Roll to the right side and sit up.

6. Come back to the breath, breathing through the CSF.

7. Feel the weight of the body and the lightness of the spine.

Pain and the Vagus Nerve

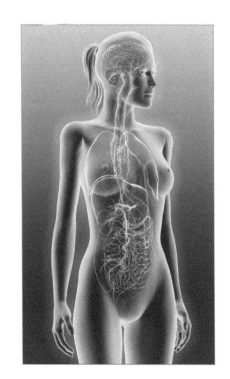

The source for our gut feelings, the vagus nerve is the nerve pulse of the body, a feeder of the parasympathetic nervous system. Stimulating the vagus nerve through yoga and breath helps with depression, digestive issues, heart rate, sweating, spinal issues, skeletal alignment, anxiety, and **pain.**

As an amputee practices more and more yoga asana and pranayama, the vagus nerve strengthens the sensory /motor parasympathetic nervous system, which bridges the mind and body of an amputee, to find his/her way back to wholeness when dealing with pain. Yogic breathing, combined with movement, such as yoga postures, deeply stimulates and nurtures the vague nerve, becoming one of the best natural methods available to manage pain and reduce its hold on a person's life.

The vagus nerve is not just roused by yoga poses and breath. Even when an amputee speaks a positive affirmation such as "I am whole" or chants "Om" the voice is activated, stimulating a chain reaction from the lower portion of the brain stem, the medulla, which in turn stimulates the diaphragm, then massages the vague nerve. This produces more space in the lung sacs, circulating more prana (or life force), throughout the mind and body.

Yogic breathing to stimulate the Vagus Nerve

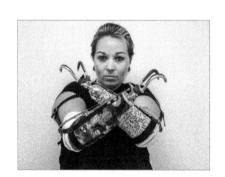

Pranayama is a life affirming tool for the person experiencing pain to feel a sense of control in life. **Ujjayi pranayama tones** and invigorates the vagus nerve. Ujjayi pranayama is unique in that it slightly constricts the airwaves which fire up the vagus nerve. The chain reaction is immediate. The blood levels shift, cellular exchange and absorption of oxygen is more complete, and the brain receives even more messages to relax the body.

Try **Ujjayi breath** to reduce pain.

Ujjayi (victoriously uprising) Breath Practice for Pain Reduction

1. Sit with the spine lengthened and the sitz bones firmly planted.

2. Try whispering 'Haaaa', as if fogging a mirror.

3. Breathe in and out as you continue to whisper 'Haaaa'.

4. Notice the quality of your breath.

5. The breath should be so effortless that there is little sensation in the throat from the vibration of the breath.

6. Eventually, close the mouth.

7. Breathe in through both nostrils for a count of four as you continue to whisper 'Haaaa'.

8. Exhale through both nostrils to a count of five while whispering 'Haaaa' with a closed mouth.

9. Continue with this breath for fifteen to twenty rounds.

10. The breath will sound like an ocean wave, soothing your nerves and your mind.

Nothing in yoga is isolated. Everything affects the WHOLE. If there is a mental block to wellness, an amputee will have a very difficult time reducing pain and suffering. Therefore, movement such as yoga is often the key to changing an amputee's mindset. Simply choosing to move can make a huge difference in redirecting the course of pain, making an amputee's mind more receptive to the possibility of reduction in pain, stress and suffering. A receptive mind invites the relaxation response, which strengthens the parasympathetic nervous system, creating more physiological resilience when facing pain.

Here's how resilience happens with yoga.

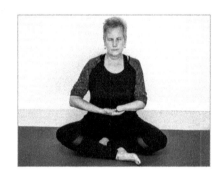

Yoga postures, breathing and meditation reduce stress, increase breath capacity, realign the skeleton, reduce muscle tension, remove toxic build up in the fascia, relax the brain, move the lymphatic fluid, increase proprioception, support the sympathetic nervous system, and strengthen the parasympathetic nervous system.

Yoga for pain reduction *does* require dedication to the practice, which can be challenging when coping with pain. Not every amputee will be ready or able to move, but she will always be able to breathe or meditate. Even a small dose of daily yoga can make a big impact on an amputee's pain.

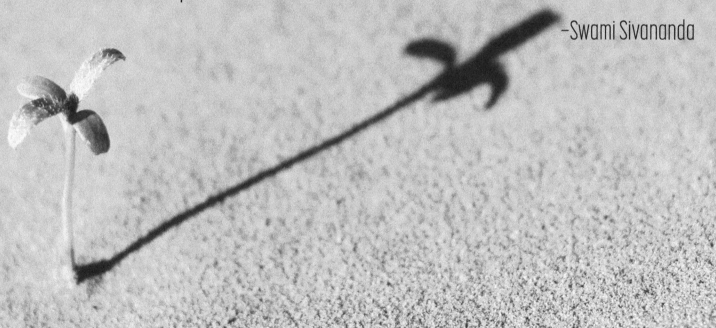

"A yogi of tapas is brilliant like a blazing fire.

Mental tapas is more powerful than physical tapas. He who bears heat and cold does physical tapas. He increases his power of endurance, but he may not be able to bear insult. To keep a balanced mind in all conditions of life, to bear insult, injury and persecutions, to be ever serene, contented and peaceful, to be cheerful in adverse conditions, to have fortitude in meeting danger, to have presence of mind and forbearance, are forms of mental tapas."

–Swami Sivananda

The 8-limbed path for pain reduction

Yamas	Moral actions that aid pain reduction
Ahimsa is the practice of non-violence, or non-harm, towards self or others.	As an amputee develops more awareness of her body and breath, a deeper respect for life occurs, encouraging her to make healthier choices.
Satya, or truth, is the ability to be completely honest with the state of one's body and pain.	It is exhausting for an amputee to have her pain dismissed by family and medical staff. She needs to be heard. On the other hand, some amputees claim they want to feel better but are addicted to the familiarity of their pain.
Aparigraha is the practice of letting go of a feeling, a thought or a memory that is no longer helpful.	When an amputee clings to a belief about past pain, she creates more pain. By practicing non –attachment, focusing on the present moment, fear is reduced, which allows the body to relax.
Asteya is non-stealing or feeling complete with what you have.	Resentment and fear due to ongoing pain steals contentment. Through yoga, an amputee can begin to experience painless moments, helping her to let go of fears and build trust in her body's ability to be pain free.
Brahmacharya is the ability to control human urges, such as obsession, promiscuity, or addiction from dominating one's life, choosing moderation instead.	When an amputee can convert the energy of anger and frustration towards motivation for well-being, pain diminishes while health improves.

Niyamas	Rituals for self-care and pain reduction
Shaucha is the practice of self-care.	When an amputee is in a lot of pain, one of the first reactions can be hopelessness, which leads to disinterest in body, mind or spirit. By teaching simple yoga techniques that can be done daily, most amputees start to value their lives more, because yoga makes them feel better.
Santosa is the practice of contentment.	Contentment is a moment to moment practice. As an amputee becomes more aware of feeling good in this moment, he has less pain and more peace.

Niyamas	Rituals for self-care and pain reduction
Tapas means burning enthusiasm for one's own self-realization.	Commitment to a healthy lifestyle which includes yoga can make all the difference to an amputee's well-being. This can help an amputee dealing with a rough patch of pain, by keeping his eyes on the prize.
Svadhyaya is the study of one's self and one's life meaning.	Finding meaning in one's limb loss and one's pain allows an amputee to move beyond the surface to live a deeper, richer life.
Iswara Pranidhana is the surrender of one's self to a larger perspective, or God.	When all else fails, surrendering to the divine or a broader purpose, gives an amputee permission to let go of his burdens and let the divine take care of them.

Other Limbs	Practices for pain reduction
Asana, or yoga posture, signifies sitting in the seat of consciousness.	Yoga has a way of telling the truth. Awareness of sensations in the body and mind, can diminish pain's hold, by practicing neutral, 'unattached to outcome' mind.
Pranayama is yogic breath, or control of life force.	The greater the ability to breathe, the more healing energy available to reduce an amputee's pain.
Pratyahara is the withdrawal of the senses to prepare for meditation.	The observation of one's inner self keeps an amputee from being distracted by pain.
Dharana is focus on a single point, to prepare for meditation.	Focusing on one point, the fluctuations of the mind, due to pain, cease.
Dhyana is absorption into meditation.	In meditation, an amputee can become deeply absorbed into the peace that meditation offers, connecting him to something bigger than himself. Knowing that he is part of all that is, he is no longer alone in his pain, but united with the divine.
Samadhi is the experience of bliss.	Bliss does not mean diminishment of pain, but a feeling of being connected to all of life and the divine, no longer separate or alone in suffering.

HEAL

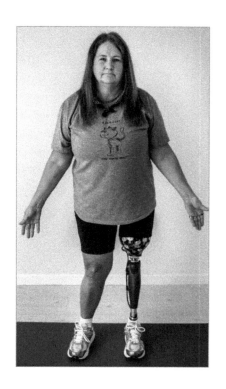

Pain management yoga practice for amputees

Immediately after amputation and beyond, pain can be a dominant force in an amputee's daily life. There are many holistic modalities employed to help amputees reduce their pain. Many single leg amputees, for example, learn the "mirror method". In the mirror method, the amputee sits facing a mirror, focusing on the remaining leg. The amputee moves the remaining leg around, while looking in the mirror, telling the brain that the amputated leg is still there. This eases the brain and body into an amputee's new reality.

For other amputees, traditional pain reduction treatments include nerve blockers, surgery, pain medication, neuromodulation, nerve stimulation and shrinker sleeves for the residual limb. Neuromodulation, similar to biofeedback, uses various proprietary techniques to access the unconscious mind, retraining it to remember pain free living.

Nerve stimulation, known as transcutaneous electrical nerve stimulation, uses a machine with two electrodes in opposing places on the skin. When the machine turns on, electrical impulses jumble up pain messages, releasing endorphins which lower pain. Additional non-invasive treatments include acupuncture, creative visualization, homeopathy and healing music. These techniques increase endorphins. Yoga, in combination with a complete wellness plan, empowers amputees suffering from pain to take back their lives. It isn't easy. Yoga requires commitment, and some very tough days to get through, but over time, results are seen and felt.

The endocrine system is severely affected by chronic pain, which in turn lessens its ability to support and balance the body and mind. Yoga is an effective endocrine balancing practice which can positively stimulate all the endocrine glands. Within a pain management yoga practice itself, it is helpful to follow the self-observation method of *breathe, relax, feel, watch and allow* to reduce pain

Endocrine balancing practice to heal pain

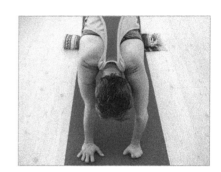

Follow this sequence of poses to help cope with chronic and phantom pain.

1. Ujjayi breath

2. Downward dog

3. Revolved triangle

4. Standing forward bend

5. Seated forward bend

6. Shoulder stand

7. Locust

8. Cobra

9. Seated spinal twist

10. Bridge

11. Fish

12. Relaxation

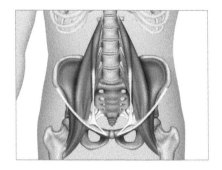

Pain and the Psoas

The psoas muscle, made up of the major and minor psoas, which rests near the vagus nerve, is directly linked to the sympathetic/parasympathetic nervous system. Located between the lumbar vertebrae and the mid-thoracic vertebrae, the psoas major serves as a shock absorber between the lower and upper body. The psoas minor is a long, string - like muscle that sits behind the psoas major, supporting lower lumbar movement. When the psoas is at rest, as can be demonstrated in a variety of yoga poses, stored tension and stored emotions relax. An amputee's psoas will tighten when coping with any kind of pain, stress or fear. More stress and tension then load up in the joint infrastructures of the body, exacerbating the fight or flight response.

The deep muscle of the psoas gets humans vertical, both physically and emotionally. We need a strong psoas to "stand up" for ourselves. Losing a limb shakes our sense of stability. A tight psoas or an overstretched psoas have all sorts of physical, psychological and emotional implications that are counterproductive to an amputee's life. Releasing, lengthening and strengthening the psoas through yoga frees up the diaphragm for deeper breathing, therefore elevating the parasympathetic response, which, rather than responding to stress or pain with "fight or flight" can respond with "tend and befriend", "relax and renew" or, "stand up and stand for".

Psoas Practice

1. Lie in easy resting pose on the back. Extend the right leg down, roll the hip out, then draw the leg back to starting point, as if in a semi –circle, dragging the ankle along the ground. Repeat on the other side. Alternately, roll the residual limb or lower right belly out to the right, then come back to easy resting pose. Repeat on the left.

2. Extend the legs. Lift the legs one at a time toward the ceiling and back down. Alternately, if wearing a prosthesis, place a strap around the prosthetic foot and lift the leg to the ceiling, returning the leg to the floor. If a prosthesis or arms are not available, practice tucking and releasing the tailbone.

3. Hug one knee into the chest (when available), then the other. If the knee is not available, draw the residual limb into the chest if able.

4. Balance on the bottom in boat pose, legs and arms, or residual limbs, lifted at a diagonal in the same direction. If the prosthesis is too heavy, place the limb on the seat of a chair, or at a wall.

5. Lie on the back. Extend the arms and legs into a star fish, reaching movements from the coccyx and crown, from the center to the periphery. If unable to lie down this can be done seated.

6. Lie on the back with a folded blanket under the lower back. Close the eyes and relax.

All movements can be enhanced by exhaling with strong sighs. This releases tension in the psoas.

An amputee's inner self can get really knocked down by ongoing or acute pain. All amputees, although dealing with pain and grief differently, do have one thing in common: they are now amputees. Moving forward in life means being able to face this new reality without letting it destroy personal happiness. Stress, rage, fear, excitement, hope and a renewed lease on life are all part of this new reality. The psoas, both the major and minor, reinforces that experience.

Yoga, ultimately, is a way to reclaim one's Highest Self in relationship with the world and with one's self. A relaxed and strong psoas, achieved through yoga practice, holds an amputee up high, to be seen and heard. Pain does not have to dominate an amputee's life. Within the forest of pain, wholeness can be found, pain can be reduced, and personal power can be restored through yoga.

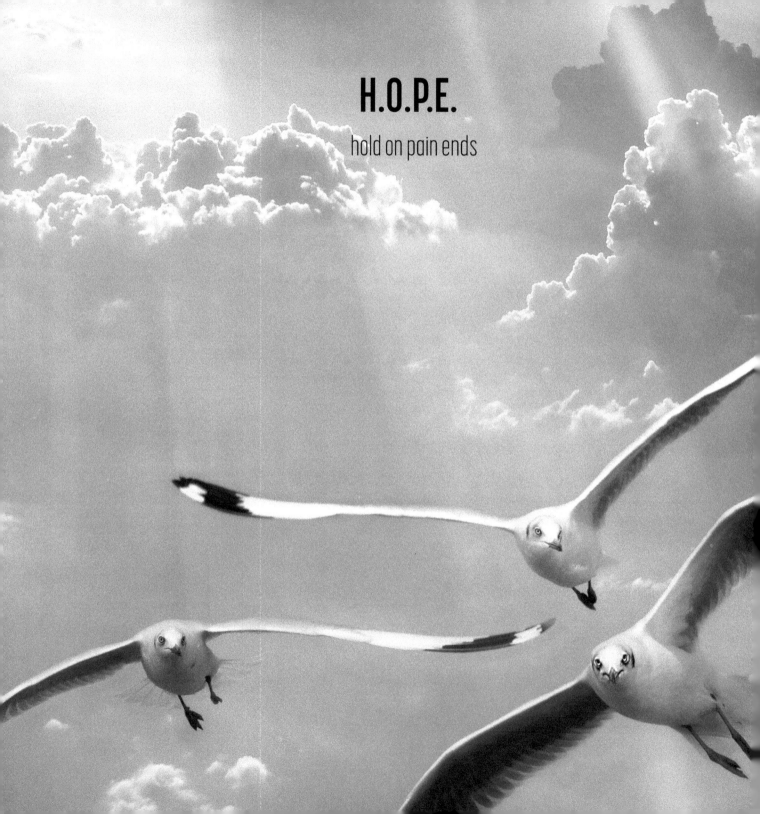

H.O.P.E.

hold on pain ends

TRAUMA

What is trauma?

The word *"trauma"* is used to describe experiences or situations that are emotionally or physically painful and distressing, overwhelming people's ability to cope, leaving them powerless. People who have been through trauma sometimes suffer from PTSD or Post Traumatic Stress Disorder. PTSD is aggravated stress brought on by muscle and brain memories that trigger a reactive response, such as disconnecting to the body, getting into a fight or being frozen in place. Some of the behaviors you will see with trauma survivors who exhibit PTSD include discouragement, agitation, disassociation and hyperarousal, or living in a constant state of fight or flight.

The amygdala, or "snake detector", which is located in the brain stem, responds to trauma with radical attempts at biological self-protection. When a person has experienced trauma, such as limb loss, or compound trauma, such as limb loss and combat stress, the amygdala protects the person by lodging the immediate trauma deep within its confines, so the person can deal with immediate needs first.

PTSD is like a repetitive loop of sensations, perceptions and body experiences that keep the trauma survivor in the original wound lodged in the amygdala, as well as other parts of the brain and the body itself, while the sufferer attempts to function in daily life.

In PTSD, three parts of the brain are affected: the amygdala, the ventromedial prefrontal cortex *(vmPFC)* and the hippocampus. The *amygdala* is at the center of the fear response (fight or flight), discriminating whether emotions are good or bad, and releasing stress hormones to cope with the immediate stressor. The amygdala is meant to settle down and recalibrate after a stressful event. In the case of PTSD, the stress hormones continue to release, and the brain is unable to distinguish the present from the past.

The *hippocampus* captures immediate memories, such as trauma, organizes them, and attempts to make sense of the progression of events. When an amputee is living in the PTSD world, the hippocampus is telling him that "this AWLAYS leads to that". If he lost his leg in a biking accident, for example, his hippocampus may constantly be telling him- "bikes are unsafe, the road is unsafe, don't ever ride a bike again because you will lose your leg."

The left side of the *hippocampus* is involved in specific memories, like a scent that evokes a feeling. If that same amputee who lost his leg in a bike accident remembers the smell of the pavement, or the sound of a

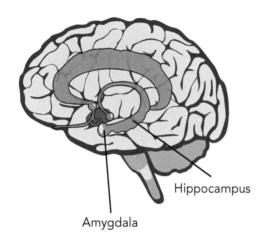

Hippocampus

Amygdala

siren as the ambulance approached, he may go into a state of PTSD any time he smells pavement or hears a siren. In other words, he is constantly on high alert, doing his best to avoid situations where his PTSD might be triggered. That is no way to live.

The right side of the *hippocampus* helps with spatial awareness, making sure a person is familiar with the space they inhabit and can move in that space safely. For an amputee, the right side of the hippocampus can often be in high gear simply because of the mental and physical focus it takes to relearn daily routines, navigating spaces at home and in the world. When an amputee is in a state of PTSD, even that navigation skill gets sluggish, confusing, and at times paralyzing.

The *vmPFC* or ventromedial *prefrontal cortex* helps in processing experiences and emotions, such as fear, grief and proper decision making. When an amputee has not processed their limb loss, and suffers from PTSD, that leads to lack of brain support, when he is faced with fear and decision making. This can bring on irrational fears or irrational fearlessness, depleting the brain and the body. An amputee with PTSD may indeed not be thinking clearly, and no amount of self-talk, therapy, or medication can change that on its own. There needs to be a connection made between the state of the mind and the state of the body. When the body begins to shift positively the mind follows, and vice versa.

Yoga and meditation have been found to reduce and change the reactions of the hyper aroused amygdala, the 'stuck" hippocampus, and the overtaxed vmPFC . Research is showing that long term yoga and meditation practices can have LASTING impact on a person living with PTSD. Through yoga and meditation, people suffering from PTSD, when faced with triggers that formerly caused stress and intense reactions, were able to both cope better and remain calm. This is because thickening of certain brain cells in the brain associated with emotion and cognitive awareness occurred. What is exciting is that yoga and meditation are non-invasive, self-directed and give people with PTSD a sense of personal control over their environment.

"Self-acceptance comes from meeting life's challenges vigorously. Don't numb yourself to your trials and difficulties, nor build mental walls to exclude pain from your life. You will find peace not by trying to escape your problems, but by confronting them courageously. You will find peace not in denial, but in victory."

– Goswami Kriyananda

How is PTSD manifested in the lives of amputees?

Post-traumatic stress can exhibit itself in many ways for amputees, the most obvious being phantom pain, which can recur years after subsiding when an amputee is put into an extremely stressful situation. Signs of PTSD such as disassociation, numbing, addiction, depression, suicidal thoughts, lack of self-care, and rage over feelings of vulnerability and helplessness, become "maladaptive behaviors" when they dominate an amputee's life.

Marriages, jobs, social networks and health may all disintegrate when the grip of PTSD takes over. External circumstances are often the triggers of ongoing PTSD. Besides certain smells or sounds, such as pops, explosions, or slammed doors, overhead lights, hospital buildings, certain people, such as a doctor involved in an amputee's care, or even the name of the city where the amputee lost his limb, can cause an amputee to plummet into PTSD.

After initial amputation, there can be more medical procedures such as revisions, limb salvage, and hospitalization for infections, skin disorders and even further amputation. Not only is there the trauma of the medical procedure itself, there is also the traumatic fear about these procedures and beyond.

In the case of veteran amputees, many have seen their exposed limb or limbs, but there was no time to process the event, and no education about life after amputation. They have endured minimal medical care in war zones before they are transferred to their main medical facility, which greatly affects their state of mind. Amputation is a violent act upon the body, and depending on how and where it happens, that violent act can be compounded.

When an amputee is in the process of recovering, feelings around sexuality, desirability, and body image can cause PTSD to recur. PTSD becomes almost a preparatory "just in case the worst happens" response to future stress. All sorts of events can cause stress for an amputee.

Aging in amputees, for example, can be stressful. The fear of heart disease, known to be higher with amputees, especially veterans, is of great concern for some amputees. In daily life, PTSD can occur when an amputee's prosthetic does not fit correctly, or insurance only covers the cheapest, least mechanically able prosthetic. Lack of a prosthetist locally is an added stress that can cause PTSD in amputees.

Many amputees with PTSD function on two levels. The first level is the level of survival. The second level is the rest of their lives, which may or may not be going well. *This is why yoga is so beneficial to amputees dealing with PTSD.* Yoga not only helps the amputee reduce stress and change the way his brain handles stress, he also gains mind/body tools to pre-emptively address PTSD before it happens. This is empowered wholeness.

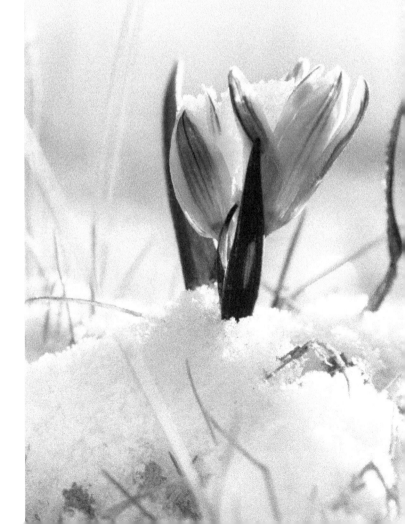

"JUST FOR TODAY, I will live through this day only. I will not brood about yesterday or obsess about tomorrow."

– Abigail Van Buren

Tips for trauma sensitive yoga practice

Amputees, both new to yoga as well as seasoned athletes, have moments when PTSD can pop up again. Yoga unpeels layers of trauma that were previously hidden, to be healed once the mind and body are ready. A prepared yogi can better handle the release of deeper traumas.

Yoga practice rituals are extremely important to the healing process. Establishing a beginning, middle, and end, as well as a context for the yoga practice, can help alleviate PTSD symptoms when they do arise. *Healthy rituals of mind, body and spirit develop new brain synapses that bring non-reactive awareness and happier healthier ways of being.* When the brain needs time to heal from trauma, yoga, especially for an amputee, can seem daunting, as it is new, requiring more adaptations of body and mind. Repeating wellness rituals such as yoga, work. A positive, life enhancing rhythm is established to rewire the brain and body after trauma.

Some basic rituals for amputees dealing with PTSD include daily yoga practice in a safe, friendly and clean space with good light. Be familiar with your space and make it your own. That way, every time you approach the space for yoga, your mind and body are already prepared to enjoy the peace and familiarity the space brings.

Commit to a daily practice at the same time each day. Repeat the yoga practice until you become familiar with it. Keep the poses simple. Add to the practice when your confidence increases, and you feel ready. A rhythm develops, with strong new positive memory synapses in the brain, which countermand the effects of PTSD. A best yoga sequence for amputees living with PTSD includes a slow steady practice with a special focus on the lower body and core strength, building a feeling of support and solid foundation.

Pranayama is the key to a fulfilling yoga practice for amputees living with PTSD. **Ujjayi breath** and simple belly breathing calm anxiety. At the end of active yoga practice, always spend at least 10 - 20 minutes or more in relaxation, giving the brain and body the ability to adjust to the idea of resting without having to revert to PTSD symptoms. When your practice is complete, review exactly what was practiced, and how you felt, to anchor the ritual into the brain and body.

Healthy rituals reassure an amputee who is suffering from PTSD to trust his body and mind as a haven. An amputee must believe at the body/mind level that nothing is going to happen to him, to trust his life again. Yoga heals.

"There is a spirit which is pure, and which is beyond old age and death; and beyond hunger and thirst and sorrow. This is Atman, one's Spirit. All desires of this Spirit are Truth. It is this Spirit that we must find and know."

– Chandogya Upanishad

"Whatever is true, whatever is honorable, whatever is right, whatever is pure, whatever is lovely, whatever is of good repute, if there is any excellence and if anything worthy of praise, let your mind dwell on these things."— Philippians 4:8

Mindfulness practice to manage PTSD symptoms

Mindfulness benefits amputees. It has been found to lessen pain and suffering without numbing or desensitizing a person to the present moment or their experience of pain.

Mindfulness is a three-step process:

1. Sitting in stillness

2. Being present with the stillness

3. Observing the stillness

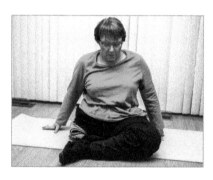

If an amputee, for example, is living with chronic nerve pain after losing an upper arm, a mindfulness practice empowers her to be able to sit in stillness, without contracting into fear of past pains, or worrying about future pain. When an amputee is in a mindful state, it is often the case that pain or any other PTSD symptoms, once observed, lose power. What freedom! This allows the amputee to rest in wholeness rather than struggle in pain.

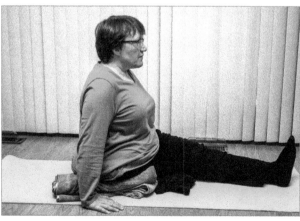

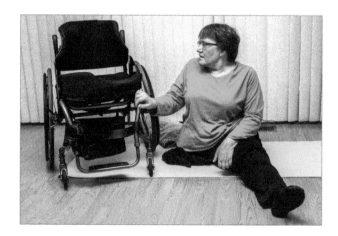

Yoga Practice for PTSD in amputees

In this simple mindfulness practice, you will learn how to use yoga to lessen your PTSD, build your inner resources and better handle the symptoms of PTSD without losing your cool.

1. Sit on your bottom with your arms either on the floor or in a chair,

2. Keep the eyes open softly.

3. If you are slouching, sit on the edge of a folded blanket, low pillow, or against a wall.

4. Scan your body as if you were a video camera, noticing how things feel physically.

5. Elongate the lower body as you inhale and exhale.

6. Elongate the spine as you inhale and exhale.

7. Begin in a seated mountain pose. Outstretch your lower limbs if seated on the floor.

8. If not wearing prosthetics and sitting on the floor, place the residual limbs on the ground or over a low folded blanket. Sink into the floor with your bottom, feeling the support of the floor.

9. Some lower limb prosthetics need extra support underneath the hips, thighs and knees. The objective is to keep the hips even. If this is you, add a folded blanket under your bottom, or under the buttocks, depending on your type of prosthetic or amputation.

10. For upper extremity amputees wearing prosthetics, be sure the prosthesis is supported by the floor or yoga block. Keep the shoulders as even as possible. For upper extremity amputees not wearing a prosthesis, place the residual limb on a chair or a pile of yoga blocks and blankets to match the armpit height. This is only if dangling the limb feels painful.

11. If available, place the palms on the floor. If your bottom is elevated, the palms can go on folded blankets 3-6" high or on low blocks.

12. Bring your focus to your belly. Take three deep breaths in and out.

13. Become aware of the sensations around you: smell, light, the floor, temperature.

14. Lengthen your spine again. Become aware of your space again: smell, light, sound, the floor, temperature, where you are in the room.

15. Twist your torso to the right. Your head will follow. Exhale. Inhale. Lengthen the spine.

16. Exhale again. Stay in a twist on the right side for at least 3-5 breaths. Notice the space around you. Note all your sensations.

17. Repeat on the other side.

18. Observe how you feel.

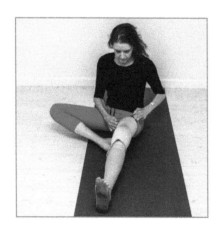

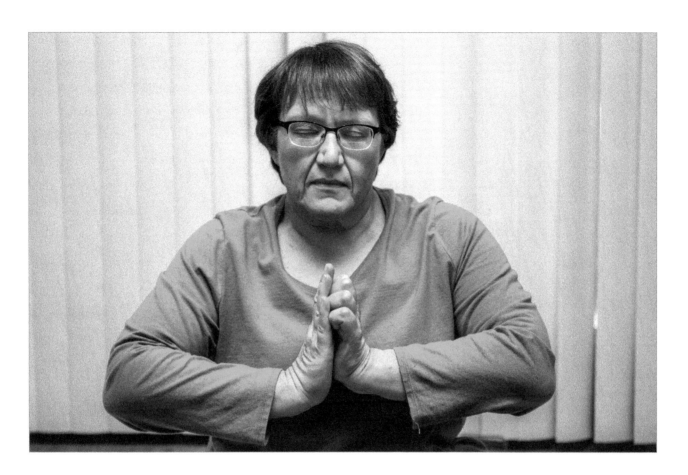

MEET LAURA

Laura is an incredible woman of spirit and strength. At the age of 39, while a practicing neurologist, she had a sarcoma (cancer of connective tissue such as bone, cartilage and muscles) at her sciatic nerve. There was no choice but to amputate not only her leg but her entire right hip and parts of the pelvis, including the right sitz bone. While she does not use a prosthesis, she loves her wheelchair. Now retired, she follows her passions of kayaking, hand cycling, quilting and being in nature. She is even a kayaking instructor!

Laura has been through a lot of trauma in her life but remains optimistic. Laura sees wholeness as fluctuating, depending on what parts of her body are working and where her mind is at, at any given time. Feeling

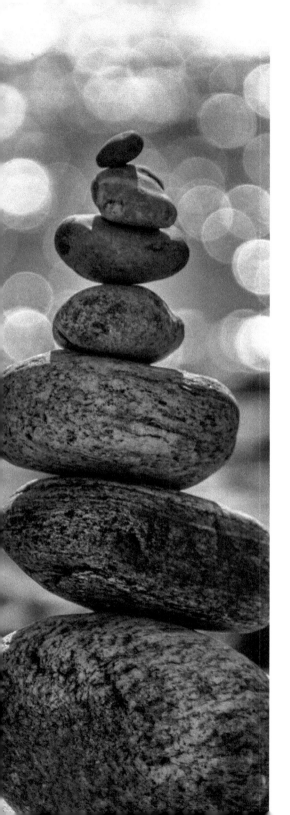

comfortable in her environment and in her spirit makes it possible for her to adapt easily, contributing to her sense of wholeness. Like many people who have endured much trauma. Laura finds it important to feel secure in her space. This reassures the brain and body. Says Laura "I had my leg for 39 years before I lost my leg. I wasn't going to adjust to it (all) in a month, a week, or even a year. You're constantly adapting and learning."

Laura, like so many in this book, has met amazing people since her amputation: people who understand her and support her. Adapting to amputation takes time and patience with oneself. Yoga can help with the process.

Laura had an extremely hectic life before losing her limb. Now, she feels she is more in touch with her body and the world around her. She would never have taken up kayaking without her limb loss. There are always threads of hope and possibility within limb loss. Laura has done her own brand of yoga for a long time, concentrating on deep stretches and pranayama (breathing) exercises to handle the mounting anxiety about her health. Even her systolic blood pressure was lowered by ten points due to her active pranayama techniques. 'A great, measurable outcome" reports Laura.

For anyone living with PTSD after amputation, Laura says "Give yourself time". Laura is proof that there is always a way to adapt to life's circumstances and follow your passions.

GRIEF

The grief of limb loss

Losing a limb is losing an essential part of who you are. Limbs are necessary for humans to perform the daily tasks required to survive and thrive. The idea of living without a limb is daunting. No longer the bread winner, the marathon runner, the dancer, the carpenter or the parent you thought you were, your limb loss requires you to look hard at what matters most in your life, what you can't control, and what you can. As the initial shock and pain of limb loss wear off, an amputee is left with the question 'Who am I? 'This is often the stage when grief takes over.

The five stages of grief as applied to limb loss

Elizabeth Kubler-Ross developed a theory called the five stages of grief, based on her close study of patients nearing death. While her five-stage system is not the only view out there on grief , and indeed many people do not go through the exact same process, in general these five stages are a helpful framework that works well with amputees enduring grief, whether low grade or debilitating. Although many times these five stages are all occurring at the same time, they are sequential. The stages are: *Denial, Anger, Bargaining, Depression and Acceptance.*

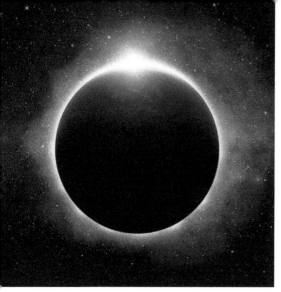

Stage One: Denial

An amputee may not feel any sense of loss about their amputation, but instead keep going, as if nothing happened. This can be a good or not so good response. Sometimes the body and mind are not ready to absorb the reality of limb loss. Sometimes the amputee is so relieved to be free of pain, or has an extra resilience chromosome, that limb loss is no big deal. Other times, the amputee consciously or unconsciously ignores and pretends that his limb loss does not exist.

An amputee can be compliant and positive, just as easily as he can be non-compliant and rebellious. In both cases, he may still be numb to the reality of his limb loss. Some amputees in the denial state may try to do what they did before losing a limb, exhausting their system and prolonging recovery. Other amputees decide not to participate in their recovery at all, succumbing to isolation and depression. These are all signs of denial about limb loss.

Denial can be a necessary step in the grief process, to protect the mind and body, psychologically and physically preparing it for the moment when the amputation becomes real to the amputee. Yoga can help support this necessary part of the grief process

Try this yoga antidote for denial.

1. Close the eyes.

2. As you breathe in, say to yourself "I ".

3. As you breathe out say "am".

4. As you breathe in say "breath".

5. As you breathe out, remain silent.

6. Repeat the sequence five to ten rounds.

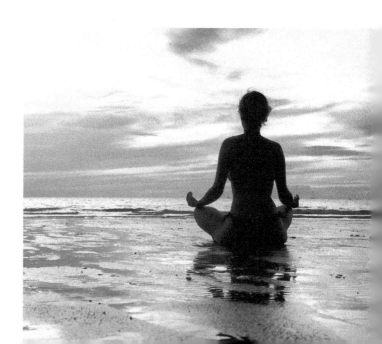

Stage Two: Anger

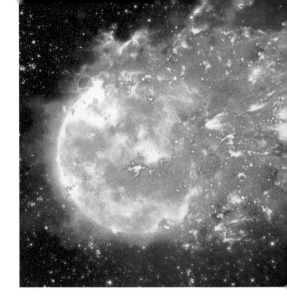

Anger can make an amputee feel lost in the wilderness, with no answers. As anger takes root, it provides some semblance of a foundation from which an amputee can find meaning. In this stage, amputees may be openly hostile, quietly seething or somewhere in between. Anger shows up by rejecting all help, and blaming others for their misery, including themselves and God. Anger can be expressed to staff, family spouses, or a stranger on the street. Amputees may also take out anger on themselves by pushing their physical limits to extremes, expecting more rapid healing, or blaming themselves or others for somehow causing their amputation. In more than a few cases, anger is justified and needs to be released.

Some amputees hold their anger in, attempting to stay positive, which initially helps the mind after loss, but ultimately negatively affects the body. Anger can be frightening for a person who is not used to expressing anger, but anger is real and valid. When anger is stored unnecessarily in the body, all sorts of physical challenges emerge, such as digestion issues, eating disorders, exhaustion, and increased blood pressure.

Hopelessness and helplessness can be signs of anger. Some amputees refuse to wear a prosthesis, without giving it a chance. They may demand the "professionals" to fix them, without making any personal effort towards their own well-being. In effect, they may throw in the towel on life, but continue to function. Anger is fuel, the "rajas" that makes a person feel alive, and somewhat in control of their grief, but it can also be what keeps a person from moving forward. When anger becomes the main emotion in a person's life, it keeps him blocked from his highest Self. With the right support and guidance, an amputee should express anger. It can propel an amputee towards positive action.

Who hasn't had an experience where they have "just had it", and made

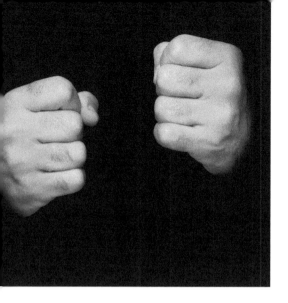

a change that made life better in the long run? Anger has a place in the healing journey and the grief process. When anger becomes the only emotion, though, it is toxic. Anger is deep down, unexpressed grief. Yoga can help integrate and process anger in a way that serves the amputee while still honoring the limb loss.

Yoga antidotes for anger

Fist breath

When a person is about to lose control through anger, she will often make a fist, as if to contain the anger and redirect her power toward a more positive outcome. This yoga practice helps an amputee harness and release anger more effectively.

1. Make fists with both hands.

2. Bend the elbows.

3. Place the right fist on top of the left fist four inches in front of the solar plexus.

4. Move the fists together up and down rapidly as you inhale through the nose, and exhale through the mouth at your own breathing pace.

5. As you continue with the inhale and exhale, make the exhale audible, and if a scream comes out, let it. Do this practice for ten rounds.

6. Rest the arms, placing hands in the lap.

7. Sit in stillness at the end, allowing the practice to settle into the body and mind.

(If fists are not available, tense the entire body, particularly the muscles of the face, on the inhale, then loosen the body on the exhale.)

Meditation to release anger

Anger is an emotion that begins in the heart, then circulates through the blood stream out into the tissues. This meditation allows the amputee to follow the waves of sensation that anger creates in the body and mind, better understanding the roots of this anger, inviting shifts in consciousness.

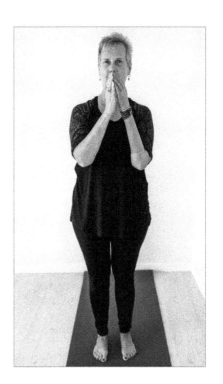

1. Take a deep breath in.

2. Exhale out.

3. Close the eyes.

4. Bring your attention to the center of the chest, the place of the heart.

5. Focus on something that makes you angry.

6. Let that anger come to the center of the chest, the heart.

7. As you continue to breathe in and out, notice the waves of sensation around the heart as you focus on this angry emotion, without changing anything.

8. Notice if the anger subsides, or if it moves to another part of the body.

9. Keep allowing the anger to flow without pushing it aside.

10. Stay with this practice for five to ten minutes.

11. To end the practice, place your hands on your heart, or if without arms, say to the center of the heart "I acknowledge you, anger. Please let me know if there is anything you need."

12. Journal for a few minutes on what you learned.

Stage Three: Bargaining

An amputee who is bargaining with others or himself is trying to fend off pain or more loss, pretending that the very real circumstance of amputation can be reversed. He is operating from a reward-based system, with thoughts such as 'I'll do this if you do this for me" or "If I do this for God or the world, then I will be rewarded for my amputation." The "if onlys" are a hallmark of an amputee bargaining. "If only I hadn't gotten into that car that night'. "If only I didn't have diabetes".

Bargaining can keep an amputee stuck in the past, before limb loss, or bypass the present by diving full force into the future, without that necessary stop at grief. He will do anything to avoid the full impact of the pain of his loss. When working with an amputee who is stuck in the bargaining stage of grief, the worst possible thing you can do is to offer pat answers or false hope. The amputation is real and will not change. Instead, offer an amputee tools to gently find his way back to his core self while at the same time building his emotional/physical/psychological strength so he can face his loss.

Yoga antidotes for bargaining

Heart opening posture flow

1. Begin seated.

2. Inhale. Roll the shoulders back as you draw the shoulder blades together.

3. Exhale. Release the shoulders. Do this three times.

4. Lift the sternum in a seated Cobra pose on inhale.

5. Exhale return to starting position. Do this three times.

6. Inhale. Exhale as you draw fists, pressing firmly into the center of the chest.

7. Round spine and tuck the chin.

8. Tighten the body. Stay in this position for three complete breath cycles.

9. Inhale. Relax the body, sitting upright.

10. Exhale. Complete three breath cycles.

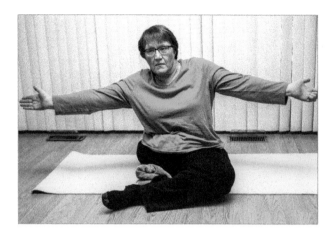

Creative visualization for acceptance

1. Inhale. Lengthen your spine.

2. Exhale. Settle into your body.

3. Tell yourself "I am still me".

4. Imagine a mirror in front of you.

5. Look into your face as you inhale and exhale, repeating the phrase "I am still me."

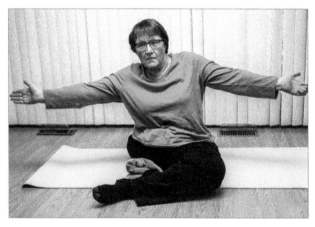

6. Feel your body heavy, sinking into the ground, feeling secure.

7. Continue this practice, enlarging the size of the mirror in your mind, until you feel comfortable looking at your entire body in the mirror.

This may take time. Notice if there is a place in your body where you stop and cannot go on Without judgement or expectation, allow yourself to feel the sensations that arise to flow through you, without pushing them away.

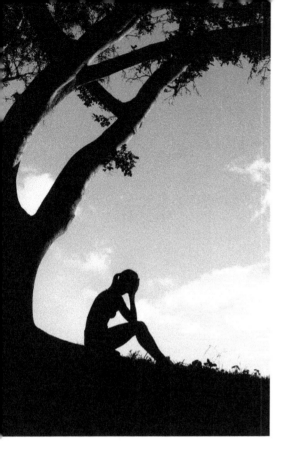

Stage Four: Depression

Hopelessness and helplessness are natural healthy responses to losing a limb. When an amputee can finally befriend the grief of sadness she is experiencing, she is one step closer to acceptance. It IS depressing to lose a limb. When grief is pushed away, however, denial, anger or bargaining sneak right back in, leading to chronic depression.

Depression is frightening to any amputee. "Will I always be depressed? Is this my new life? Why bother anyway?" These are normal questions after amputation. Naturally, there is a physiological process which protects an amputee at the beginning of limb loss from facing too many traumatic realities at once, but chronic depression is different, hovering over an amputee's life without letting up. When an amputee is also taking pain medications, has multiple amputations or compounded stress from family dynamics, poor medical care, or loss of identity, depression can become a way of life.

For example, soldiers who lose multiple limbs may feel that they are no longer the heroic protectors they once were. A mother may wonder how she will ever be able to care for her children again and fall into a deep state of depression.

For some amputees, symptoms of depression include retreating, listlessness, a sense of giving up. This type of depression is tamasic, or stagnant. Other amputees living with depression may become overachievers, high on life all the time, unable to sit still or be present. This type of depression is rajasic, or excitable. ***There is a way out.***

Yoga antidote for tamasic depressives (low energy)

1. Breath of fire: Inhale through the nose. Exhale strongly through the nose as if pumping the belly in. Repeat five rounds.

2. Punching breath: As you practice breath of fire, punch out and in with each round. *

3. Eye gazing: Focus on one object for five complete rounds of breath.

4. Mountain pose.

5. Downward facing dog.

6. Bridge pose.

If arms are not available, continue to practice Breath of Fire, adding a strong "Ha!" in the exhale.

Yoga antidote for rajasic depressives (manic)

1. Counting breath: Close the eyes. Inhale for a count of three. Exhale for a count of four. Complete ten rounds.

2. Seated or standing forward bend with ten complete rounds of breath.

3. Mountain pose with eyes closed and palms in prayer pose at the heart, if available.

4. Childs pose.

Stage Five: Acceptance

Acceptance is a lot like yoga relaxation. Relaxing into the truth of being an amputee gives an amputee the freedom she has been longing to find again. Acceptance is not giving up. Acceptance is embracing

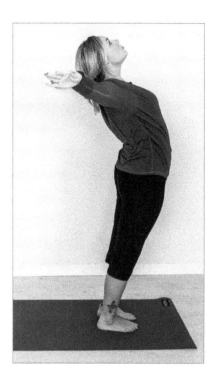

"Self-acceptance is my refusal to be in an adversarial relationship to myself."
— *Nathaniel Branden*

reality, working with the loss and moving forward into wholeness. Here, in acceptance, the amputee can finally see herself as whole. That does not mean she is necessarily happy about her amputation, but she is able to accept it.

Healing occurs when grief is acknowledged, Throughout an amputee's life, grief will pop up: when an amputee has a phantom pain incident, when she drives by the hospital where she had her amputation, when she can't do something she used to do. Acceptance means an amputee can have these moments, without being dragged down into hopelessness. A body/mind approach to grief is the best way to support an amputee's grief.

Below are some yoga and breath practices particularly for grief.

YOGA PRACTICES FOR GRIEF

Pranayama: Nadi Shodhana: Alternate nostril breathing

1. Begin by taking your right hand in to Vishnu (or sustainer) mudra: thumb up, index finger and middle finger down, ring and pinky finger up. Alternately, focus on breathing through the right then left nostril.

2. Take a deep breath in through both nostrils.

3. Now bring the right thumb to the right nostril and exhale GENTLY from the left. Now inhale through the left, close off this nostril with your pinky and ring finger as you open the right nostril to exhale.

4. Exchange back and forth for a few rounds, ending with an exhale on the left side.

Warm ups: Spine stretch

1. Cat/Cow

Asana: Poses

1. **Warriors I & II:** Virabhadrasana

2. **Intense Stretch:** Parsvottanasana

3. **Cobra:** Bhujangasana

4. **Upward Dog:** Urdhva mukha svanasana

5. **Fish:** Matsyasana

6. **Bridge Pose:** Setu bandhasana

7. **Relaxation:** Savasana

8. **Yoga Nidra**

Meditation on the heart's wisdom

This meditation invites healing when grief has been all consuming or hidden under a blanket of "busyness".

1. Get comfortable, sitting upright.

2. Bring your focus to the heart area, including the mid chest, ribs and collarbone. Keep breathing in and out until your focus is drawn to a single point in the center of the chest.

3. Notice any sensations in this central point.

4. If available, press the thumb into the center of the chest. If a thumb is not available, use visualization, or do the exercise on the floor, face down, resting the chest on a folded blanket or low pillow.

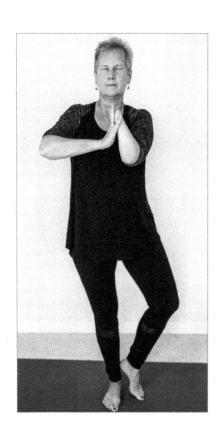

5. With firm but gentle pressure, continue to breathe in and out, focusing exclusively on this center of the heart. This center of the heart is known in Chinese medicine as the sea of tranquility. Allow yourself to feel all the feelings and sensations that arise, whether tranquil or not.

6. As you stay with this central point of the heart, the firm pressure of the thumb, and the breath, you are giving yourself permission to remove layers of protection, both physical and emotional, without losing control of yourself.

7. Keep repeating "I receive the wisdom of my heart, which is pure."

8. Continue with this practice as long as you can. Let out three deep sighs.

9. Feel the heart become more spacious, receptive, and alive. There is an exchange happening, between grief and the joy of life, all taking place in the wise heart.

Yoga to Allow Life to Unfold

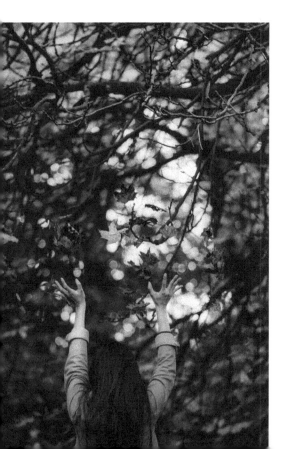

When I lost my left leg to bone cancer, all I wanted to do was get my prosthesis and walk again. I wasn't expecting leg sores, prosthetic adjustments, bone spurs, callouses, and misalignments to be part of the plan. It has been a long road for me, with so many challenges. My patience with myself has always been slim. I have found, though, that when I allow my life to happen, rather than force it to happen, more gifts emerge than I ever thought possible.

Patience is challenging, and necessary for amputees! A good day can be followed by a slippery fall, or a broken prosthetic. Travel plans can change because facilities are not accessible. The list is endless.

By inviting life to co-create with us and through us, we as amputees take back our power and our peace of mind, no matter what is happening.

Letting go of the outcome, inviting new awareness in body, mind and spirit to take hold, we amputees become even stronger in our faith and acceptance of the life we now have. The yoga sequence below encourages amputees to stay present and open to fresh possibilities.

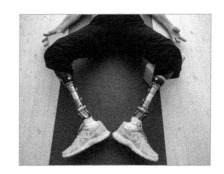

Supine Butterfly: Supta Baddha Konasana

1. Sit with the legs extended, hands to the side of the hips.

2. Lean into the elbows and roll onto the back, knees bent, feet flat on the floor.

3. Keep the tailbone drawn under slightly until reaching the floor (place a bolster or two rolled yoga blankets lengthwise under the spine for a variation).

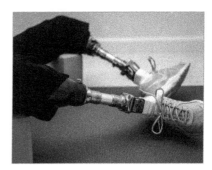

4. Once down on the back, roll the knees open in a diamond shape, the heels touching. The outside edge of the knees can rest on yoga blocks.

5. To release from the pose when ready, roll to one side and use the hands to press up to a seated position.

BK and AK amputees

- With a prosthesis, place a folded blanket under the left or right hip to even out the pelvis, if needed.

- Bring the yoga mat to the wall, pressing the toes into the wall.

- Place yoga straps around the thighs, gently tugging on the outer edge of each strap to roll the thighs in, keeping the knees from splaying. At the same time roll the calves out slightly.

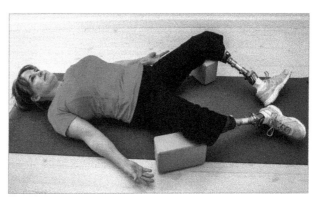

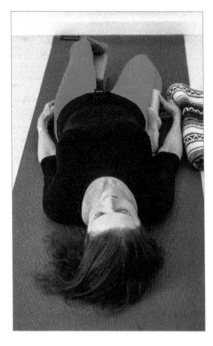

- Without a prosthesis, elevate the residual limb on a folded blanket so the hip is even with the other hip.

- Draw the buttocks down toward the feet to expand the sacrum.

UE amputees

- Have props set up before rolling down. Roll to the side to come onto the back.

- Place pillows and/or folded blankets under the arms/residual limbs to even out the shoulders.

Reclined hero: Supta Virasana

1. Begin in hero pose.

2. To come into the supine variation, be sure the knees are safe to do so.

3. Place the finger tips under the top of the sacrum and draw the flesh down towards the thighs.

4. Lengthen the sacrum and begin to lean the torso back towards the floor, first leaning on the elbows then eventually coming all the way down, resting the entire back on the floor.

5. If the knees are off the floor, come up higher onto the elbows to work on lengthening the torso.

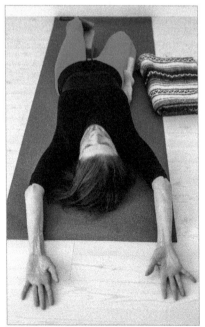

BK and AK amputees

- Place a yoga bolster lengthwise beneath the spine and back of the head.

- Put a folded blanket under the residual limb.

- If a below knee amputee, do not practice this pose with a prosthesis if the knee does not fold completely.

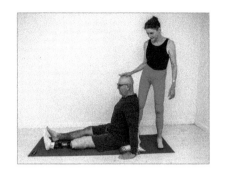

UE amputee

- If the forearm is available, lean on the forearms rather than go all the way back.

- Roll to the side and roll the back onto a bolster to open the chest.

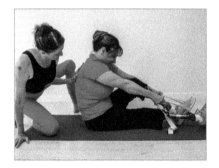

Seated Staff: Dandasana

1. Start in easy sitting pose.

2. Extend the legs out in front.

3. Draw the buttocks flesh away and spread the sitz bones.

4. If the lower back is tucking under, sit on the edge of a pillow, yoga mat or rolled up blanket.

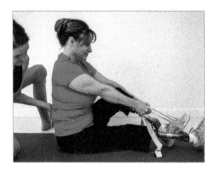

5. Flex the feet.

6. Roll the pelvis forward.

7. Place the hands beside the hips, reaching the palms or finger tips into the ground.

8. Press the bottom down and reach the crown up.

9. Draw the abdominal muscles gently in to elevate the spine.

10. Gaze at the toes.

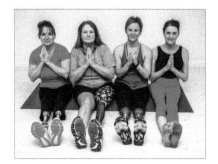

HEAL

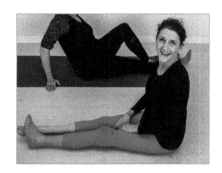

11. Keep the chin parallel to the ground.

12. Reach the heels and sitz bones in opposite directions.

13. Draw the back muscles and the hip muscles in to the center.

14. Press the palms or fingertips firmly into the ground.

BK and AK amputees

- Place the hands on yoga blocks. Sit with the back against the wall.

- Sit with the feet pressing into the wall.

- Practice with the knees bent and a rolled towel or yoga mat underneath.

- Practice with a yoga block between the thighs for greater leg strength.

UE amputee

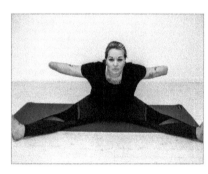

- Practice the chin lock (jalandhara bandha) for added inner core stability.

- Sit against a wall while practicing the pose.

- Press the feet into a wall and lengthen the spine.

Seated Wide Angle: Upavista Konasana

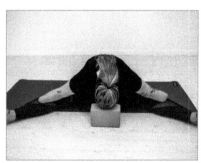

1. Sit with the legs outstretched in a "V".

2. Inhale.

3. Grab hold of the big toes.

4. Exhale.

5. Roll from the hips forward with the torso.

6. Inhale.

7. Lengthen the spine.

8. Exhale.

9. Fold forward.

10. Inhale.

11. Press into the legs.

12. Lift back up.

13. Release.

BK and AK amputees

- Place a rolled towel under the prosthetic knee.

- Sit on a folded blanket.

- Sit with the back to the wall.

- Sit with the feet pressing into the wall.

- Place a yoga block 1-2 feet in front under the hands.

- Place straps around both feet and hold, sitting up tall.

UE amputees

- Think about expanding from the heart.

- Rest the residual limb on a chair if needed.

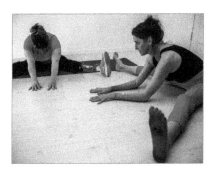

"Only people who are capable of loving strongly can also suffer great sorrow, but this same necessity of loving serves to counteract their grief and heals them." — Leo Tolstoy

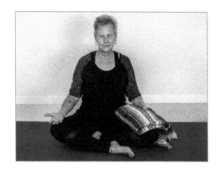

Easy Sitting Pose: Sukhasana

1. Find your sitz bones. Pull the flesh of your buttocks away diagonally so the sitz bones can drop further down into the ground.

2. Press the crown of the head up to the sky.

3. Roll the shoulders back and relax them down.

4. Have a soft gaze towards the floor or close the eyes.

BK and AK amputees

- Place folded blankets or bolsters under the knees.

- Sit on a yoga block, meditation pillow or folded blankets.

- If needed, place a folded blanket under the residual limb for even hips.

- Lean against a wall.

- Extend the legs rather than sit cross legged.

- Sit in a chair.

UE Amputees

- Place yoga blocks under the elbows if available.

- Lean the upper arm on a chair seat if needed.

- Lean back against a wall and draw the shoulders back if available.

Easy Resting Pose/Crocodile: Makarasana

*See Chapter 5 for complete steps to this pose.

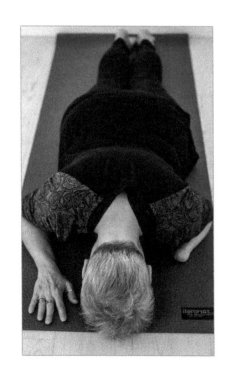

Psychological hurdles for amputees and their teachers

Amputees are dealing with a myriad of issues from the physical loss of a limb, pain, grief, rage, denial, body image perception, self-esteem, personal empowerment and sexuality issues. For amputees who have been in poor health for a while and may be expecting an amputation, they may be more likely to accept their limb loss. For amputees who have lost a limb suddenly or because of the quick onslaught of an illness, they may be less likely to accept their situation. Amputees may be concerned about many underlying fears as well, such as falling, dependency on others, helplessness, re-injury, embarrassment, damage to the prosthesis and re-traumatization. Amputees coming to yoga class may want the yoga teacher to fix them, heal them, argue with them, leave them alone, love them, help them, teach them, believe in them, and give them hope. All and everything apply.

Amputees aren't the only ones who could be dealing with psychological hurdles. Yoga teachers and clinicians may have their own psychological hurdles to teaching amputees as well. Some of these hurdles may include fear of injuring an amputee, fear of assisting an amputee, shock at seeing the actual residual limb, a need to fix or save an amputee, personal trauma being retriggered, over-assisting, under-motivating due to fear of harm, false expectations, ignorance and arrogance. Once both student and teacher develop a trusting relationship by asking and allowing open ended questions and experiences, many psychological hurdles can be overcome. In all cases, as Sri K. Pattabhi Jois promised "Do your practice and all is coming."

Try this yoga sequence to embrace your hurdles and go beyond them.

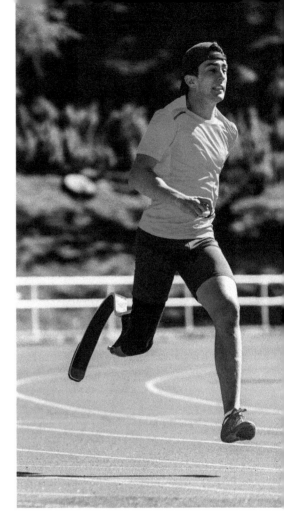

Psychological Hurdles Practice

1. **Pranayama:** Three Part Breath

2. **Warm up:** Circle joints in the body

3. **Asana:** Poses

a. **Warrior II:** Virabhadrasana II

b. **Side Angle:** Parsvokonasana

c. **Tree:** Vrikshasana

d. **Warrior III:** Virabhadrasana III

e. **Mountain:** Tadasana

f. **Chair:** Utkatasana

g. **Downward Facing Dog:** Adho Mukha Svanasana

h. **Childs:** Garbhasana

i. **Relaxation:** Savasana

YOGA BLISS: BODY IMAGE AND SEXUALITY
Body image

We are born divine and whole. The path of our life leads us back, again and again, to that wholeness. Within that framework, yoga lives. We practice yoga to return to our wholeness. Self-esteem, in particular, is a reflection of our wholeness, especially challenging when our bodies change dramatically due to limb loss. Valuing the new you is a process. Yoga can help.

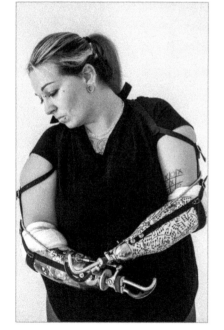

"Grief does not change you... It reveals you."
— John Green

Self-observation is foundational to yoga. The techniques of yoga provide us with the impetus to flush out untruths about our self-worth, and cling to the truth of our infinite nature. Listening to ourselves takes practice. Our outer world does not always match our inner world, but it is the inner world that tells us who we really are, beyond our amputation. Trusting your body's messages, then acting to honor those messages, restores our self-esteem. The simple practice of Beingness is an excellent start to embracing yourself exactly as you are. There is no future or past. Now is now. With or without limbs YOU ARE YOU.

The following activity will aid your self-esteem.

1. On at least five individual index cards, write down a unique strength that you possess. *If unable to write, record your list.*

2. On the back of each card, describe an event that demonstrated that strength.

3. Stack the cards or listen to yourself describe each strength.

4. Notice sensations in your body, the quality of your breath and the state of your mind.

5. This the real you, the one that shows up in the world, without self-judgment or self-criticism.

Accepting yourself as you are is the gateway to intimacy. Be patient with yourself. You deserve to be happy, just like everyone else. Claim that happiness for yourself by staying present.

Sexuality

Amputees deal with a multitude of challenges after limb loss, but body image and sexuality are often the biggest. Amputation, after all, is permanent. It's not like getting a bad haircut. Hair will grow back. Amputation affects amputees on every level, but especially our

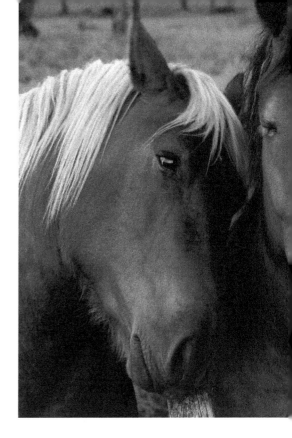

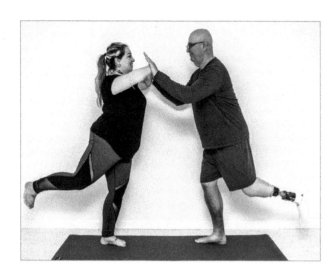

"You yourself, as much as anybody in the entire universe, deserve your love and affection."
— Sharon Salzberg

sense of identity. New amputees may be too busy adjusting, relearning basic life skills, before feeling the full impact of their loss. After the initial shock of amputation sets in, an amputee is left with her own inner journey to reclaim her identity and her personal power.

Sexuality is a huge part of that personal power. Our identity, although we might claim it isn't, is very much tied in to body image. After amputation, who are we, and will we be attractive to a current or potential partner?

Self-consciousness may not have been on a person's radar before limb loss. After limb loss, any reaction is possible. Losing a limb is extremely vulnerable. An amputee can feel uncomfortable talking about sexuality with others, dismissing it as unimportant or embarrassing. She might not seek help for something that is at the very core of her identity.

Looking honestly at the body after losing a limb takes time. Some people can't look at their residual limb at all, the reality too painful to bear. Healing from limb loss means coming to terms with this new body and this new identity: easy for some, not so easy for others.

As an amputee, a healthy body image begins with self-acceptance on all levels; body, mind and spirit. Being seen for who you are, not for what you have overcome, or what you lack, is a daily practice of self-awareness. The truth is, there will always be people who are not comfortable being in a relationship with an amputee. Others won't care.

Men and women amputees, in general, may deal with body image and sexuality quite differently. For a man whose identity was tied to his ability to provide, or his physical strength, his sense of desirability can diminish if he must change his job, be on disability, or needs help to walk. For women who pride themselves on looking their best, their sense of personal beauty can change. They may not be able to wear clothing they could wear before, such as heels. They may feel that they are "damaged goods". Prosthetics can be unattractive, and with insurance limits not everyone can get the prosthetic they want.

Couples experience big changes, adjusting to a new sexual life, dealing with what it means to be desired and to desire each other. They may be concerned how their marriage or partnership will change. The amputee may feel suddenly ashamed of her body and try to hide it during sex. Singles may worry about whether they will be able to meet anyone as a "disabled" person, wondering if they should share the truth of their amputation, or hide it. If they do share their amputation they open themselves to a whole world of amputee devotees, which can be upsetting, or exciting, depending on the amputee.

Some amputees make assumptions about their partners' perception of them that are incorrect, limiting them in their full expression of their sexuality. Not all amputees will know how to adapt their body to sex, and indeed may feel awkward with intimacy. Sexual drive can change after amputation, due to fatigue or pain.

Sexuality can be even more complicated for an amputee missing multiple limbs. These significant body modifications can't be hidden but are plainly visible anywhere a multiple limb amputee goes, which makes some amputees feel endlessly vulnerable, and "abnormal". Some multiple limb amputees find movement difficult, ending up isolated and alone too much of the time. It takes persistence and commitment to one's wholeness to come to terms with so many body and sexuality changes. Yoga practice offers many effective ways to build body confidence, combat fatigue, and increase libido.

In yoga terms, sexuality is vitality, creativity, life force and union with the divine. Yoga awakens kundalini, which refers to the latent sexual energy available to expand the consciousness and experience bliss. Kundalini

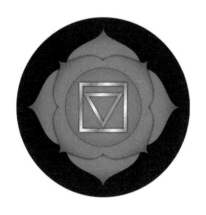

is meant to stay dormant in the body when it is not needed. The bandhas keep kundalini energy contained until needed. Sexual fluids are the nectar of an awakened sexuality, the result of divine bliss, not to be used unconsciously. Whether a person has limbs or not, this divine energy is always available. Imagination is a wonderful thing.

As discussed in earlier chapters, compassion and self-acceptance are hallmarks of the Royal Path of Yoga. Learning how to love yourself is the foundation to any good sex life and to a healthy body image.

Self-consciousness can be exacerbated in the bedroom after amputation. Change that phrase to **SELF-awareness,** and you have a whole new way of experiencing your own body and your sex life. Being present during sex gives an amputee and partner permission to open to new levels of passion, a timeless moment of unity and ecstasy.

The following yoga sequence increases sexual energy.

Yoga Bliss for Increased Sexual Energy

Pranayama

1. Sit on the floor, if able.

2. Breath in and out forcefully through the mouth as you practice Mulabandha.

3. Close your eyes. Relax.

4. Inhale deeply through the nose.

5. Suspend the breath as you pump the muscles of the pubic area in mulabandha, inviting the energy to rise to the third eye, or center of the forehead.

6. If it helps, imagine the energy as a color, swirling from the pubic area through the sexual organs, up through the spine to the third eye and back down again.

7. Allow that energy to fill you.

8. Exhale and release.

Asana

1. Cat/Cow pose

2. Cobra pose

3. Butterfly pose

4. Head to knee pose

5. Seated wide angle pose

6. Bridge pose

7. Childs pose

8. Seated meditation

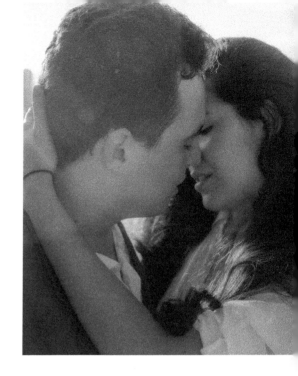

Yoga restores self-confidence naturally, which in turn builds self-esteem. Daily practices of positive self-talk, deep listening to the body's needs, and meditation to reduce stress mean a more fulfilling time in the bedroom. The benefits of the physical practices of yoga; flexibility, strength, and stamina can make the bedroom more fun. Who knows how an amputee can twist and turn his body by adding yoga to the mix! Yoga's focus on relaxation reduces stress hormones, increases focus, and strengthens breath capacity. This in turn raises the libido, creating better orgasms. In a 2015 Harvard research study, yoga was found to enhance sex significantly.

Many people have heard of Tantra (rituals of enlightenment in body, mind and spirit) and the Kama Sutra (rules of desire), ancient texts that offer various yoga techniques to not only increase sexual pleasure, but ultimately to offer encounters with the Divine. In fact, Raja Yoga has its roots in various aspects of Tantra Yoga. The foundation of these

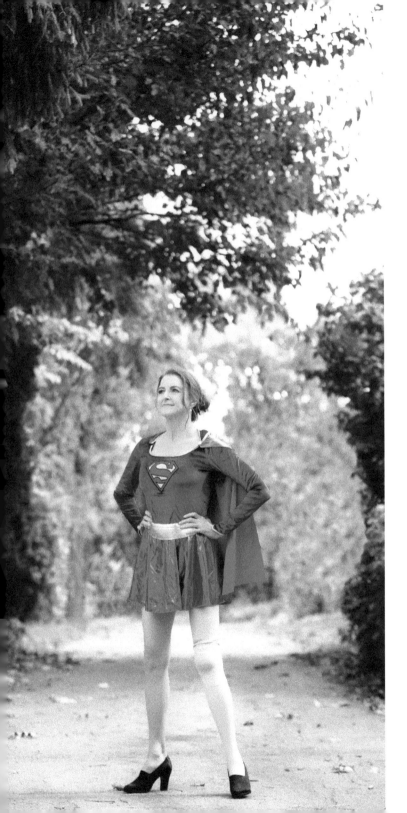

practices is the ability to love one's self, and the Divine Self that lives within.

Navigating sexuality is one more challenge to face for an amputee. Rest assured, when you commit to yoga, you are also committing to your self-esteem and your divine right to a fulfilling sex life. By practicing yoga and becoming the blessed recipient of its benefits, you become master of your own sexuality. Now get to it!

CHAPTER EIGHT

THE MANY FACES OF AMPUTEE YOGA

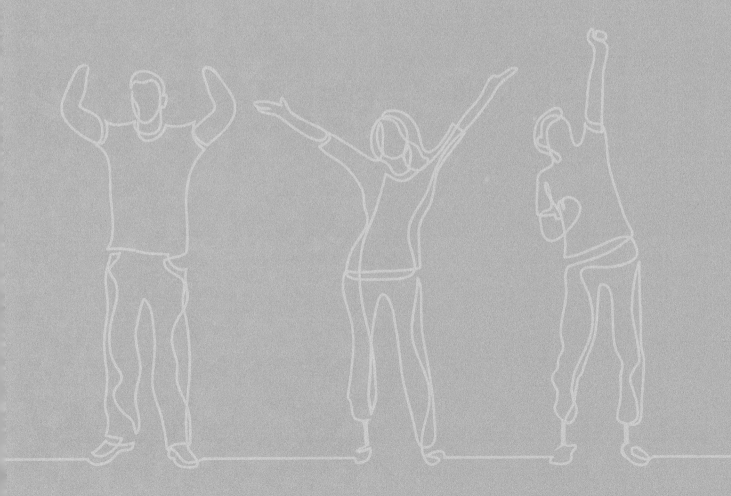

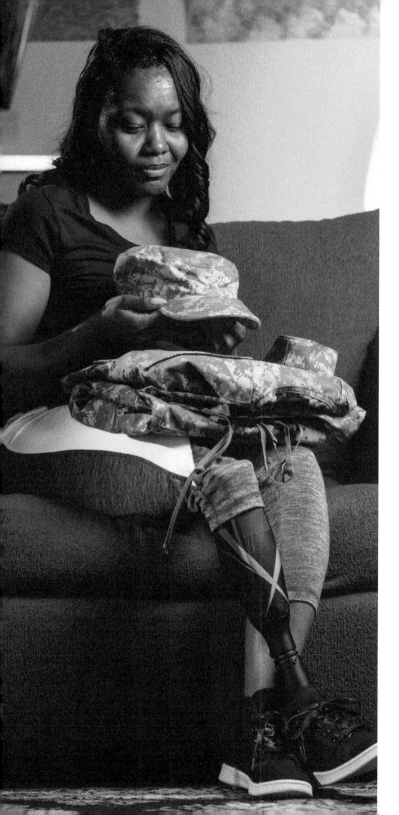

Amputees come in all shapes and sizes, from newborn infants to centenarians. Not only are there generalized needs for amputees which can be addressed through yoga, there are specific yoga tools that help a variety of amputees. We begin with veterans.

VETERANS

Veteran amputees are a unique and complex group due to the variety of injuries and psychological needs. Many veterans are returning from war with major limb loss, in addition to torso, pelvic and genital/urinary damage. Because protective gear does not adequately guard the head and extremities, Bomb blasts, IEDs (improvised explosive devices), land mines, as well as active combat, contribute to these limb losses and injuries. The main source of limb loss in these situations happens on foot, usually due to IED's.

Many veterans returning home have lost multiple limbs. Veteran amputees from previous wars such as the Vietnam War, have additional complications such as cardiovascular illness, addiction, age-related illness and diabetes.

Conditions in which amputations occur are extreme, and in the majority of cases, the rehabilitation is long. Not only is the veteran learning how to handle the limb loss, and all that goes with it, there are also flashbacks, head injury, side effects of chemicals worn or inhaled, ongoing post-traumatic stress and combat stress disorder. Recovery for veterans is a battle unto itself. When a veteran loses a limb or limbs, restoring the warrior spirit central to his/her identity takes time. Immediate concerns take over. Yoga is an invaluable aid for veterans.

Many of the advances in prosthetics emerge from an urgent need within the military community, but that does not mean that a veteran will necessarily have access to a state of the art prosthetic. Due to scar tissue, tissue damage, disease, long term medical care, and budget cuts, advanced prosthetics with more functionality are not always available, nor are they always comfortable to wear.

Yoga specifically for amputees addresses multiple issues on multiple levels, because yoga is not just about strengthening a quad muscle or reducing stress. Yoga is about developing a relationship with the highest aspect of one's self. This offers hope in the quagmire of veteran recovery from amputation.

Some veterans will respond to yoga very quickly because of their age or fitness level. Others will need a lot more physical and mental support before they ever do a yoga pose. Yoga for an amputee veteran must lift her spirit as well strengthen her body. Combat wounds create trauma and injury on all levels. Yoga is an antidote to get amputee veterans back to wholeness.

Pain, for many veteran amputees, is compounded by emotional loss and suffering. When independence seems to be stripped away, yoga gives the veteran some sense of control and power. A gentle, simple strengthening yoga practice is the best approach. Pain, exacerbated by PTSD (post-traumatic stress disorder) and CSD (civilian stress disorder), is counteracted by the parasympathetic response that yoga provides. Yoga pulls a veteran out of a constant contracted state of pain, suffering, hopelessness and depression into an expanded, relaxed, hopeful state of being. For many veterans who have years and years of stress, the contracted state feels familiar and "safe" for survival. Yoga shows veterans how to feel the difference between being empowered by inner peace rather than fueled by negativity.

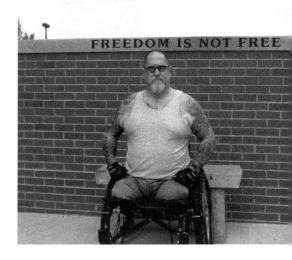

"Think thou also of thy duty and do not waver. There is no greater good for a warrior than to fight in a righteous war." —
Bhagavad Gita 2:31

Yoga is a life management skill for amputee veterans.

Emotional and mental wellness is key to yoga for amputee veterans. In any yoga practice for veterans, accessing deep breath right away can make a veteran feel better in seconds. This sends a message to the amputee veteran that he has the power in his breath to create his own positive experience.

A yoga practice for amputee veterans will be more trauma sensitive. Repetitive yoga drills work best, especially drills that the amputee can repeat on his own, to handle daily stressors. Yoga is a life management skill for amputee veterans.

The approach focuses on three key principles:

1. **Strength**

2. **Stamina**

3. **Serenity**

What is strength? Strength is power, vitality, immovability in the face of difficulty, ability to withstand or resist, determination, commitment, compassion, courage and love. It takes strength, both physical and mental, to live life as an amputee. Yoga builds up that strength.

What is stamina? Stamina is endurance, focus, steady strength, staying power and vital life force. For amputees, daily routines require stamina they may not have needed before limb loss. From the act of walking, to the necessity of performing everyday tasks, a certain physical stamina is required. It takes stamina to endure pain or endure the vulnerability of being an amputee in a world set up for the able-bodied. Yoga builds stamina inside and out.

What is serenity? Serenity is a sense of being complete, at one with your life and circumstances, content as is, and tranquil within. Through the various aspects of yoga practice, from breathing to relaxation, serenity becomes a way of life, not a temporary fix. This is achieved through the many physical, mental and spiritual benefits that yoga offers.

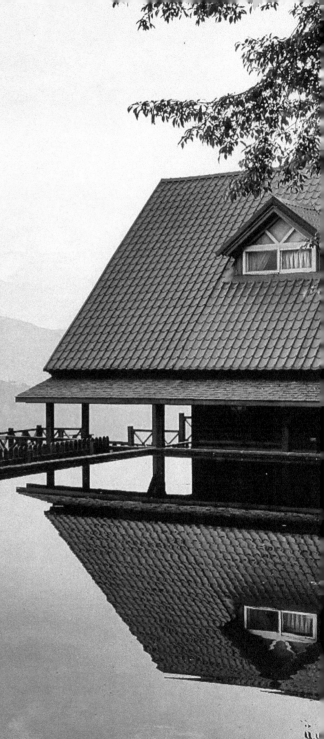

The Guest House

This being human is a guest house.
Every morning a new arrival.

A joy, a depression, a meanness, some momentary
awareness comes as an unexpected visitor.

Welcome and entertain them all!
Even if they are a crowd of sorrows, who violently
sweep your house empty of its furniture, still, treat
each guest honorably.
He may be clearing you out for some new delight.

The dark thought, the shame, the malice.
Meet them at the door laughing and invite them in.

Be grateful for whatever comes. Because each has
been sent as a guide from beyond.

— Rumi

An emotionally strong person has greater resolve to handle limb loss and rehabilitation. A person of brute physical strength may be physically able to withstand physical pain, but less able to handle the emotional impact of amputation and the changes to personal identity. In both cases yoga attends to exactly what the person needs at that time. A serene person may be better able to handle all the ups and downs of amputation and recovery. A discontented person will feel frustrated, anxious and angry about losing a limb. Both perspectives are welcome in yoga. The magic touch of yoga is the compassion it offers for one's own journey.

Learning how to trust life again is the focus for amputee veterans. This means trusting the body to heal itself and learn a new way of being, trusting those who care for you professionally and personally, trusting the prosthetics, trusting that life can and will get better, trusting that the world can be safe, trusting that life can be productive, fulfilling and capable of offering the freedom to be independent and whole.

Amputee veterans work best with a program that gently builds body awareness while at the same time creates a safety net of support. Veterans need to challenge the "limitations" of amputation, illness or mindset to feel that they have won in life. Counterintuitively, they do this by embracing their new "limitations" rather than dismissing them. Minimizing pain naturally and mindfully through yoga empowers the veteran amputee. A veteran amputee needs to know that she is in control.

Veterans have been trained to use their body to employ strength, endurance, courage, and mental acuity. Below is a yoga practice which addresses the three core elements of yoga for veterans: **strength, stamina, serenity.** Each aspect of this practice nourishes and sustains a veteran in her wholeness. This practice can be done standing or in a chair. *(standing can mean holding on to parallel bars, a walker, two canes or leaning against a wall.)*

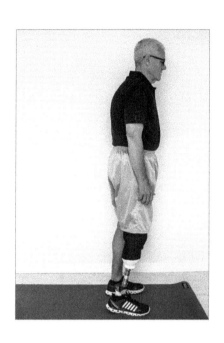

Veteran Amputee Yoga Practice

1. Inner Mountain

   a. **Find your inner mountain.** Align your spine, draw your abdominals in, and lengthen the sides of your body. Strength

   b. **Find your focus.** Gaze at one spot while you breathe in and out. Stamina

   c. **Find your outer mountain.** Stand feet hip width apart. Follow directions for finding your inner mountain. Find your focus. Relax the skin and nervous system as you breathe in and exhale deeply. Serenity

2. Lifting

   a. **Pelvic floor lift.** Draw the groin and perineum into the center of the pelvis as you tone the abdominals towards the spine. Strength

   b. **Pelvic floor lift.** Continue with this inner lift as you inhale and exhale deeply. Stamina

   c. **Relax your shoulders** as you continue to lift from the inner core. Serenity

3. Twist seated in a chair

   a. **Seated twist with arms upstretched.** Draw the navel in towards the spine. Lift the arms up overhead, parallel to the shoulders, palms facing each other. Alternately, lengthen the sides of the torso. Move the whole torso to the right, center, then left. Strength

   b. **Repeat the seated twist** to the right. Stay to the right as you lengthen the spine, inhale and exhale. Twist to the right a little more for three inhales and exhales. Repeat to the left. Stamina

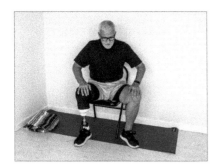

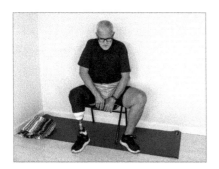

c. **Seated twist.** Unwind. Sit comfortably, relax the shoulders and feel the benefits of the deep twist. Serenity

4. Standing/seated mountain

a. **Imagine planting roots** into the ground from your navel to the soles of your feet, sitz bones or bottom. Strength

b. **Standing/seated mountain.** Continue with standing mountain, reaching the arms or sides of the torso high, breathing in and out three times. Stamina

c. **Standing/seated mountain.** Release the arms, soften the sides of the body, close the eyes, and breathe gently, feeling the echoes of the pose. Serenity

5. Chair pose

a. **Stand in mountain pose.** Bend the knees as you tilt your torso forward to a forty-five-degree angle. Lift the arms up overhead. Alternately lengthen the sternum. Draw your navel into your spine. Strength

b. **Chair.** Maintain the pose for three to five long breaths with a focus straight ahead on a spot or object. Stamina

c. **Standing forward bend.** Release the arms, bend forward and relax the neck. Serenity

6. Downward Dog

a. Come to the hands and knees. Press into the hands as you lift the knees off the ground, folding at the hips into an upside down 'V'. Strength

b. **Downward Dog.** Hold this position for three breaths, increasing to ten with practice. Stamina

c. **Childs pose.** Release the knees to the floor, extend the arms in front, round the lower back tucking the tailbone under, and sit back on the heels if possible. Serenity

7. Push up to a standing position from child's pose

   a. **Stand** in Mountain pose. Strength

   b. **Warrior II.** Step the feet wide. Turn the right foot straight ahead, and the left foot in about fifteen degrees. Bend the front knee. Extend the arms out parallel to the legs. Stay three to five breaths. Repeat on the left. Stamina

   c. **Standing Mountain.** Step the feet back together. Relax the arms to the sides. Soften the eyes and the shoulders. Relax. Serenity

8. Focus your breath on your heart as you lengthen your spine.

   a. **Feel** the power and strength of your heart. Strength

   b. **Continue** to breathe in and out focusing on the heart eight to ten times. Stamina

   c. **Meditate** on the courage of your heart. Serenity

9. Stand in Mountain

   a. **Send compassion** to every cell of your body. Strength.

   b. **Meditate** on that which makes you grateful today. Stamina.

   c. **Chant** OM. Serenity

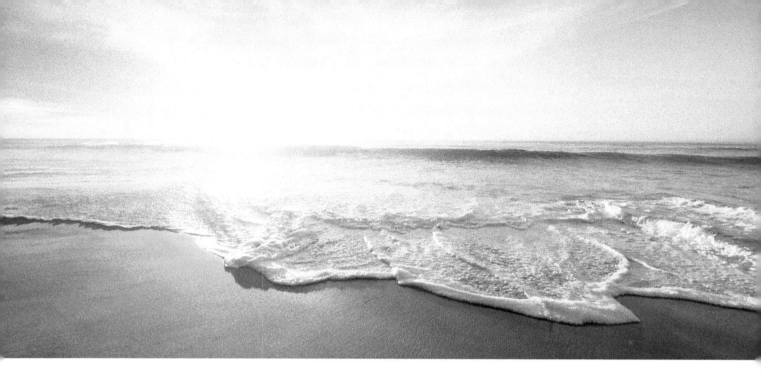

Learn How to Breathe Again

Breathing is fundamental to a veteran's sense of well-being. Stress, especially intensified stress ,chronic stress due to PTSD, CSD, and pain, affects the mechanisms of the body involved in breathing in significant ways. Stress due to war has deep psychological and physical ramifications, including violent outbursts, sleep disorders, paranoia, chronic disease and depression.

Movement, especially movement with breath, can positively influence the outcome of a veteran's self-esteem. When a veteran is experiencing PTSD, his heart beats rapidly, his breath shortens, his eyes can move rapidly or stay fixated, he can have vertigo, and live with low back pain. When any or all those symptoms occur, the muscles around the ribs contract, the lower belly begins to grip, the chest collapses, the jaw tightens, the diaphragm moves with less elasticity, the psoas shortens, and breathing is limited to the upper chest.

Getting the breath to regulate and drop into the lower belly lets the psoas soften just a little, giving more space for the diaphragm to move easily, and in turn, bring in more prana, or life force. For many amputee veterans, learning how to breathe again re-establishes a core sense of self, a self which can cope with life's challenges more easily. Several breathing techniques that unite movement in the psoas with deep abdominal breathing can truly help the amputee veteran.

A great place to start is on the back (supine), with the knees bent. For amputees not wearing prosthetics, the residual limbs should rest over a blanket, with a slight tilt in the pelvis. New amputees (within one year) should not elevate the residual limb. Lying supine with bent knees relaxes the psoas, making diaphragmatic breath easier. In some cases, adding a weighted bag, five to ten pounds, over the lower belly, allows the veteran to surrender into the floor.

Steps to supine breathing

1. Lie on the back with the knees bent or supported over pillows / rolled blankets.

2. Lengthen the tailbone.

3. Relax the lower back into the floor.

4. Take ten to twenty deep breaths, bringing focus to the lower belly as the source of the breath.

5. For variation, lift the arms above the head on the inhale, then float the arms back to the side on the exhale.

Supine breathing with leg extension

1. Prepare as above.

2. Inhale.

3. Exhale. Extend the right leg if able.

4. Inhale. Slowly return the leg to the original position.

5. Repeat on the left.

6. If this movement triggers phantom pain, return to the original supine breathing practice.

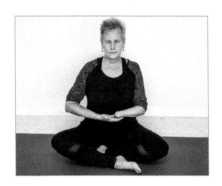

Diaphragmatic breathing

1. Sit up, the spine elongated, the chin parallel to the floor.

2. Place the hands over the side ribs. Alternately bring your awareness to the side ribs.

3. Breathe in, feeling the ribs expand.

4. Breathe out, feeling the ribs draw in.

5. Place the hands on the lower belly.

6. Breathe in. Feel the belly drop.

7. Breathe out. Feel the belly lift.

Simple presence breath

1. Sit up as in diaphragmatic breathing.

2. Breathe in, saying to one's self, "I am".

3. Breathe out, saying "Here".

4. Breathe in saying "I am"

5. Breathe out saying "Here now."

6. Repeat five to ten rounds.

Amputee veterans deserve our appreciation. Veteran amputees have battled to protect basic human rights often at the expense of their limbs and lives. In fact, **Vishpala**, one of the most famous warriors in Hindu myth, was a female amputee who wore iron prosthesis. Losing a limb does not have to stop veterans from thriving in life. With yoga by his side, a veteran can heal losses and learn to live abundantly.

CHILDREN

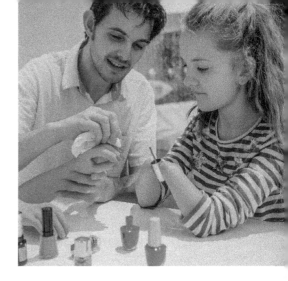

Children's amputations and prosthetics are different from those of adults. Children will normally get their first prosthetic when they are able to stand on their own. They will need many prosthetics throughout their childhood to adapt to their growth spurts. Sockets, which are molded to the shape of a child's residual limb, need to be changed at least once per year, sometimes more. Many prosthetists develop additional prosthetics for children who are interested in different sports and activities, such as running, football and gymnastics. It is far better to start children off with prosthetics at a very young age, so their prosthesis feels like second skin. Like adults, they will need physical therapy to aid in developing healthy gait and stability. Just as children learn languages more easily when they are young, prosthetic use in general is easier for children than adults. A child's prosthesis is designed to enhance freedom of movement. If the prosthesis gets in the way of that freedom, such as children who are still crawling, then the prosthesis will be avoided. Developmental stages in children have a lot to do with whether a child wears a prosthesis or not.

Situations for which children need prosthetics

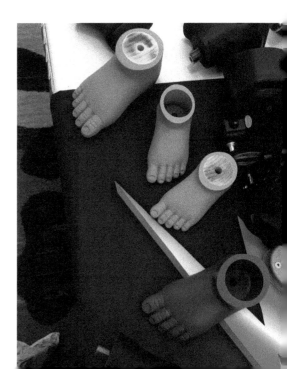

Children need prosthetics for several reasons. Congenital limb deficiencies, serious illness such as cancer or infection, and traumatic injury are the three main causes of amputation in children. Children born with congenital limb deficiencies may have elective amputation because the deformities they were born with would keep them from doing everyday activities. In those cases, amputations are done early in life, and prosthetics become their new limbs. Most children use functional prosthetics, as the wear and tear are quite extensive.

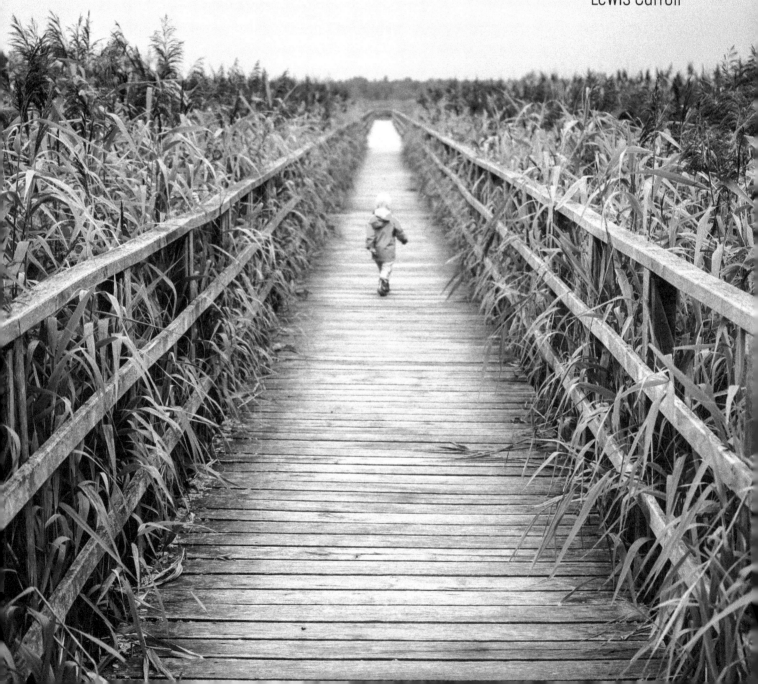

"No, no! The adventures first. Explanations take such a dreadful time."

–Lewis Carroll

Cosmetic prosthetics are used more for children with upper limb amputations, to avoid unnecessary discrimination or for reasons of self-consciousness.

Yoga for Child Amputees

Yoga for child amputees can begin around 3 years of age. Children learning yoga will be all over the spectrum of mobility, stability and development. In the best-case scenario, the child learns to use her prosthesis during yoga practice to best learn standing poses and flow poses at an early age.

Vulnerability and body image can still be a factor for child amputees in children's yoga classes, whether in an all amputee class or an all body type yoga class.

Education and awareness about disability has certainly grown in the past twenty years, but children can still feel out of place in a non-amputee world. In most cases, once an amputee child in yoga class is accepted and understood for his/her differences, most non-amputee children just want to get back to yoga and have fun.

Some children, non-amputee and amputee alike, do have a hard time with their amputee yoga friend. They can be afraid, upset, or overly curious to the detriment of the flow of the yoga class. There is nothing wrong with any of that. A child's reaction is her reaction. Openness, teachable moments and celebration of our unique differences is the way to handle a child's reaction. It is important, though, that children of all abilities do not play with, hit, kick or otherwise damage the prosthesis of a child. It is not a yoga prop!

In general, yoga practice for amputee children will be far more physical with very few modifications. Most child amputees are quick to find an alternate way to move if one way is not available. A children's amputee yoga practice follows the same formula as any yoga practice, with a few modifications. Yoga props need to be available, but somewhat hidden for the safety of the child. Children have an uncanny way of making yoga props into something other than yoga props. Injuries and damaged property take less than one full yogic breath! Some children are not able to move to the floor, so practicing in a chair works just as well.

Any amputee child doing yoga needs to know that she is safe. What that means for a child is structure, follow through, attention and the freedom to express herself without shame or embarrassment. The challenge for an amputee child can be the "visibility" of being different, and in some cases, wanting attention because of this difference. While most children do use prosthetics for yoga, there are some cases where prosthetic use in yoga is not recommended.

It is important to get a base line for range of motion in the knees and hips. Not all knees bend deeply. Not all prosthetic feet are stable enough to stand for long periods of time, especially those built for more athletic activity such as running or soccer. Kids get excited, sometimes overexcited, in yoga class. If they are not being mindful, they can land on their residual limb, or torque their prosthesis. Yoga teaches kids to listen to their bodies first.. Yoga is such a wonderful way to help amputee kids learn how to mindfully move through life, not with trepidation and fear, but with confidence, poise and body awareness.

Centering	5 minutes	Namaste Bow
Breathing	5 minutes	3-part breath
Warm Ups	10 minutes	Stretch and jiggle the body
Poses	20-25 minutes	10 poses
Relaxation	5 minutes	Use props for comfort
Closing chant	5 minutes	Namaste or Om

A children's yoga practice formula

Children love to practice yoga using affirmations with their movements. The words create rhythms to connect to the movement, which makes the yoga practice memorable and approachable. All amputee children can do the sequence in either a chair, standing or on the floor. There is always a way for everyone to do yoga.

An amputee children's yoga practice helps them remember who they are by teaching the body, mind, spirit tools of yoga that are so foundational to an integrated, whole life. Teach them how to **Be, Breathe, and Bend** early in life, and they will be unstoppable as adults.

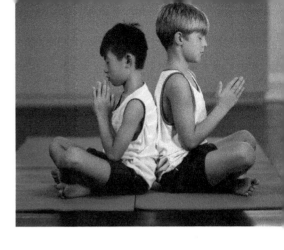

A kid's yoga practice, children ages 5-12

1. Namaste. Bow to the teacher.

2. Namaste. Bow to each other.

3. 3-part breath.

4. Affirmations: I am Fearless, I am Humble, I am Kind, I am Powerful, I am Compassionate, I am Self-Controlled, I am Wise, and I am Harmonious. Repeat this mantra series three times.

5. Stretch and jiggle the entire body.

6. Begin **Asana** practice. With each yoga pose, say the mantra that accompanies that pose.

7. **Tadasana: Mountain:** I am compassionate.

8. **Virabhdrasana: Warrior II:** I am fearless.

9. **Utkatasana: Chair Pose:** I am powerful.

10. **Uttanasana:** Standing Forward Bend: I am humble.

11. **Adho Mukha Svanasana: Downward Dog:** I am wise.

12. **Udrhva Mukha Svananasana: Upward Dog:** I am kind.

13. **Adho Mukha Svanasana: Downward Dog:** I am wise.

14. **Uttanasana: Standing Forward Bend:** I am humble.

15. **Utkatasana: Chair:** I am self-controlled.

16. **Tadasana: Mountain:** I am harmonious.

17. Belly breath.

18. Relaxation.

19. Namaste. Bow to the teacher.

20. Namaste. Bow to each other.

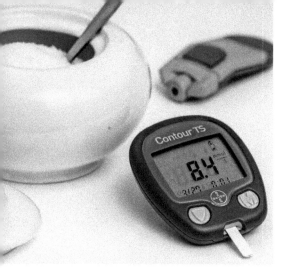

DIABETES

What is diabetes?

Diabetes is a metabolic disorder in which insulin is no longer produced normally in the body, causing elevation in glucose levels. When the glucose in the blood stream is elevated and not properly controlled by diet and exercise, the body endures many health conditions, such as heart disease, eye problems, kidney disease, skin disorders, diminished cognition and other complications, including amputation.

Diabetic limb loss

Often due to the changes in the normal functioning of the endocrine system, the skin goes through many evolutions. Skin can become thin. Injury to the skin can heal slowly, and in some cases, cause ulcers or open wounds, leading to infection and ultimately gangrene, or dead tissue. First, toes or fingers are amputated, then the lower leg or arm may need to be amputated as well.

One significant way that this skin weakness can be reduced is to build up the oxygen in the body through pranayama. A committed pranayama practice can change the chemistry of the skin over time, reducing the risk of ulcers. If a person has already lost a limb, yoga becomes an important preventative medicine for the future.

Yoga for diabetic amputees

Some yoga poses can directly stimulate the pancreas to produce insulin. There has also been research showing that yoga can improve glucose and cholesterol measurements. Pranayama combined with abdominal lock practices invigorate the pancreas and restore balance. When digestion and elimination are naturally stimulated, the body can more easily release toxins.

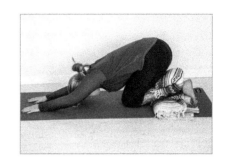

Safety precautions for diabetic amputees

If you have an active skin wound, practice wearing shoes and diabetic socks that have grip. Do not use yoga mats provided by the yoga studio. Invest in your own yoga mat and keep it clean with a vinegar and water spritz. Take a carbohydrate snack before exercise to avoid blood sugar drops, vertigo or fainting. Keep the intensity of your yoga practice low rather than high. Avoid hot yoga as too much sweating can lead to dehydration followed by poor wound healing and sugar imbalances. Inversions such as headstand and shoulder stand should only be practiced by an advanced yoga practitioner.

Seated Yoga Practice for Diabetic Amputees

1. **Kapalabhati:** Breath of Fire for five to ten minutes.

2. **Ardha Matsyendrasana:** Seated Twist.

3. **Bhujangasana:** Cobra.

4. **Shalabasana:** Locust.

5. **Maha Mudra:** The Great Seal.

6. **Halasana:** Plow.

7. **Makarasana:** Supine Crocodile.

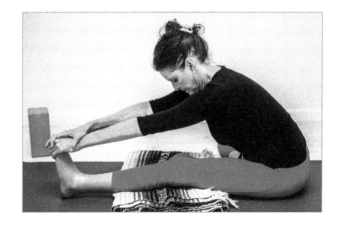

Cardiovascular Disease

Cardiovascular disease is many things, from high blood pressure to peripheral arterial sclerosis. The body can be hit hard when cardiovascular disease is present in the body due to the systemic nature of the disease. While there are many reasons for cardiovascular issues, from lifestyle choices to genetics, the fact remains that cardiovascular disease is the number one disease in the US, causing 80% of amputations. Yoga has been found to positively affect people with cardiovascular conditions.

Cardiovascular limb loss

Peripheral artery disease is the main cause of limb loss for people with cardiovascular diseases. The arteries are narrowed or blocked, causing poor circulation to the limbs, leading to neuropathy, and deterioration of limb tissue.

Yoga for amputees with cardiovascular conditions

Hip openers like Bound Angle, Tree, Triangle and Warrior II get more blood flow through the pelvis, but if the amputee suffers from serious heart disease, avoid Triangle and all Warrior poses. Backbends like Cobra and Upward Facing Dog stimulate the respiratory system. Vinyasa flow gets the blood moving through the extremities but is not recommended for people with uncontrollable high blood pressure or recent heart surgery, such as a pacemaker. Forward bends calm the heart and reduce stress in the system, but the head should not be below the heart if the amputee suffers from unmedicated high blood pressure. Head to knee pose stimulates the core and releases the hips.

"Take care of your body. It's the only place you have to live." —
Jim Rohn

Supine knee to chest pose cleans the digestive system and opens the hamstrings. Bridge pose opens the chest and pelvis.

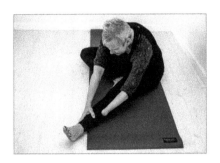

Precautions for amputees with heart disease

It is not good to sit on the heels and limit blood flow to the feet, in poses such as Hero pose, or Heron pose. Boat pose can elevate blood pressure too quickly. Inversions such as legs up the wall, Shoulderstand, Handstand and Headstand should be avoided for people with vertigo, and uncontrolled blood pressure.

A Yoga Practice for Amputees with Cardiovascular Conditions

1. **Nadi Shodhana:** Alternate nostril breathing.

2. **Savasana:** Relaxation.

3. **Janu Sirsasana:** Head to knee.

4. **Pavana Muktasana:** Knees to chest.

5. **Garbhasana:** Childs.

6. **Virasana:** Hero.

7. **Yoga Nidra:** Yogic rest.

CANCER

What is cancer?

Cancer is a disease that can affect any body system. Body cells split and quickly reproduce, invading healthy tissue. They spread both rapidly and slowly, usually developing into tumors, or hostile growths. Cancer treatment can include a combination of Western approaches, such as chemotherapy, radiation and surgery, and complementary treatments such as raw food diets, cleanses, and Eastern practices such as yoga and acupuncture. Amputation is also considered a cancer treatment. Nearly 7% of amputations are a result of cancer. The most common forms of cancer that produce limb loss are bone cancer, melanoma, and soft tissue sarcomas.

Amputee cancer survivors have many added concerns in addition to the limb loss. Dealing with the uncertainty of cancer's cure or recurrence can leave a hovering anxiety which influences daily life. Yoga's focus on seeking contentment in the present moment helps an amputee cancer survivor cope better with this internal anxiety. Yoga keeps a cancer patient fit and active, stimulating immune response and releasing the build-up of toxins from cancer medications. The mind relaxes, the emotional load lightened and pain lessened as moments of harmony return.

The following gentle yoga practice supports those who have been diagnosed or survived cancer.

Please practice care if you experience any of the following: bone loss, fluid retention, heart issues, dizziness, generalized fatigue, abdominal surgeries, neuropathy, nausea, or severe anxiety.

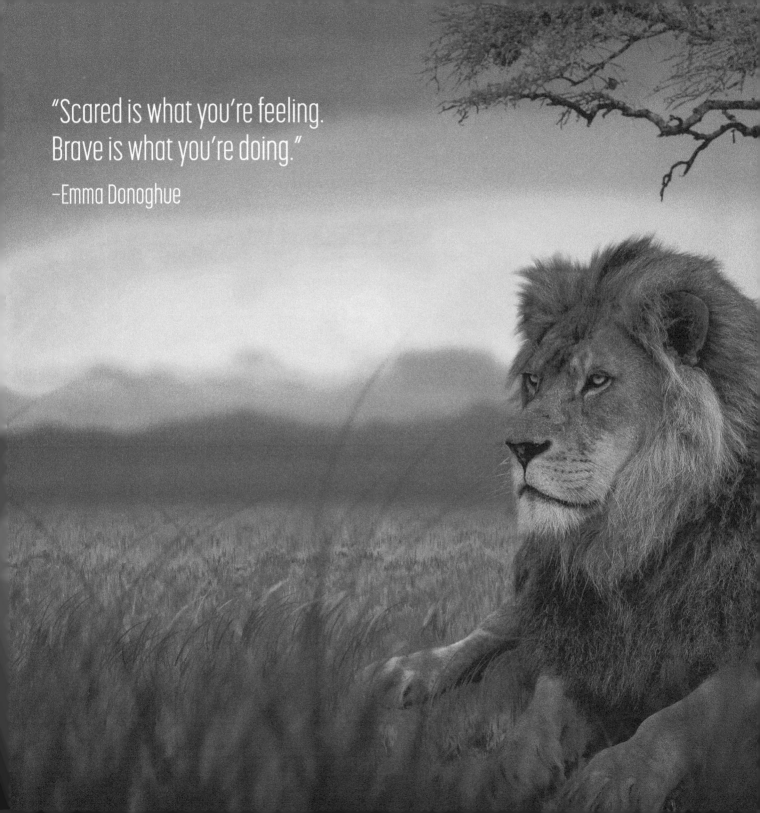

"Scared is what you're feeling.
Brave is what you're doing."

–Emma Donoghue

A yoga practice for amputee cancer survivors

1. Meditate on the present moment.

   a. I am here now.

   b. I receive the goodness that each breath brings to me.

   c. I receive the goodness of this moment,

2. Sighing breath with the tongue sticking out.

3. **Half Downward Dog** pressing hands into the wall, or resting the forehead on a chair.

4. Standing Cat/cow with hands or back at the wall.

5. **Ardha Matsyendrasana:** Seated twist.

6. **Bidalasana:** Cat/cow.

7. **Supta Baddha Konasana:** Supine bound angle.

8. **Savasana:** Relaxation.

9. **Sukhasana:** Easy Sitting Pose.

10. **Nadi Shodhana:** Alternate Nostril Breathing.

11. Affirmation-I receive the goodness of life in each moment.

12. OM

SCOLIOSIS

Scoliosis, a curvature of the spine, affects some amputees. Mild or severe, it can change through time. In most cases, scoliosis is a result of rapid bone growth in childhood, resulting in curvatures. In the case of amputees, the use of crutches, wheelchairs, or certain prosthetics can misalign the spine, and over time, result in permanent curvature.

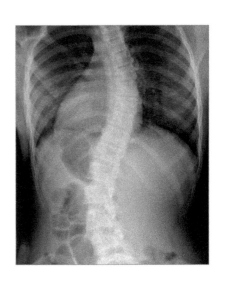

A scoliotic spine is S or C curved, causing various health challenges for amputees. These challenges include lower back pain, neck pain, restricted breathing, a forward drooping head, shoulder hunches, a collapsed chest, misalignment of the shoulders, back and hips, spinal bone spurs, exhaustion, a shortened gait and stiff arms with gait.

When an amputee begins to stiffen the arms to the side, as can happen with scoliosis sufferers, there is less momentum to propel the body forward which, over time, limits range of motion. Amputees with scoliosis no longer have the support of the muscles, tendons, nerves, bones and ligaments of their former limbs to give them the baseline they need for stability in walking, standing and everyday tasks. The spine, in turn, can take the brunt of those misalignments. Amputees can develop bad habits in how they walk and stand that exacerbate, rather than correct, scoliosis. Yoga shows amputees how to re-align their spine, use underused muscles and develop strong abdominals to build and support the back.

There are general guidelines for an amputee to follow. First, the side of the body that is not curved needs to be stretched and strengthened. Depending on the severity of the scoliosis, spinal flexes can help balance the less used and more used sides of the body. **Hip opening poses, leg strengthening poses** and **abdominal exercises** help amputees develop solid lower bodies for better gait, so the spine, especially the mid-back, does not take up the slack inappropriately. Alternate nostril breathing helps teach both sides of the lungs to fill up evenly which is very helpful for amputees living with scoliosis.

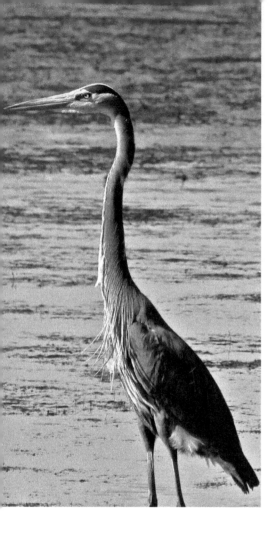

Amputees with prominent scoliosis should avoid backbends, twists, shoulder stand and any neck pressure poses such as fish pose. The spine can become more brittle and truncated in certain areas, therefore more fragile.

Upper extremity amputees **should work on filling up both sides of the lungs** evenly, raising the upper chest underneath the collarbone during breath work, aligning the sitz bones in seated chairs, and massaging the lower belly for grounding.

Below knee amputees should focus on foot placement in each pose for maximum alignment. **Warrior poses, eagle pose, tree, child** and **forward bend** all help amputees with scoliosis.

Above knee amputees should focus on **wide angle poses,** such as seated or standing wide angle, triangle and warrior I pose. **Downward dog** with the prosthetic heels pressed into the wall is also excellent. During pranayama, the shoulder opposite the curvature should be elevated to balance the two sides. For amputees with hemipelvectomies, focusing on bringing the ribs forward from the back can help even out the breath. Swaying the spine from side to side with breath, bending forward halfway and practicing mountain pose restore balance and contribute to a healthy spine.

Yoga practices for amputees living with scoliosis

Practice One

1. Stand, using crutches or a prosthesis. Alternately sit in a chair focusing on the sitz bones.

2. Observe the muscles, joints, spine, breath, position of the head and neck, arm and shoulder position.

3. Now take a step forward. Or slide one sitz bone forward.

4. How do you organize this movement?

5. What do you notice?

6. Come back to your starting position.

7. Write in a journal about your findings. Observe your emotional and physical state.

Practice Two

1. Sit in a chair.

2. Notice the placement of the legs. Alternately notice the placement of the lower back and pubic bone.

3. Observe the hip placement, spine, breath, neck, arms, and shoulders.

4. Now lift the arms up overhead. Or lengthen the sternum and sides of the ribs.

5. How do you organize this movement?

6. What do you notice?

7. Come back to your starting point.

8. Journal. Report any findings, including emotions.

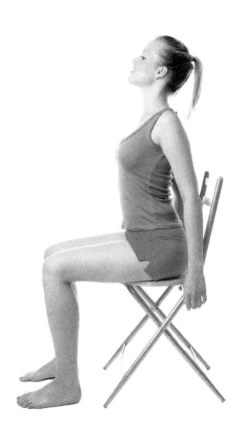

Scoliosis, while it can feel like yet another complication from limb loss, does not have to limit an amputee from living life fully. Introducing yoga into daily life helps amputees with scoliosis thrive even more.

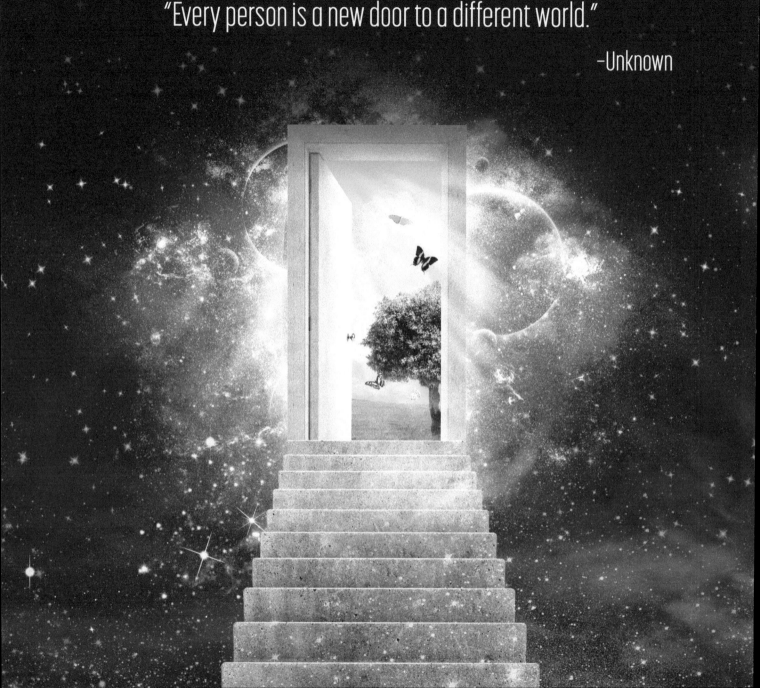

YOGA TO CHANGE
YOUR PERSPECTIVE

CHAPTER
NINE

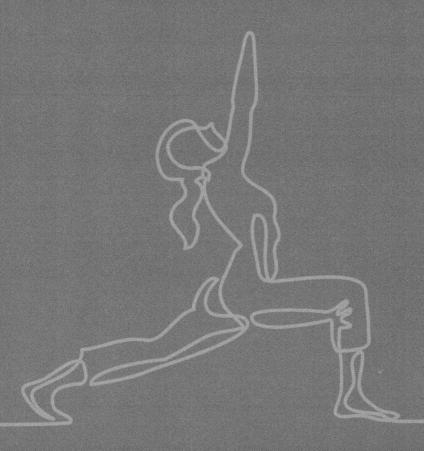

"For the soul there is neither birth nor death. The soul that is will never cease to be. It is unborn, eternal, ever existing, undying and primeval. One's essence does not die when the body dies."

–Bhagavad Gita 2.20

The sacred journey

*What if we **are** our body, and that's okay?*

Most amputees are determined to create a fulfilling life for themselves, no matter the circumstances. I have often heard statements such as "I don't let my amputation define me" and "I am so much more than my amputations." As an amputee, I certainly understand where these statements come from. However, as a yoga and movement therapist, I believe that mindset can hinder us from the full spectrum of our life experience. I would like to offer a different approach.

What if losing a limb DOES indeed define a person? What if ignoring the reality of amputation rather than embracing it fully creates *more*, not less, separation, from our highest selves? If beliefs form our own version of our reality, are amputees who "don't let their amputation define them" doing themselves a disfavor?

Think about it. An amputee must learn a new way of living life. That new way adds layers of personal strength, determination, and body wisdom an amputee may never knew she had before her amputation. Rejecting "the limitation" of the amputation may mean she is pushing away the greatest personal transformation opportunity she could have. Integrated wholeness means embracing everything that is real (amputation and prosthetics) as is and choosing to live a full authentic life deeply connected with oneself and the world.

What if we ARE our body and our thoughts? What if yoga practice for an amputee IS about welcoming what is clearly physically, psychologically and emotionally true?

Many yoga traditions claim that "we are not our body, we are not our thoughts", but I say, as an amputee, our very limb loss represents not only who we are individually, but a microcosm of who we are collectively. What indeed makes a person whole? What makes a society whole?

"Who is it that loves and who that suffers? He alone stages a play with Himself; who exists save Him? The individual suffers because he perceives duality. It is duality which causes all sorrow and grief. Find the One everywhere and in everything and there will be an end to pain and suffering." — *Anandamayi Ma*

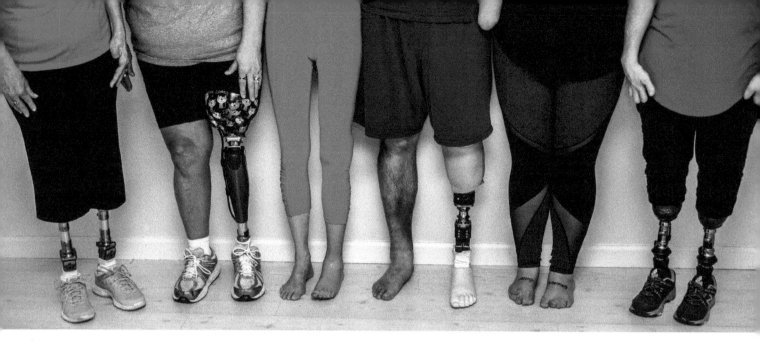

What makes our environment whole? Certainly health, both mental and physical, can present the appearance of wholeness. All of us have known people who seem healthy, but are lacking love, compassion, or any sense of social responsibility. Are they whole? What about the amputee who gets around in a wheelchair? Is she less whole, or does her limb loss give her a deeper purpose and more empathy towards those who struggle?

Take my example. Once I fully acknowledged my prosthetic leg as part of my wholeness, rather than a constant reminder of my limb loss, my yoga practice and my life became more interconnected. I no longer felt alone. My compassion increased one hundred-fold. We are all on our own path to love.

It is time to look differently at the body, particularly for an amputee. This body is the vessel of the spirit, the way that enlightenment shows up - through a body, not outside of it. The material reality of the body is intricately woven into the pranic (or energy) field of every human being which is believed to have its starting point in the akasha, or ethers (according to yogic texts). In other words, everything has its own vibe which is part of the vibratory pulse of the Divine. In quantum mechanics, this would be known as the **zero–point– energy–field.** This energy field is a network of tracks. In yoga, we call these tracks, or circuits, nadis, or rivers. For an amputee, this amazing circuitry gets rewired to adjust to the limb loss. The body is a vessel of divine light. Awaken the circuitry (or energy body) with yoga, and union with all of life happens.

Quantum physics has made the bridge between yogic science and modern science conceivable. In terms of amputation, the physical reality of the limb missing a body and the body missing a limb are the starting point for healing and integration. The missing limb and the body who had it are part of the same energy field.

Quantum physics and indeed many yoga texts, assert that preset reality is illusory, based solely on the brain's perception.

What if the next step to healing is to teach amputees that the road back to oneness is the energetic re-grafting, through yoga, of the "separated" parts, or limbs? The amputated limbs have never been separate at all but are existing in a different energetic form which may be able to someday materialize.

Interestingly, there are new prosthetics being developed controlled by the wearer's thoughts. Researchers are also studying the re-vitalization of cadaveric tissue for organ transplants, thereby re-teaching cellular memory to 'dead' organs. Who knows what future bridge can be forged between yoga and science, or "heaven and earth"?

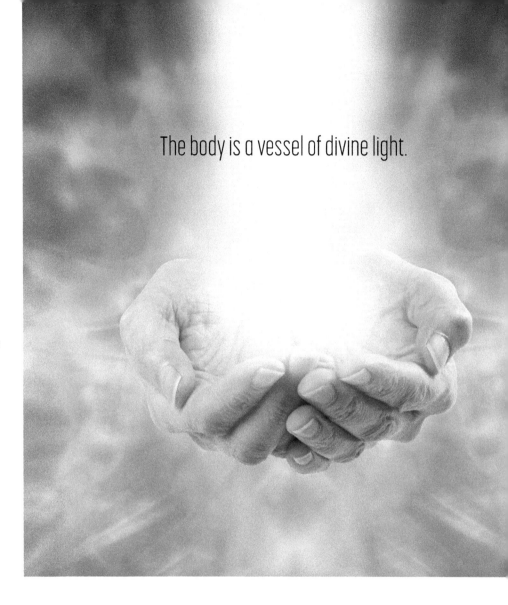

The body is a vessel of divine light.

Everything is energy. When an amputee can recognize that his/her limb or limbs lost a body too, an expansive understanding of healing, compassion and wholeness takes place. Like losing a beloved, the spirit of the beloved doesn't die with death. The memory lives with the living. Consciousness goes way beyond physical reality. It transcends reality, grows beyond the ordinary realms, and brings a yogi to that state of divine union. Acknowledging the limb's loss of its home may reassure the limb and the amputee that their physical separation is only temporary.

While I am no quantum physicist, as an amputee and a yogi, I know that we are ultimately pure consciousness. According to one yogi, "Everything you need to know about the cosmos is right here (here as in the body)." The yogis called that Satchitananda: truth, consciousness, bliss. I call it wholeness.

Yoga as a life path

Yoga sees the body as having many dimensions, the koshas, as discussed in the chapter on pain management. As a reminder, the five koshas are: **Anamaya Kosha** or Body Sheath, the **Pranamaya Kosha** or Breath Sheath, the **Manomaya Kosha** or Mental Sheath, the **Vijnanamaya Kosha** or Intellect Sheath, and the **Anandamaya Kosha** or Bliss Sheath. Understanding these sheaths from a larger spiritual perspective can help an amputee see beyond the loss of the limb to their own wholeness.

The sheaths are like holographic imprints which reflect the make-up of all human beings, in body, mind and spirit. Harmony in one sheath means harmony in all sheaths. The same is true for disharmony. For example, when an amputee increases his flexibility through ongoing yoga practice, he finds that he is more flexible in his attitude towards others and himself.

In review, the **Anamaya** sheath is the gross body sheath, the densest sheath, which includes all physical systems and tissues of the body, such as bone and the skeletal system. The **Pranamaya** sheath or breath sheath is like the battery of the body. Low prana means low energy and poor health. High prana means high energy and good health. The pranamaya kosha holds the body sheath together. Each kosha, or layer, is less dense than the last. The **Manomaya** sheath is the mental or thought body that rules the five senses. Thoughts become things in the manomaya kosha. When we fill our minds with good

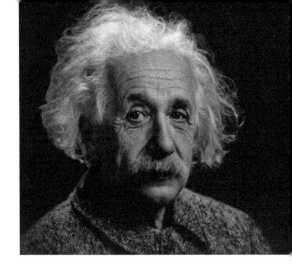

thoughts, our nervous system functions best, releasing necessary feel good hormones to the brain and body. The **Vignamaya** sheath is the intellect sheath. This is the aspect of us that discerns, refines thoughts, operates free will, and acts from a higher state of consciousness. The **Anandamaya,** bliss sheath, represents the mystic in all of us. This is the most thinly layered kosha, blurring the edges between our daily life and our highest selves, or divine nature. The experience of pure bliss encapsulates this body.

Through deep yoga practices, the **anandamaya** or bliss sheath gets awakened regularly, sustained for longer periods of time. The bliss sheath offers us those profound moments of oneness and love with all of life. We have all experienced this, in nature, with orgasm, loving our children, falling in love. For amputees, tapping into all five sheaths reminds us that we are more than just our physical selves. We are as broad and wide as the universe itself.

Yoga teaches us that we are all vibrational beings, held together by sound. When the sound or vibration of the body, mind and spirit is resonant, everything feels good. When the vibration is dissonant, everything feels off. A perfect example is an ultrasound test. If there is an incongruent vibration such as a tumor, the ultrasound machine will pick it up. If all is congruent, the ultrasound will show no problems. When a yogi is vibrating harmoniously, he has a sound body, mind, and spirit, and all the sheaths are in alignment, whether with a limb or without.

How is harmony achieved? With daily yoga practice, whether for five minutes for fifty minutes. Ancient yogis' observations of the world around them as well as their consciousness within led them to the conclusion that SOUND is the generator of all living things, the web and glue that sustains and IS life. To quote Albert Einstein "Everything in life is vibration".

"Everything in life is vibration"
— Albert Einstein

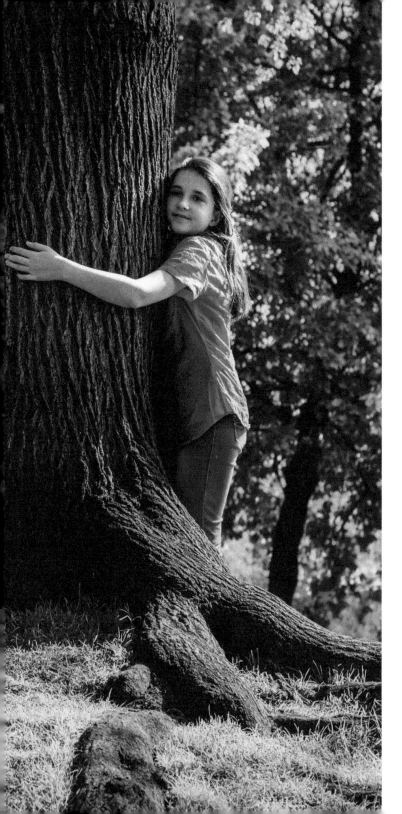

Amputation can often bring an amputee back to their sense of wholeness, where once they lived an incongruent life. The practice of yoga shows amputees that wholeness has nothing to do with whether a limb is missing. Rather it has everything to do with remembering that you are an important part of the web of life. Living harmoniously in body, mind and spirit elevates all of us.

Ultimately, we are all connected. If you think of a tree, everything about the tree's existence is interdependent with everything else. There is no tree without a seed, sun, wind, water, hibernation time, ground, insects and animals to nurture the tree, space and a world where the tree can find roots. Once the tree is full grown, it offers human beings its own oxygen, and in return we feed it with our carbon dioxide. Even if the tree loses limbs, or is simply a stump, it is still a tree. The tree is a constant reminder to every human being that there is no human being without a tree, and vice versa. Everything is part of the collective whole. Nothing is separate.

In quantum physics, when two or more objects have been connected, they influence each other's cells and energetic structure, even when separated by thousands of miles. An amputee may have had his limb amputated, but he will never truly lose his connection with the essence of that limb. It is simply in a different form.

All the connective tissues of a limb provide information for that interrelationship of the body/mind/spirit in the subtlest of ways. For example, bones have a strong connection to the breath, blood and endocrine system because of the production of blood cells through the bone marrow. Blood cells, in turn, nourish the organs necessary for breath, and organs do best when the endocrine system is functioning well. When a limb is amputated, it has lost that vital connection to blood flow and the body has lost its ability to send blood to that limb. However, through the eyes of quantum physics and yoga, the limb is still there, but in a different form. In other words, the limb is never really without its maker.

It has recently been "discovered" that there is an additional type of lymphatic system, or connective tissue system, which swathes the nervous system. This means that for an amputee, practicing deep movement such as yoga, does indeed positively affect the nervous system, and consequently all systems, of the body, mind and spirit. After amputation, nerves, especially, take a hit, due to pain and the confusion of phantom limb sensations. Nerves retrain themselves to adjust to the amputee body they now inhabit. That process adds to an amputee's stress and body image challenges. Nurturing the lymphatic system with yoga has a direct positive impact on an amputee's life, helping him stay connected to this quality of oneness that unifies all life.

Connective tissue bathed in the lymphatic system includes muscles, skin, and joints. Muscles not only allow the movement of the bone, they are also the catalyst for flushing the system of acid buildup. Muscle groups in amputees can atrophy from underuse or build up too much from overuse. Yoga helps amputees balance muscles, taking advantage of smaller deeper muscles to support the health of the system, cleansing the connective tissue of built up acid.

Skin, which is an organ as well as connective tissue, is like a crystalline grid around the body, reflecting the health of the body, holding the container of the body together. An amputee deals with a variety of skin issues, such as skin breakdown, callouses, and scar tissue. Yoga can soften, strengthen and flush the skin of toxic buildup and inflammation.

Joints are cushioned by synovial fluid, a thick viscous substance, which not only supports the movement of the joints, but serves as a boundary protecting the joints. Synovial fluid carries nutrition to the body, including the cartilage. Amputees' joints equally can be over or underused, especially the non-amputated limbs. Supporting and healing the joints is essential to long term prosthetic wear and aging.

Harmony for an amputee involves the physiological balance of the body and its psycho-spiritual balance. Going back to the koshas, or layers of the body, yoga provides the balance. Yoga brings consciousness to the body, mind and spirit of an amputee. Each aspect of yoga is a sound vibration at a different frequency. Yoga postures, breath, withdrawal of senses, focused meditation; devotion, self-inquiry and disciplined commitment all have their own sound.

An amputee is always whole. Any deviation from that truth is simply that; a forgetting. Yoga practice is multi-dimensional. An amputee may begin yoga to get more flexible, stronger, and less stressed. Asana, or posture, and pranayama, or breath, are ways to achieve that. Over time, with frequent yoga practice, the mind and emotions begin to make small but significant shifts in perspective as well. Flexibility, for example, no longer becomes the goal, but a wonderful benefit.

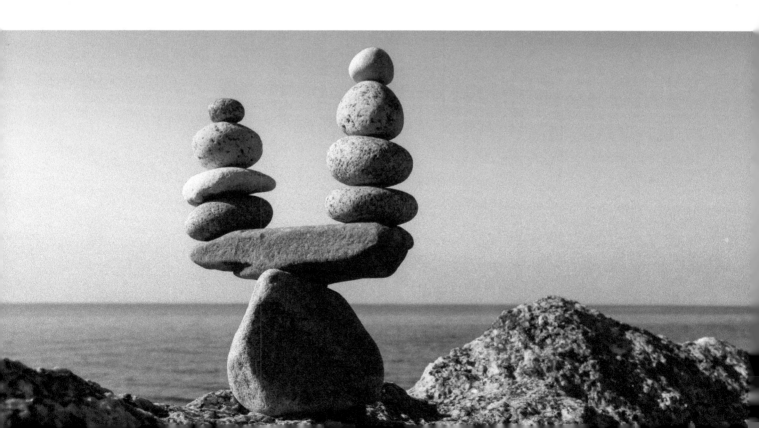

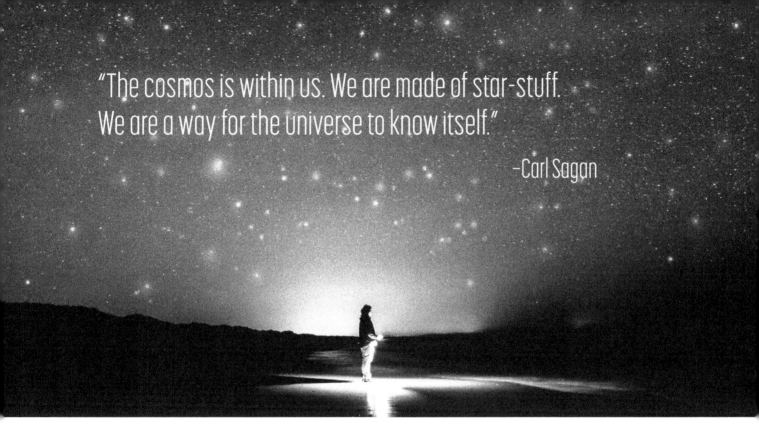

"The cosmos is within us. We are made of star-stuff. We are a way for the universe to know itself."

–Carl Sagan

There are countless stories of amputees becoming motivational speakers, achieving amazing physical feats with or without prosthetic limbs. These are testimonies to the human spirit, and to the awakened potential of a person who has been inside all along. The difference with yoga is, amazing physical feats won't satisfy the long-term yoga practitioner, who finds his only desire is to have no desires, to reside in that place of union with All on a regular basis, the source of divinity itself. Nothing else compares.

Many amputees practice yoga asana. They are beautiful and amazing amputees who have overcome so much. But, what about those amputees digging deeper into their self-realization, bravely getting comfortable with the discomfort of their losses, coming to grips with what wholeness really is in body, mind and spirit? Not every amputee will be able to do an advanced yoga pose, but every amputee is able to connect to the divine within. Consciousness of that essential oneness through the practice of yoga brings about a profound contentment that has nothing to prove or achieve; only known deep down into every cell of the body.

This is yoga.

The limb misses its body: A healing yoga practice

1. Sit comfortably with the eyes closed.

2. Tell yourself "All is well. I am secure. I am surrounded by love and light."

3. Repeat this phrase until you feel relaxed.

4. Bring your attention to your residual limb.

5. Tell your residual limb that you would like to help heal the missing limb that lost its body.

6. Sense body sensations to see if you have permission to do that.

7. If so, continue.

8. Bring your attention to your missing limb.

9. Tell your missing limb "All is well, my love. You are secure. You are surrounded by love and light. "

10. Repeat this phrase as many times as needed.

11. Notice sensations and emotions arising in your body.

12. Are they specific to the residual limb?

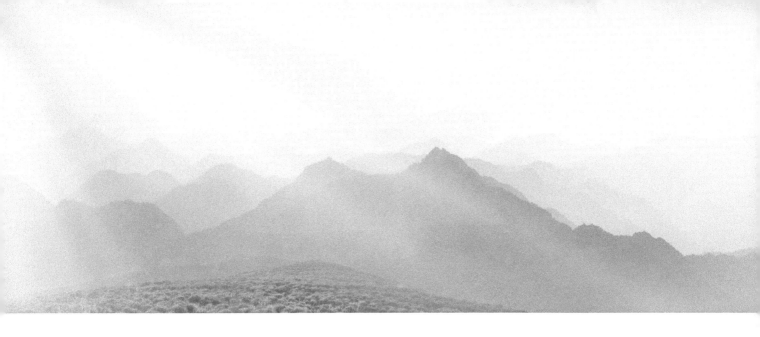

13. Are they moving through the body, or staying in a part of the body?

14. If you feel safe, ask your missing limb if there is anything it would like to tell you.

15. Wait for any messages.

16. Then ask your missing limb if there is anything it would like to hear from you.

17. Wait for any messages.

18. Stay with this process if you like.

19. If it becomes too physically or emotionally painful, stop immediately.

20. Even if stopping immediately, or stopping slowly when ready, thank your missing limb and your body for being so brave.

21. Tell your missing limb and your body "I love you.

22. Let out a sighing breath when your practice is complete.

23. Open your eyes.

24. Journal about what you observed.

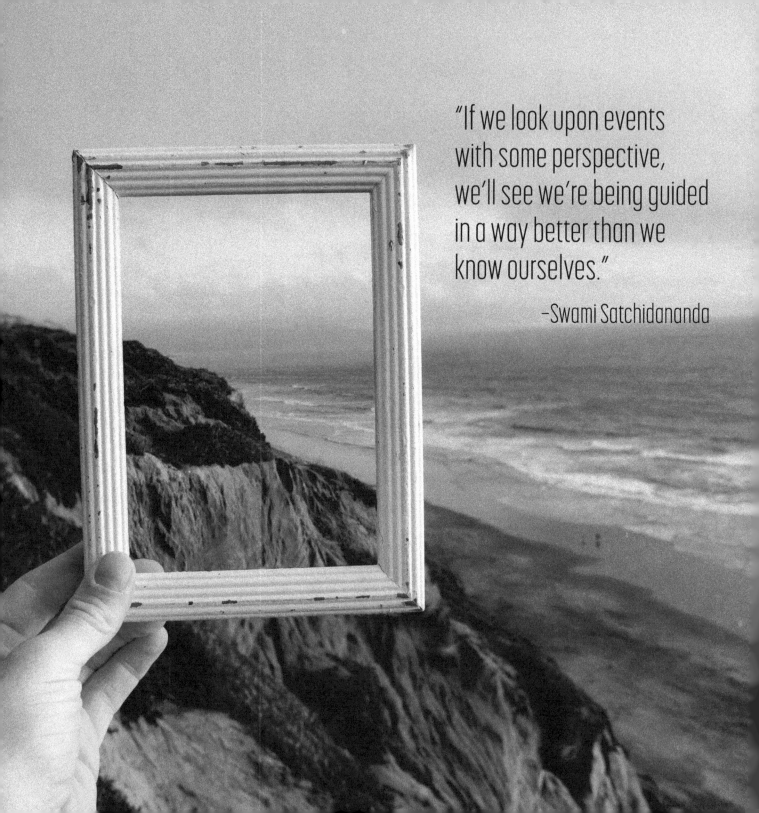

"If we look upon events with some perspective, we'll see we're being guided in a way better than we know ourselves."

–Swami Satchidananda

Yoga to Change Your Perspective

As a younger woman I lived near a beach in California. Some days, at sunrise, when no-one was around, I would sit at the beach to restore my spirit. I had been practicing the art of being open to magical experiences, but I wasn't prepared for the one that came my way one morning. My only companions were some seagulls and the random piece of seaweed. I relished in my spiritual solitude, and my 'get closer to God moments.' Soon, a fellow who I thought was' weird' and 'probably homeless', dressed in scuba gear, complete with flippers and scuba mask, walked right up to me and sat down by my side.

For a moment, I was scared, wondering if he was high on drugs, going to hurt me, or ask me for money. Instead, I decided to put my practice of being open, to work. As it turned out, the man went on early morning dives before his work as the director of a major medical clinic in Los Angeles. Not only did my perceptions change that day, but I ended up volunteering at his clinic and experiencing much emotional healing as I finally dealt with my limb loss and childhood cancer. Magic!

Losing limbs can tarnish or enhance our perception of a purposeful life. The practice of yoga has specific guidelines to help us shift our perspective and gain deeper insight into our vast selves. **Non-attachment** is one such guideline. The **witness self** is the other. Non-attachment is the practice of staying present with every moment as it is, with no expected outcome. This frees us from the confines of our fears, false beliefs and repetitive patterns. The witness self observes one's self in each moment without judgment or expectation.

The following yoga practice is designed to open your mind and spirit to a bigger vision of yourself and your wholeness using the methods of non-attachment and the witness self. Allow yourself to stay in the moment and watch the magic unfold!

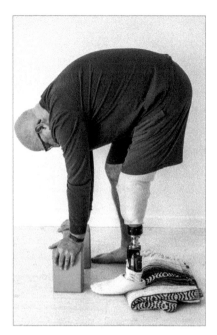

Wide Angle Forward Bend: Upavista Konasana

1. Stand in mountain pose.

2. Step or jump the feet out wide 3 - 3 ½ feet apart.

3. Place the hands at the hips.

4. Breathe in, lengthening the spine.

5. Press into the feet, lifting the arches.

6. Exhale, fold at the hip creases.

7. Reach the palms towards the floor or blocks.

8. Open the inner thighs as you draw the feet towards each other isometrically.

9. Place the hands on the hips as you rise.

10. Come back to mountain.

BK and AK amputees

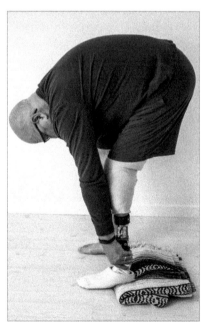

- Do this pose with the back at the wall.

- Stand in front of a chair seat and fold over the edge of chair.

- Loop a yoga strap around both thighs and resist the thighs into the strap.

- Place a rolled towel or the edge of a yoga mat under the prosthetic heel.

- Bend the prosthetic leg if needed for hip evenness.

- Place yoga blocks under the hands.

- Do the pose seated on the floor.

UE amputees

- Hug the shoulder blades in.

- Fold over the edge of a chair with a blanket on top.

- Bend the knees as you fold over to stay secure.

- Place the hand of non-residual limb over the opposite shoulder.

Side Angle: Utthita Parsvokonasana

(See page 146).

Revolved Triangle: Parivritta Trikonasana

1. Stand in mountain pose at the top of the mat.

2. Step the right foot back about three feet, with the right foot turned in towards the center 45 degrees. Your left foot is turned 90 degrees.

3. Keep the knees soft but extended.

4. Lift the right arm to the sky, the upper arm skimming the right ear.

5. Inhale.

6. Elongate forward over the right extended leg with a flat back until the torso is parallel to the floor.

7. Exhale.

8. Place the right hand to the inside or outside of the right ankle.

9. Revolve the belly and torso towards the left.

10. Extend the left arm up to the sky.

11. Turn the head to look up at the left hand.

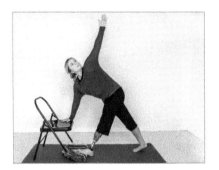

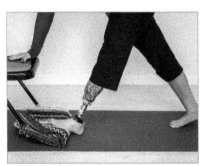

12. Continue to inhale. Lengthen and twist the torso.

13. Exhale. Relax into the twist.

14. When complete, lift the left arm up and arch it back behind you.

15. Press into the feet, hug the belly to the spine and come upright with the torso.

16. Rest both arms to the side.

17. Bend the left knee.

18. Tuck the tailbone and chin.

19. Gently step the right foot forward to meet the left in mountain pose.

20. Repeat on the other side.

BK and AK amputees

• Place a yoga block to the side of the ankle in front. Reach for the yoga block, rather than the floor, with the opposite hand.

• Practice revolved triangle at the wall. To twist to the right side, step the right leg forward, leaning it towards the wall. Twist the torso to the right, placing the hands on the wall.

• Practice revolved triangle in front of the back of a chair. Step forward with the right foot. Bend the torso forward towards the chair, resting the hands on the chair. Place the left hand at the center back of the chair. Turn the torso to the right. Repeat, switching sides.

• Use both a chair and the wall. Stand facing the chair, with the side of the body at the wall, right foot forward, left foot behind. Place the left hand on the center back of the chair, and the right hand at the wall. Repeat on the other side.

- Practice revolved triangle seated in a chair. Sit with the legs closed, feet resting on the floor. Slide the back of the hand to the outside of the right knee. Open the right arm up to the sky. Twist the torso to the right. Repeat to the left.

- Try revolved triangle on the floor. Lie on the back. Slide the left leg across the right upper thigh (when available). Slide the right hand to the outside of the left thigh or left side. Turn the head to the right. Switch sides and repeat.

UE amputee

- Focus on stabilizing the feet and revolving from the lower to mid torso.

- Use a wall. Step the left foot forward and the right foot back three feet. Leaning against a wall with the back of the shoulders, revolve the torso to the left. This opens the chest more. Repeat, switching sides.

Seated Twist: Ardha Matsyendrasana

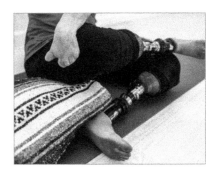

1. Sit with the legs outstretched, spine long, head reaching up to the sky and bottom pressing down into the earth.

2. Flex the feet.

3. Bend the right knee, then place the right foot on the outside left thigh.

4. Wrap the left elbow around the right knee, and then twist from the lower torso to the right, placing the right hand behind on the floor.

5. Allow the head and eyes to twist last.

6. Release from the pose by drawing the belly into the spine and unwind the spine back to center.

7. Repeat on the other side.

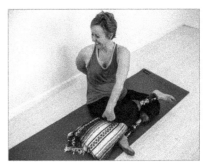

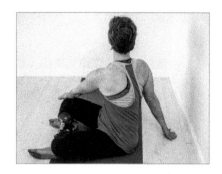

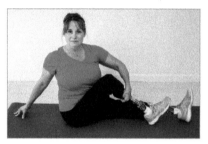

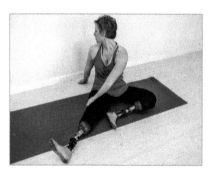

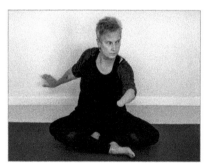

BK and AK amputees

- With prosthesis, bend the knee as much as able, with the option to place the prosthetic foot to the inside of the extended leg.

- Elevate the hips on a yoga block or bolster.

- Sit lengthwise at the wall. Keep the bent knee to the inside of the extended leg, twist to the wall, and press the hands to the wall.

- Sit at the wall with the extended leg pressing into the wall.

- Place the hand that is outside the hip on a block.

- Without the prosthesis, wrap the strap around the residual limb including the bent knee (when possible) to twist.

- Rest the residual limb on the opposite thigh, then twist.

- Keep the residual limb forward (or the prosthetic limb when needed). Rest on a folded blanket to remain even with the extended leg. Place the fingertips or hands on the outside of the extended leg and twist.

UE amputees

- Sit with the back against the wall. Draw the navel to the spine and twist the torso to one side then the other.

- If able to bend the knee and place it on the outside of the extended leg, focus on lifting the sternum and twist.

- If unable to lift the bent knee, slide the foot flat on the floor until parallel with the calf or thigh of the extended leg, then twist the torso.

- Place a folded blanket on top of the thigh of the bent knee and lean into the thigh with the torso as you twist.

Supine Knee Down Twist:
Supta Matsyendrasana

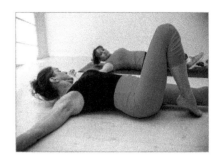

1. Lay with the legs outstretched, spine long, head resting on the floor.

2. Flex your feet. Bend your right knee, and then place your right foot on the outside of your left thigh or the top of your left knee.

3. Extend your arms into a 'T' position.

4. Roll the right knee over to the left while keeping the left buttocks towards the floor.

5. Look toward the right hand.

6. Roll back to the center and reverse sides.

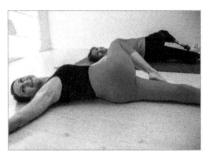

BK and AK amputees

- Place a yoga block underneath the bent knee.

- Press the extended leg (with the prosthesis on) into a wall.

- Roll the body completely over to one side, and hug a yoga bolster, wrapping the residual limb over the bolster when available.

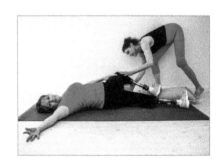

- Lie on the belly with the residual limb turned in one direction, the head turned in the other. Or do the same thing resting the entire torso over a yoga bolster or lengthwise folded blankets.

- With the prosthesis on, press the prosthetic knee, in the twist, into a wall.

- Do the pose seated. Concentrate on twisting the torso in one direction while the head twists in the other direction.

- Do this seated in a chair, crossing the legs where available. Twist in the same direction as the top leg.

- Roll the pelvis to one side, then the other.

- UE amputees

- Roll the pelvis to one side while pressing the center of the shoulders firmly into the ground.

- Roll the head to one side then the other.

- Expand from the center of the heart out as you roll the hips to one side then the other.

- Do this pose seated in a chair, focusing on twisting the torso in one direction while the head goes in the other direction.

Childs: Garbhasana

(See page *195*).

Upward Facing Dog: Urdhva Mukha Svanasana

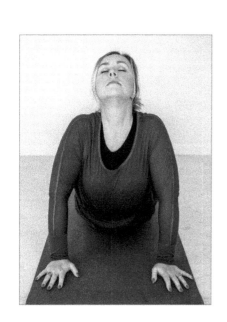

1. Lie on the belly.

2. Place the hands under the shoulders.

3. Firm the thigh bones to the back of the thighs.

4. Broaden the collarbone.

5. Draw the fingers and palms isometrically back towards the ribs to create lift in the spine.

6. Slightly rotate the thighs inward.

7. Tuck the tailbone under slightly.

8. Elongate the belly and draw the chest upwards in an arch.

9. Open the back of the neck.

10. Press into the tops of the toes and lift the legs off the floor.

11. Create space between the ears and shoulders.

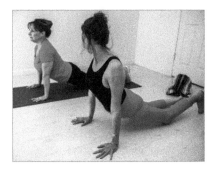

BK and AK amputees

- Place a yoga block under the thighs or knees.

- Wrap a yoga strap around the upper thighs.

- Put a rolled yoga mat or blanket under the thighs or pubic bone.

- Place blocks under the hands.

- Curl the toes under.

- Place a yoga block between the knees or thighs and lean the forehead on a yoga block.

- Press the feet into a wall.

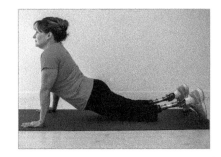

UE Amputees

- Place folded blankets under the residual limb to match the height of the other arm.

- Place a foam roller lengthwise from the sternum towards the top of the mat.

- Lean the side of the torso against a wall to create length.

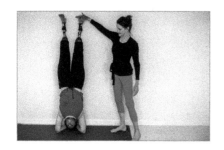

Headstand: Sirsasana

1. Come to all fours.

2. Come down to the forearms, lining the elbows up with the shoulders.

3. Interlock the hands creating a cradle for the crown of the head.

4. Lean the crown of the head into the floor as the knees lift and the feet walk towards the body.

5. Bend the knees if needed and continue to balance on the crown.

6. The legs lift parallel to the shoulders.

7. To come down, bend the knees towards the chest and release the feet to the floor.

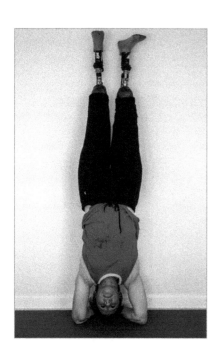

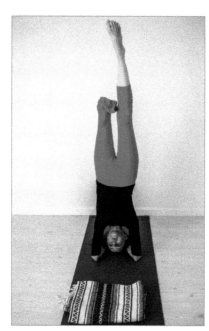

BK and AK amputees

- Do this pose at the wall, so the back-body rests on the wall in the pose.

- Practice this pose without prosthesis.

- Instead of interlocking the hands, bend the elbows placing the hands on the floor towards the front of the body, like a pedestal. Place one shin on each upper arm then lift one leg at a time.

UE amputee

- If fully stable on the crown, place a yoga block under the residual limb and lift.

*** Research is indicating that headstand and other yoga inversions may be counterproductive and unsafe for most adults, especially those with degenerative disks. Please check with your doctor and listen to your body before doing headstand. Use discernment!*

Shoulderstand: Sarvangasana

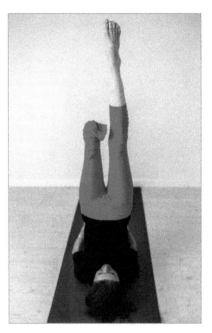

1. Lie on the back, hands to the sides.

2. Bend the knees in to the chest.

3. Support the buttocks and lower back with the hands and roll up onto the midback or upper back.

4. Draw the belly button in and down towards the heart.

5. Keep the thighs glued together.

6. Stretch the legs up to the sky or at a 45-degree angle.

7. Bend the knees to the chest and release.

BK and AK amputees

- Do this pose with the legs resting up the wall, hips flush to the wall.

- Place the legs on the front edge of a chair.

- Rest on the back 2 feet from the wall. Lift the legs with the knees bent so the feet and knees are parallel. Press the feet into the wall.

- Fold a blanket under the upper back to the edge of the neck for extra neck support.

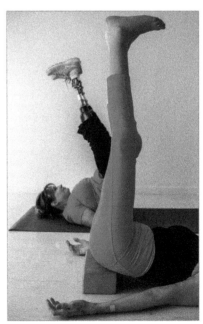

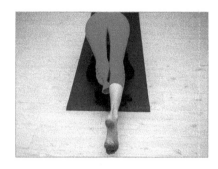

- Loop a strap around the thighs and lift.

- Do a downward dog if too difficult to lift the prosthetic limb.

- Practice reverse crunches until able to lift the lower back off the floor, resting the lower back in the hands.

- Place a yoga block under the lower back while the legs float above.

- Do the pose without prosthesis.

UE amputees

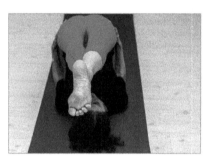

- Develop core strength and stability to be able to lift the legs up to the sky without momentum.

- Do this pose with the legs to the wall.

- Rest the upper back over a folded blanket.

- Place a blanket under the residual limb for balanced shoulders.

Pigeon: Kapotasana

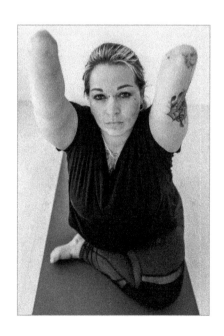

1. Start in downward facing dog or table pose, on all fours.

2. 2Lift the right leg up behind you.

3. Bend the right knee, drawing it close to the chest and right shoulder and press forward into a modified plank pose.

4. Keep lifting through the abdominals and gently place the outside of the right knee to the floor, near the right hand, and the outside of the right foot at the left hip.

5. Balance the hips, keeping both hip bones facing forward and extend the left leg behind, the top of the left thigh and shin resting on the floor.

6. The torso faces forward.

7. Press into the floor and lengthen from the pubic bone to the upper chest, creating a small backbend.

8. Alternately fold the torso forward over the front bent right knee, hands resting one on top of the other under the forehead.

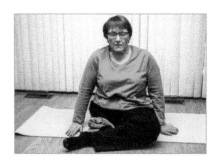

BK and AK amputees

- If unable to bend the knee, lift the prosthesis, or rest the outside of the knee on the floor, try a lunge on the edge of a chair, or come onto the back for a modified pigeon pose.

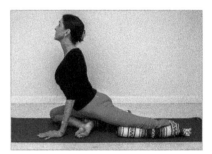

- To do pigeon pose on the back, place the left foot on the floor, with the left knee bent. Lift the right leg up, bend the right knee and turn the right hip out to the right. Cradle the right knee with the right hand. Lift the right knee, letting it rest in a yoga strap or place the outer edge of the right foot on top of the left thigh. If the foot on the floor is slipping, do this pose against a wall, pressing the left foot into the wall. Switch sides.

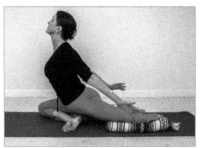

- Alternately, with the right hip at the wall, lie to the side of the wall. Lift the right knee and press it into the wall, creating a hip opener in the inner right hip. (Thank you Larisa) Switch sides.

- Sit in a chair, feet hip width apart. Lift the right foot off the floor, turn the right hip out to the right and rest the outer right foot on top of the left thigh.

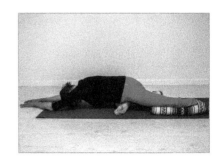

- If doing pigeon without prosthesis, use pillows or folded blankets to prop up the residual limb, either under the extended leg or the hip. The main objectives are to keep the hips square, create a slight backbend and open the hips and groin.

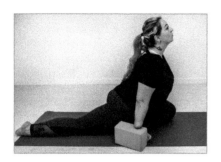

UE amputee

- If able, do downward dog with one arm and proceed as above. This requires tremendous skill and strength to keep the torso balanced.

- Try pigeon from table pose. Slide the right knee forward and through. When finished with the right, change to the left.

- Do the pose on the edge of a chair, a modified lunge with more hip turnout in the front hip.

- Do pigeon pose in a chair as described above for AK/BK amputees.

- Sit on the floor with the legs extended. Come into half lotus on the right, extending the left leg out and letting the outside of the right foot rest on top of the left thigh as the right hip opens. A pillow or folded blanket may be needed underneath the knee. Switch sides.

Seated Forward Bend: Paschimottanasana

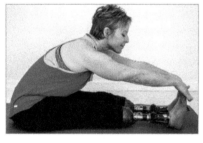

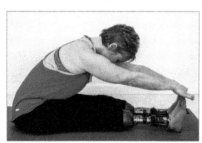

1. Start in Dandasana (legs extended in front, feet flexed).

2. Roll the sitz bones diagonally back by pulling the buttocks flesh out and to the sides.

3. Lift the arms up overhead, parallel to the shoulders, reaching through the fingertips.

4. Roll the hips forward.

5. Inhale. Lengthen the spine.

6. Exhale drop forward keeping the spine aligned without rounding the shoulders.

7. When feeling the 'edge' of sensation, release the hands to the toes, shins, or thighs.

8. Draw the collarbone open as the shoulders drop.

9. Reach down into the sitz bones.

BK and AK amputees

- Wrap a strap around the feet as you bend forward to keep the spine lengthened.

- Press feet against a wall.

- Roll a yoga mat under the edge of the buttocks (closest to thighs) to tilt the pelvis more.

- Place a yoga block between the legs so the head can rest on it when forward.

- Straddle a chair and allow the head to rest on the chair.

- Place the hands on the side of the hips, pressing into the fingertips to move forward.

- Place a folded blanket lengthwise under the prosthetic limb.

- Do the pose at the edge of a chair, feet pressing into a wall.

UE amputees

- Sit against a wall and lean forward.

- Place folded blankets and a bolster under the torso.

- Place a yoga strap around the feet, and then grab hold of the strap with the remaining limb, pulling the strap toward the center and bend forward.

Head to Knee Pose: Janu Sirsasana

(See page *193*).

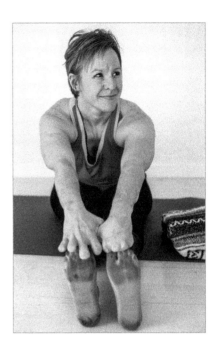

Perspective invites us to see our world both closely and far away. The present moment practices of yoga, combined with its eternal principles, remind amputees to live from a larger viewpoint, and yet find magic in the tiniest moment.

MEET JENNY

Jenny is a deeply spiritual woman who has used many holistic tools, including yoga, to enrich her life. Jenny was born with a congenital limb difference in her left hand. As a child, finger buds were surgically removed, keeping the rest of the limb intact. Amniotic bands caused her limb difference. Amniotic bands are vascular constrictions around developing fetuses, usually limbs. Jenny was a passionately dedicated English high school teacher until her early retirement, when she was diagnosed with ovarian cancer. While her cancer returned a few times, she is now doing well. She wears a cosmetic suction prosthetic while in public but never at home. She functions better without her prosthetic.

For Jenny, being yoked in mind, body and spirit is wholeness. She feels her spirit in church, her body when she runs and her mind when she reads. Wholeness, she believes, is maintaining a core sense of self, at peace within and without, even if life is challenging. Cancer brought Jenny back to who she really is in her depth of being. She draws on her practices of Qigong, yoga, creative visualization, her service to a women's cancer support network and her grandchildren to stay whole.

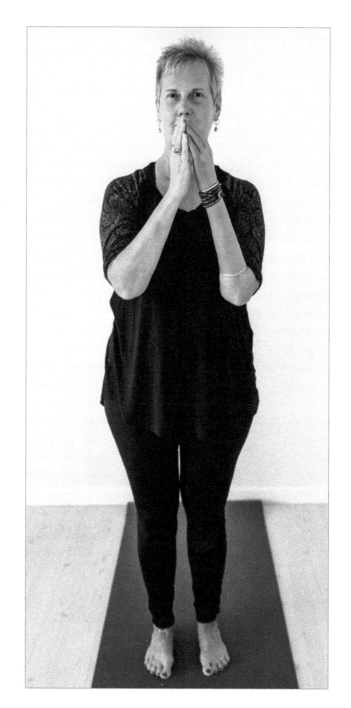

Living with a limb difference has taught Jenny a lot over the years. While her mother, a strong, determined career woman in a generation when most women didn't work, saw no difference in Jenny, Jenny still had questions. Jenny recalls asking her mother once "What's it like to have two hands? ". "Well Jenny "replied her mother "What's it like to have one hand?" Jenny's mother pushed for insurance to cover a cosmetic prosthesis. Her mother wrote to the government, at a time when only prosthetic hooks were used. Her mother wanted to give Jenny a chance to be seen for who she is, not for her limb difference. Her parents nurtured Jenny to be independent and self-sufficient, believing that something good would come out of her limb difference. Indeed, much good has come from Jenny's journey. Jenny has great empathy for people who otherwise might be discounted or discriminated against.

Yoga has been an anchor for her over the years. Offering her peace, fullness, wholeness and even tears when necessary, yoga is both cathartic and uplifting. When she went through ovarian cancer, it was yoga that allowed her grief to release. Yoga isn't just about the physical for her. As Jenny puts it "If I had just been working from the body, I would fall to pieces. When the body rests in the mind and spirit, then you can deal with any news." Yoga reminds Jenny that she is not just her body but so much more.

Even with all that awareness, it has taken Jenny a long time to show up in a short sleeve top. Her cancer journey gave her the courage to be seen as she is. Her presence in this book is a testimony to how far she has come.

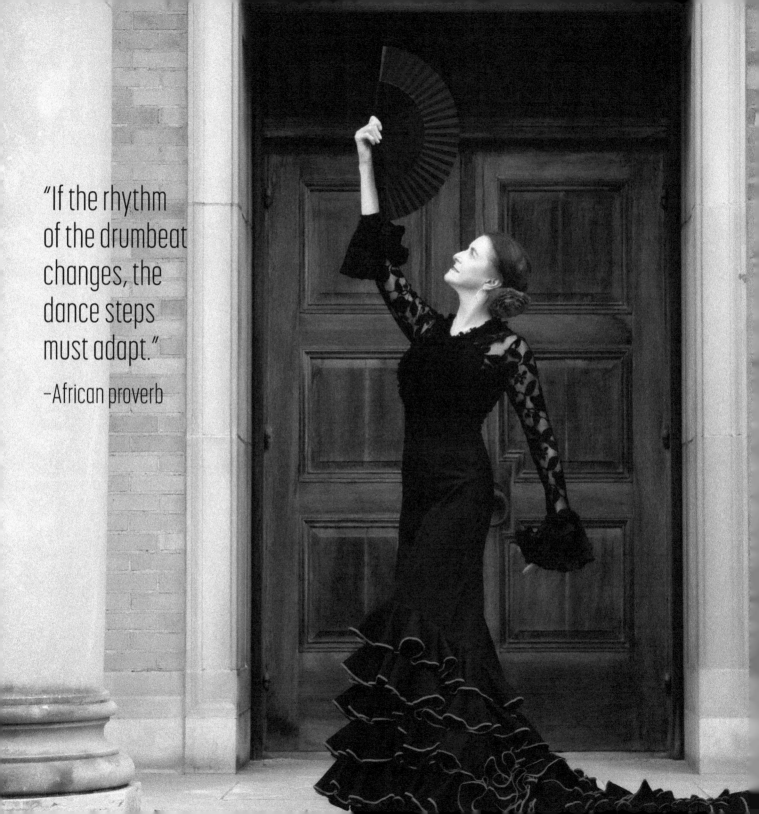

"If the rhythm of the drumbeat changes, the dance steps must adapt."

–African proverb

CHAPTER TEN | YOGA FOR THE REST OF YOUR LIFE

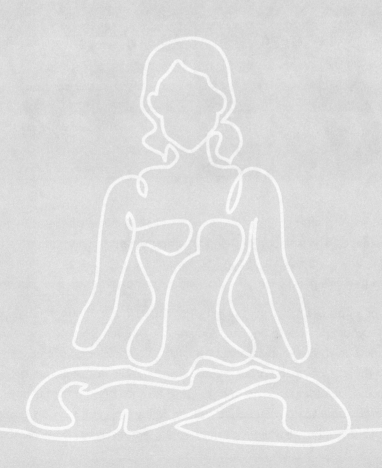

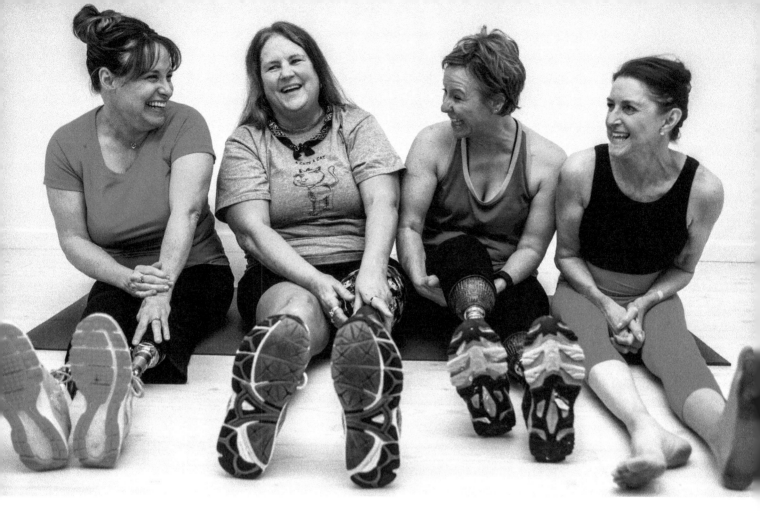

Many amputees leave the hospital after amputation, unaware of all that is available to them, from support groups, to grants for prosthetics. The isolation of being an amputee among non-amputee family members and friends can be overwhelming. As much as those who love us try their best to understand, no-one can "get" us like a fellow amputee. We need each other to validate our experience and give us hope.

A yoga class exclusively for amputees has many benefits, not found in a traditional public yoga class. First, there is no need to explain your limb loss to anyone. You are who you are, your group is there to get you through the tough times and celebrate your victories. You also gain knowledge such as the best prosthetic socks, what to wear when there is ice on the ground, and how to handle invasive staring. Seeing another amputee standing, balancing, or folding forward in a standing forward bend provides hope for the amputee who wonders if he will ever be able to do what he did before. Many amputee support groups are branching out to include more physical activities, all while allowing pent up emotions to be released and accepted.

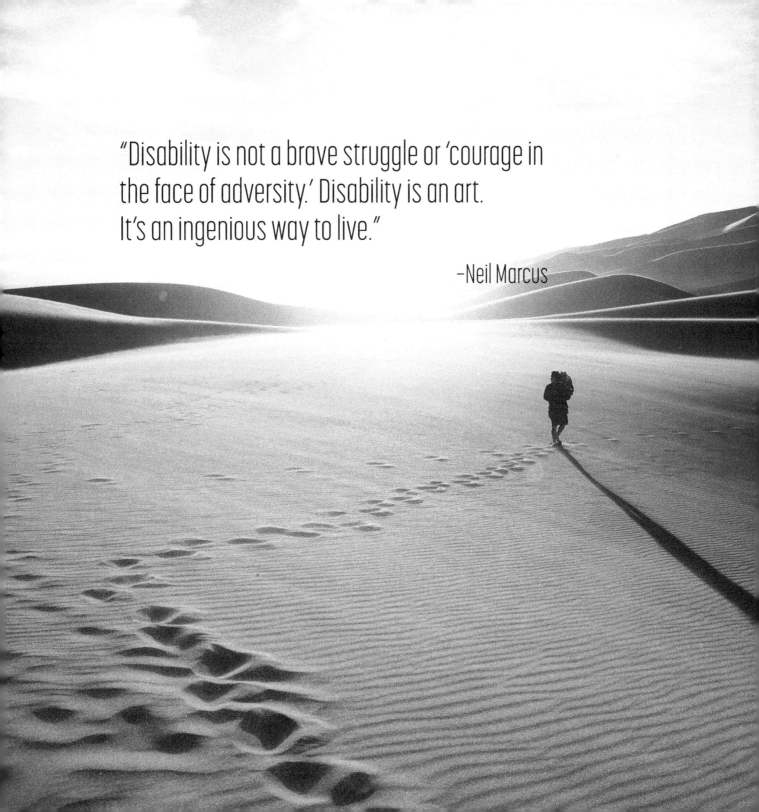

"Disability is not a brave struggle or 'courage in the face of adversity.' Disability is an art. It's an ingenious way to live."

–Neil Marcus

I was gonna buy artificial limbs, but they would cost me an arm and a leg.

"Forgiveness is the fragrance the violet sheds on the heel that has crushed It" — attributed to Mark Twain

Humor is an important aspect of an amputee yogi class. All amputees have been subject to comments like "It's too bad. You're so pretty/ handsome." "You are so brave to wear your bathing suit at the beach" and a personal favorite" I don't think I could handle it. I would want to kill myself." Laughter certainly empowers us to better handle those awkward moments we, as amputees, often face.

Forgiveness is another facet of a yoga class for amputees. Many amputees have trouble forgiving themselves, their bodies, their families or their situation. Emotional hurt lingers, feeding our sympathetic nervous system, and keeping us stressed. Ahimsa, or loving compassion, shows us how to be kind to ourselves and our bodies, which reduces hurt feelings and lowers our stress. We are not obliged to forgive ourselves and our amputation, but we do have the power to become disentangled from the hold unforgiveness has on our lives. Sometimes, "letting it go" is too much work. Letting it be may be the most compassionate response to our suffering. Compassion for the process of healing, self-acceptance, our circumstances and our weaknesses can be better supported among amputee peers. It all starts with a breath.

Become your own warrior. To live your best life as an amputee, you must constantly advocate on your own behalf. A team of fellow amputee warriors is powerful. When one falls, another can pick him up. In preparation for the group practice described below, transform yourself into your own warrior, who will do what it takes to live a life of abundance.

Warrior II: Virabhadrasana II

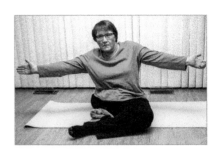

1. Stand sideways in Tadasana in the center of the mat.

2. Step the feet wide 3 ½ feet.

3. Open the arms wide.

4. Turn the right foot straight ahead

5. Turn the left in about 15 degrees. The left foot will follow.

6. Bend the right knee to a 90-degree angle, knee parallel to the ankle.

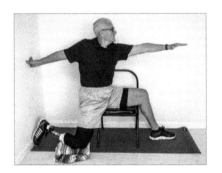

7. Line up shoulders and hips.

8. Arms are in line with the shoulders, palms down.

9. Gaze over the right fingertips.

10. Reverse sides.

BK and AK amputees

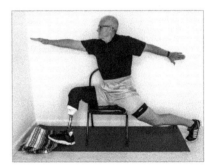

- Do this pose with the back to the wall.

- Rest the front bent knee over the chair with added support under the front foot if needed.

- Press the back heel into the wall.

- Practice sitting at the edge of a chair, turning sideways.

- Place yoga blocks under the extended back leg thigh or knee.

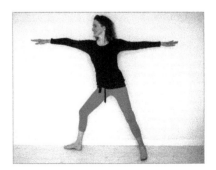

- Wrap a strap around the thigh of the front leg and lift the strap up as the thigh resists down.

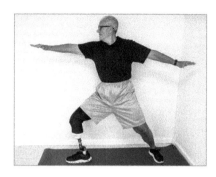

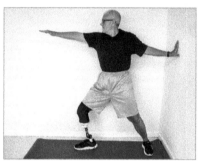

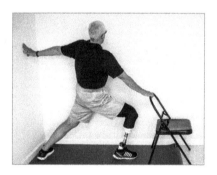

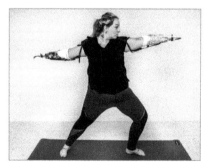

- Stand 3 feet from the wall, step forward, lean the bent knee into the wall and press the fingertips of the front hand into the wall. Reverse facing away from the wall, pressing fingertips into wall for stability.

- Loop the strap around the lower shins and step out wide.

- Do this pose in front of the back of a chair, holding onto the edge.

UE amputees

- Do this pose against a wall to feel the shoulders opening.

- If unable to lift the residual limb, rest it by the side and lift the armpits.

- Lift in and up from the lower belly to the crown of the head.

- Expand from the center of the chest.

The group practice below is designed exclusively for amputees. Adaptations are found in earlier chapters. Set up the class by placing chairs in a semi-circle so everyone feels seen and connected to the entire group. Students can alternate between standing and seated. Some students will be able to get to the floor in seated poses, while others will need to stay in a chair.

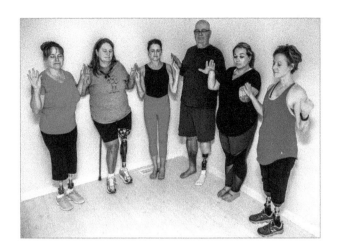

Group meditation on wholeness

- Turn to the person on your left and tell them "You are whole and full of possibility."

- Follow with Namaste, bowing to each other.

CENTERING

- Each person in the circle presses palms into her neighbor's palms. If the neighbor is without arms but is wearing a prosthetic arm, press the palm into the prosthetic hand. If the arm amputee is not wearing a prosthesis, place a yoga strap around the lower ribs, and have the neighbor gently hold the end of the yoga strap.

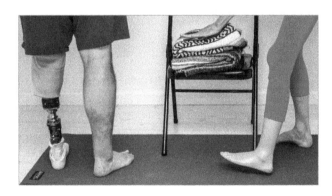

- Close the eyes.

- Imagine sending the breath from person to person.

- Inhale as if inhaling through the left side of the body.

- Exhale as if exhaling through the right side of the body.

- Allow this breath chain to circulate 3-5 times.

- Finish with the first person in the chain coming into Namaste, with or without hands, by taking a bow towards the heart.

WARM UPS

- Six movements of the spine.

POSES

Seated or Standing Mountain

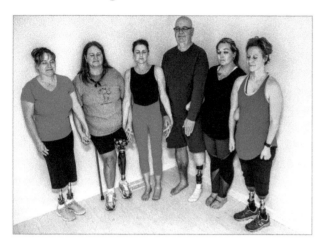

Seated or Standing Warrior II

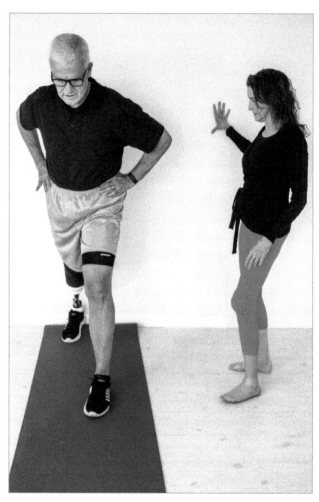

Seated or Standing Tree

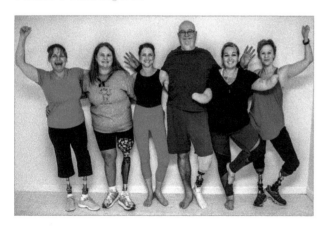

Seated or Standing Goddess

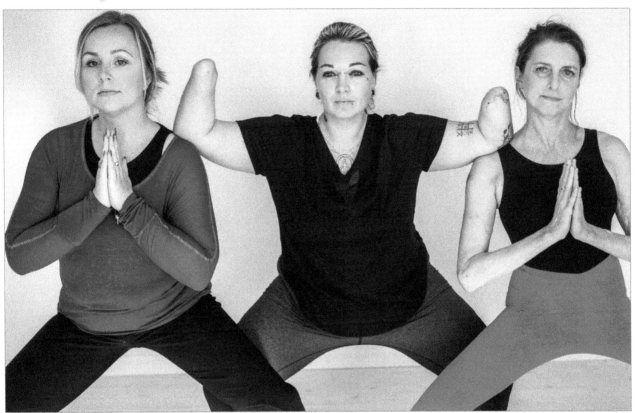

Seated or Standing Downward Dog

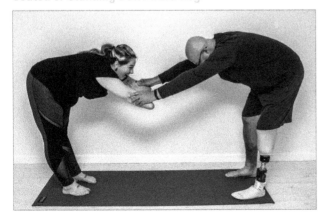

Plank or Seated Mountain

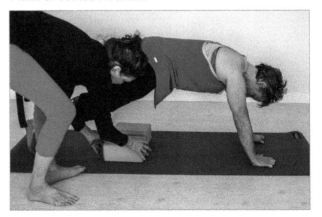

Seated Staff in Chair or on the Floor

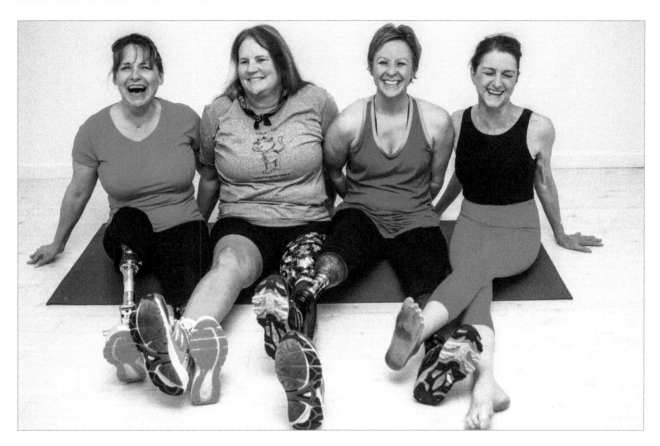

Seated or Prone Cobra

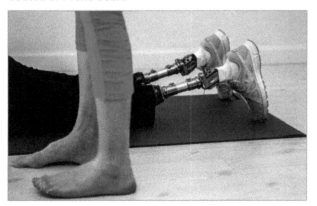

Easy Sitting Pose

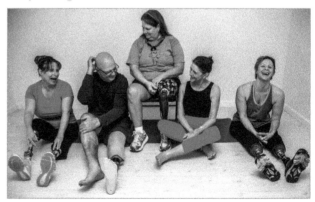

- When relaxation pose is completed, come back to a seated position on the floor or in a chair.

- Close the class with 3 rounds of 'Om'.

- Namaste to everyone in the class.

- Allow time for socializing.

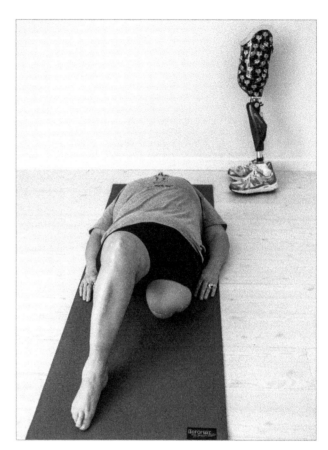

Adapting to our bodies as amputees is a lifelong process. Our bodies change, our age changes, and in some cases, our finances or health change. With each new change along the way, yoga can make life easier.

Accompanying yoga is **Ayurveda,** the science of life, which improves quality of life for amputee yogis. Each of us has a primary constitution of air, water or fire, that directs our actions and reactions. These constitutions, known as **doshas,** influence us at different periods of life.

At the beginning of life's journey, we are in the **Kapha (water)** phase. From infancy to age 21, we experience tremendous tissue growth and mental /emotional development. This time of our lives requires vigorous exercise, plenty of sleep, calming foods and warmth. Yoga practice must light a fire "under our feet" and keep us focused, as we can easily be distracted by the incredible world around us. Creating harmony rather than drama sustains a growing person in the kapha years.

Our middle years, from 21 to 65, are known as the **Pitta (fire)** years. During this time, we build careers, families, work long hours, accomplish goals and make money. We need high intensity workouts, including yoga, physical and mental challenges, spicy foods, and expansive foods, like lettuce and kale. We also need a schedule to keep from burning out.

The later years, from 65 onward, are the **Vata (wind)** years. Daily rituals at specific times help to tame the excess air in the body, which causes dry skin, brittle bones and fear of the future. Rest is essential, with early sleep times

"Life is a promise. Fulfill it." —
Mother Theresa

and early rising times, to accommodate the varying waves of energy available throughout the day. More fats are needed, along with calming soups and root vegetables. Vata time is slowing down time.

Each stage of an amputee yogi's life will be reflected in her practice. By following this natural rhythm of the doshas, she can maintain good health into her later years, while respecting the needs within each stage of her life. Therefore, a Vinyasa practice is excellent for someone in their middle years, while a restorative practice nurtures a person in later years.

It IS possible to have a beautiful, long life as an amputee. A healthy daily routine that includes meditation, pranayama and asana keeps the body and mind vibrant. Resting is essential for high metabolism, good skin and mental clarity. Make sure you have a solid social life and support network which positively affects your mood as well as the strength of your heart. Practice self-care by nurturing your body with clean, unprocessed foods and good thoughts. Honor your difficult emotions but choose to have a good day anyway. Take risks. This keeps your life fresh and interesting. Stay active every day: movement is vital to our wellbeing. Set your mind to what you do want, rather than what you don't want. Keep your preventative care up to date. And finally, laugh often and deeply. Laughter boosts your immune system and reduces stress.

Let yoga be a focal point of your day. You will see and know the benefits immediately. You are worthy of a fulfilling life. As Mother Theresa said "Life is a promise. Fulfill it."

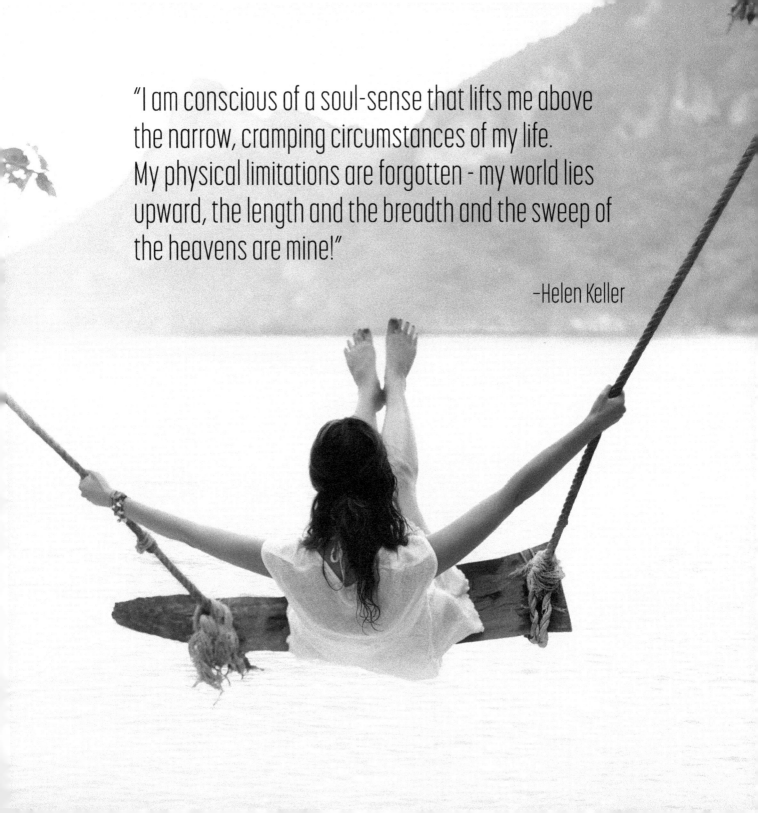

"I am conscious of a soul-sense that lifts me above the narrow, cramping circumstances of my life. My physical limitations are forgotten - my world lies upward, the length and the breadth and the sweep of the heavens are mine!"

–Helen Keller

AFTERWORD

Having shared this journey of yoga for amputees with you, my hope is that you can see how much yoga can make your life better. The more you practice, the more you benefit. The deep healing experiences that yoga offers shape your destiny to be one of fulfillment, and personal wholeness. Each time you come to the yoga mat, you can witness your own divine essence, reminding yourself that you are much more than the sum of your parts.

I myself revisited my yoga practice more intensely in writing this book. I was reminded once again that yoga makes everything new, challenging me to see beyond my perceived limits and reacquaint myself with my endless possibilities.

This realization has been important for me at this stage of my life. With new challenges, a move across the country, and a major shift in my career, I was once again a complete beginner. The rewards have far outweighed the losses. As I dug deep into my life through yoga, memories and dreams flooded in. People from my past, some I hadn't heard from in forty plus years, began to show up. Staying open to the new, something yoga has taught me repeatedly, paved the way for exciting opportunities. One such opportunity was the chance to teach yoga at a national amputee convention.

As I walked around the convention, I was surrounded by people like me, people who had lost one, two, three and even four limbs, all coming together to collaborate, inspire, support and learn from each other. It was very empowering to be among this tribe of amputees, rather than being the lone wolf in a crowd of yogis. I didn't have to explain my limb loss. Most people didn't even notice my prosthetic leg. The attendees were positive and encouraging. They knew, like I did, what it takes to move forward after amputation.

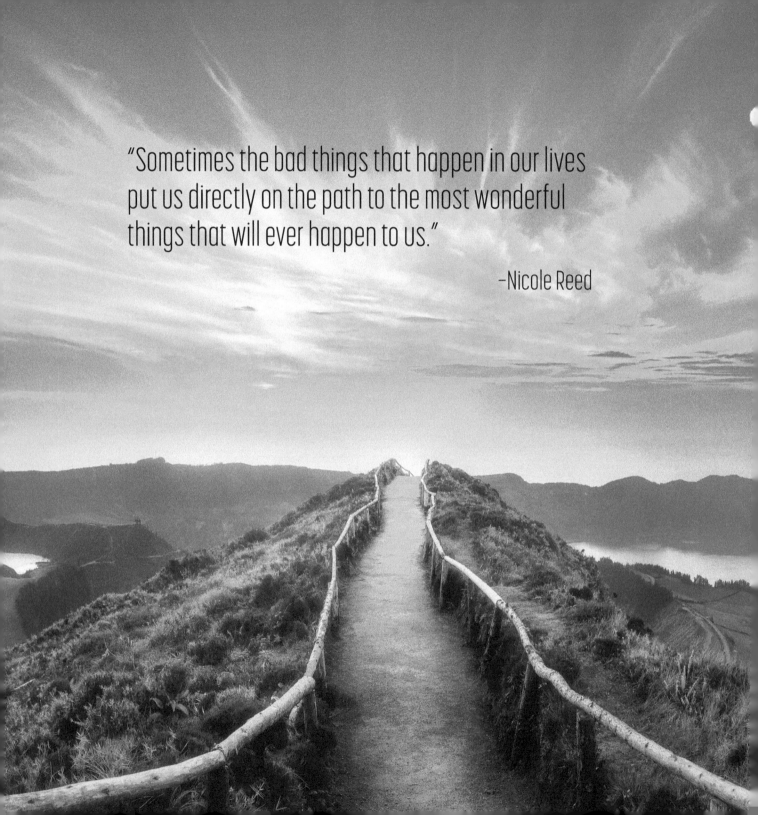

"Sometimes the bad things that happen in our lives put us directly on the path to the most wonderful things that will ever happen to us."

–Nicole Reed

"Blackbird singing in
the dead of night
Take these broken wings
and learn to fly
All your life
You were only waiting
for this moment to arise."
— John Lennon
and Paul McCartney

One morning while at the conference, I taught yoga to a rather large group of amputees. For the average yoga teacher, that alone would have been demanding. Each student was so unique, from those who moved quite well to those who struggled to get from the door to a seat in the room.

An adorable woman wheeled herself in to the class. She was not wearing a prosthesis. Her delight was infectious. Without any help, she determinedly lifted her heavy body off the chair and found her way to the floor. She had never done that before. Her determination to practice yoga with the group overrode any perceived limits. I believe she tapped into her divine essence, the part of her soul that knows who she is and knows what she can do.

Yoga is like that. As we drop our fears and listen to the deeper truth of our wholeness, we break through our limits. 'Lead me from the unreal to the real'. The truth is that we as amputees are always whole. May you know and experience this divine wholeness emanating from your entire being in every moment. Namaste.

Love, Marsha

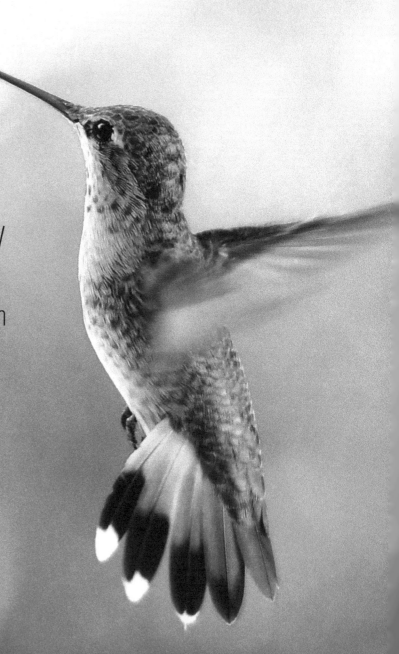

"Today I choose life. Every morning when I wake up I can choose joy, happiness, negativity, pain... To feel the freedom that comes from being able to continue to make mistakes and choices - today I choose to feel life, not to deny my humanity but embrace it."

–Kevyn Aucoin

YOGA SOLUTIONS

Practice for diabetes

Ujjayi breath, childs, hero, seated forward bend, seated sage, cow, bridge, legs up the wall, supine twist, childs, downward facing dog, standing forward bend big toe hold, childs, fish, relaxation.

Practice for heart disease

Dirgha breath, easy sitting pose, butterfly, lunge, mountain, chair, warrior II, triangle, standing spinal twist, hero, cobra, wind relieving pose, relaxation.

Practice for scar tissue

Easy sitting pose, hissing breath, cat/cow, seated spinal twist, wind relieving series, relaxation.

Practice for sciatica

Supine leg extension with strap, staff, seated twist, half cow, knee to chest, standing twist, standing leg extension with strap, warrior II.

Practice for pain reduction

Sighing breath, nadi shodana, joint freeing series, 6 movements of the spine, spinal twist, cobra, butterfly, childs, relaxation.

Practice for strength

Ha breath, root lock, mountain, warrior II & III, triangle, big toe hold standing forward bend, crow, boat, hero, relaxation.

Practice for depression

Rajasic-nadi shodhana, ujjayi, childs pose, locust, standing forward bend, headstand. Tamasic-ujjayi, breath of fire, cobra, camel, fish, headstand

Practice for core

Ujjayi breath, breath of fire, butterfly pose, seated twist, cobra, locust, downward dog, plank, upward dog, four limbed pose, childs, supine twist, abdominal crunches, relaxation.

AK/BK gentle practice

Centering, dirgha pranayama ,cat/cow, downward dog, mountain pose, half moon, seated twist, sphinx, locust, knees to chest, relaxation.
Upper Extremity Yoga Practice Centering, dirgha pranayama, neck rolls, shoulder circles, seated twist, bridge, knees to chest, mountain, warrior I, warrior II, five-pointed star, chair, supine leg lifts, relaxation.

Stress reduction

Centering, sighing breath, spinal twist, cat /cow pose, half moon, relaxation.

PTSD yoga practice

Full body scan, sun breath, easy sitting pose with eyes open, staff, twist.

Athlete amputee practice

Centering, dirgha breath, six movements of the spine , mountain, warrior I, warrior II, side angle, chair, standing forward bend, salutation to the sun, crow, side crow, plank, four limbed, cobra, childs, relaxation.

BENEFITS AND CONTRAINDICATIONS

Pranayama

Alternate Nostril Breath : Nadi Shodhana

Benefits: Nadi means channel and Shodhana means cleansing. This breath restores balance to the body, stimulating alternate sides of the brain. It is very calming, soft, and extremely gentle. Nadi Shodhana is very helpful in reducing anxiety.

Contraindications: Sinus infection, recent rhinoplasty

Belly breath

Benefits: Belly breath familiarizes practitioners with long deep breaths. This breath oxygenates the farthest reaches of the lungs. It calms and soothes the mind and introduces deep breathing. It is very meditative.

Contraindications: Recent abdominal surgery, Herniated disc, recent back surgery

Breath of Fire (Kapalabhati)

Benefits: Moves toxins out quickly. Clears the brain. Clears sinuses. Flushes the organs. Tones the abdominal muscles. Strengthens the lower back. Develops core strength.

Contraindications: Detached retina, recent abdominal surgery, vertigo, high blood pressure, neck injury, anxiety disorder.

Breath of JOY   **Benefits:** Expands the lungs. Moves trapped energy in the body. Increases oxygen. Uplifts the spirit.

Contraindications: Detached retina, shoulder injury, neck injury, TMJ, high blood pressure, vertigo

Ocean (Ujjayi) breath   **Benefits:** Ujjayi breath warms the body, focuses the mind and helps to deepen yoga postures. The constriction of the throat heats the air coming in, increasing circulation, digestion.

Contraindications: Sinusitis, claustrophobia, neck injury, vertigo, tracheotomy

Dirgha and Ujjayi breath can be combined.

Sun Breath   **Benefits:** This breath prepares you for warm-ups and is an excellent to way stretch the side body, expanding lung capacity and opening the intercostal muscles.

Contraindications: Shoulder injury, unmedicated high blood pressure (do not lift arms above shoulder)

Three Part (Dirgha) Breath   **Benefits:** Three-part breath teaches you to breathe deeply in to your diaphragm. It cleanses the lungs of stale air and uses all three parts of the lungs.

Contraindications: Recent abdominal surgery or injury

Asana

Boat

Benefits: Strengthens core abdominal muscles, stretches hamstrings, strengthens lower back, strengthens and stretches spine, improves digestion, tones abdominal organs, improves posture, stretches arches and toes, improves balance.

Contraindications: Pregnancy, low back injury, recent abdominal surgery or inflammation, low blood pressure, neck pain (practice with upper shoulders to the wall).

Bound Angle

Benefits: Opens hips, tones ovaries , kidneys, bladder, supports healthy menses, can help ease labor, stretches hamstrings and inner thighs, elevates mood, lengthens spine, tones abdominals, increases blood flow to pelvic region, strengthens lower back, relieves sciatica.

Contraindications: Groin injury, knee injury, sexual trauma (proceed with caution), do not practice post-partum or with a prolapsed uterus, neck injuries, serious back injuries, recent shoulder injury.

Bridge

Benefits: Strengthens legs, strengthens ankles, opens chest, increases spinal flexibility, regulates thyroid, tones kidneys, stretches front of body, reduces fatigue, and regulates kidneys.

Contraindications: Shoulder or back injury, knee injury, neck injury, wrist injury, unmedicated high blood pressure.

Camel

Benefits: Helps correct posture, increases lung capacity, improves blood circulation to all organs of the body, tones back and spinal muscles, removes stiffness in shoulders, back and ankles, relieves abdominal cramps, regulates menstruation, opens the throat.

Contraindications: Constipation, diarrhea, headache, migraine, hypertension, recent heart attack, lower back injury, knee injury, spinal injury, neck injury, low blood pressure, vertigo.

Cat/Cow   **Benefits:** Releases neck, spine and lower back tension, opens the back body, back body awareness, opens the back ribs and the lungs.

Contraindications: Lower back pain, shoulder surgery, wrist or hand surgery, and tendinitis in the shoulders.

Chair   **Benefits:** Focus, strength, power Blood flows more easily to hips, legs and ankles. Can help with arthritis in knees and ankles, lumbago and disc problems alleviated, increase digestion and elimination, reduce constipation, tones the abdominals, provides more space in the diaphragm for breath, and relieves stiffness.

Contraindications: KNEES!!! Surgery, problems, injuries shoulder surgery (have arms by side), high blood pressure (shorter hold), Achilles tendon injury (do only after completely healed and with great caution), weak ankles (just a little bend in the knees), lower back injuries. Use extreme caution getting OUT of the pose, using a wall or chair to protect the back.

Childs   **Benefits:** Calms body and mind, counter stretch for backbends, flexibility in hips and legs, stimulates digestion, tones abdominal organs, relieves gas, relieves constipation, strengthens ankles, knees and hips, opens back body, alleviates head, neck, chest.

Contraindications: Inflammation of knees, severe constipation, pregnancy, claustrophobia.

Cobra   **Benefits:** Reduces stress, relieves depression and anxiety, improves spinal alignment, cleanses lymphatic system, tones digestive organs, lengthens spine, opens chest, uplifts the heart, strengthens arms, stretches lower back, shoulders, legs, tones calves, cleanses kidneys, reduces fatigue.

Contraindications: Pregnancy, unmedicated high blood pressure, severe spinal or neck injury, recent abdominal injury, injury to hip flexors, abdominal inflammation, lower back injury, shoulder injury.

Cow   **Benefits:** Improves stiff neck, releases shoulder tension, opens knees, strengthens, opens chest. Stretches thighs and arms, opens lower back, stretches back.

Contraindications: Shoulder injury or inflammation, injury in the hip, ankle or knee .

Crane   **Benefits:** Reduces anxiety and depression, lengthens hamstring, stimulates lymphatic system, stretches chest, shoulders, improves digestion, relieves menstrual cramps, tones kidneys, liver, reproduction, energizes body, relieves headache.

Contraindications: Insomnia, pregnancy, knee injury, ankle injury, hip injury, asthma.

Crocodile   **Benefits:** Strengthens legs, strengthens ankles, opens chest, increases spinal flexibility, regulates thyroid, tones kidneys, stretches front of body, reduces fatigue, regulates kidneys, and restores balance.

Contraindications: Shoulder or back injury, knee injury, neck injury, wrist injury, un-medicated high blood pressure, angina (keep the head above the heart).

Crow   **Benefits:** Improves balance and coordination, strengthens arms strengthens abdominal muscles, opens hips, increases focus and concentration.

Contraindications: Carpal tunnel syndrome, wrist or shoulder injury, elbow injury.

Downward Facing Dog   **Benefits:** Lengthening of the spine, calm and decongest nervous system, greater flow to lymphatic system. Stimulates circulation, stimulates and regulates the glands, stimulates hair growth, can help with sciatica, helps stimulate brain function.

Contraindications: Unmedicated high blood pressure, detached retina, conjunctivitis, injury or surgery in shoulders, severe sciatica, recent toe or foot surgery.

Eagle	**Benefits:** Strengthens ankles, relieves leg cramps, improves focus, improves balance, opens shoulders, chest, and hips, and strengthens ankles, knees, hips.
	Contraindications: Knee injury, shoulder injury, elbow injury, lower back injury.
Eight Angle Pose	**Benefits:** Strengthens abdominals and arms, builds resilience, creates a sense of play, and strengthens the wrists.
	Contraindications: High blood pressure, carpal tunnel syndrome, arm, shoulder and wrist injuries, recent abdominal surgery, hamstring injury.
Easy Resting Pose	**Benefits:** Strengthens legs, strengthens ankles, opens chest, increases spinal flexibility, regulates thyroid, tones kidneys, stretches front of body, reduces fatigue, regulates kidneys, and restores balance.
	Contraindications: Shoulder or back injury, knee injury, neck injury, wrist injury, un-medicated high blood pressure, angina (keep the head above the heart).
Easy Sitting Pose	**Benefits:** Opens the hips, relaxes the shoulders, helps develop good posture, grounds the body, increases breath capacity, calms the mind, and prepares the body, mind and spirit for meditation.
	Contraindications: Knee or lower back problems, fatigue in sitting for too long, arthritis causing stiffness or difficulty being on the floor.
Extended Side Angle	**Benefits:** Corrects misalignment of shoulders and shoulder blades, relieves backache and neck sprains, makes spine supple, strengthens the legs, stretches hamstrings, opens hips and hip flexors, tones abdominal and pelvic organs, stimulates digestion, relives acid in the system, relieves sciatica.
	Contraindications: Stress related headaches, migraines, osteoarthritis of the knees, rheumatic fever, varicose veins, low BP, chronic fatigue syndrome, diarrhea, psoriasis, insomnia, depression, and bulimia.

Extended Stretch

Benefits: Corrects slooping shoulders, increases hip flexibility, strengthens arms, relieves joint stress, stretches hamstrings, improves digestion and circulation, increases respiration, stimulates thyroid and parathyroid, soothes nervous system, relieves menstrual cramps, tones liver, spleen and pancreas, nourishes and lengthens spine, strengthens thighs.

Contraindications: Pregnancy, shoulder injury, ankle injury, low blood pressure, high blood pressure, recent abdominal surgery, abdominal hernia.

Firefly

Benefits: Strengthens abdominals, increases focus, strengthens wrists and forearms, opens hips, opens hamstrings, tones lungs and abdominal organs, develops balance and strength.

Contraindications: Wrist injury, recent abdominal surgery, hand injury, lower back or neck injury, weak wrists or forearms.

Fish

Benefits: Chest opener for better breathing, more space in the heart, releasing grief and anxiety, opens upper lobes of lungs, stretches psoas and intercostals, nourishes and stimulates organs of the belly to help with regulating and even preventing diabetes and hypoglycemia, strengthens upper back muscles, balances adrenals with deep contraction in mid back, increases e flexibility in neck and spine, thyroid and parathyroid stimulator and regulator, calms nerves, aids in respiratory conditions such as asthma, releases stiff shoulders .

Contraindications: High or low blood pressure, injury in neck, shoulders or lower back, insomnia, for weak back muscles place palms under sacrum and a prop under head.

Forward Bend

Benefits: Stretches hamstrings, strengthens ankles, lengthens spine, relaxes neck, increases blood flow to the brain, calms the mind, creates inward focus, improves digestions, tones inner organs, may help reverse osteoporosis, clears sinuses.

Contraindications: High blood pressure, low blood pressure, lower back injury, ankle injury, detached retina, torn hamstrings or tight hamstrings (practice with knees bent), menses, pregnancy.

Gate **Benefits:** Lengthens side of body, strengthens abdominal organs, stretches and strengthens ankles, opens inner thighs, opens hips, opens chest, stretches shoulders.

Contraindications: Knee injury, lower back injury, high blood pressure, sciatica, groin injury, SI injury, ankle injury.

Goddess **Benefits:** Decongests the nerves, encourages strength and resolve, tones inner thighs and ankles, increases blood flow to the pelvis.

Contraindications: Detached retina or weak eye capillaries, severe knee problems or knee surgery.

Great Seal **Benefits:** Stretch to the entire back body, opens hamstrings, stimulates digestion, increases vitality and sexual energy, relieves hemorrhoids, and strengthens the immune system.

Contraindications: Back injury, sciatica, pregnancy.

Half Bound Angle Forward Bend **Benefits:** Tones the spleen, liver, and colon, helps with ulcers, opens the hamstrings, rejuvenates the body, and calms the nervous system.

Contraindications: Knee issues, overly tight hips, lower back injury, shoulder injury.

Half Moon **Benefits:** Improves circulation, increases energy to low back and spine, strengthens ankles, stretches hamstring, opens chest and hips, relieves menstrual cramps, relieves sciatica, improves balance and coordination, focus, willpower, relieves backache, improves circulation in the feet, relieves acidity, removes fatigue.

Contraindications: Knee injury, neck injury, low blood pressure, vertigo, stress headaches, migraines, eye issues, varicose veins, insomnia, high blood pressure; look straight ahead, not up or down.

Headstand	**Benefits:** Reduces varicose veins, increases blood flow to the head, relaxes lower back and pelvis, clears the brain, reduces stress, reduces signs of depression, may help increase fertility, relaxes nerves, stimulates glands improves digestion, reduces bad breath, supports transition to menopause, may help cure migraines.
	Contraindications: High blood pressure, neck injury, rotator cuff injury, detached retina, menses, conjunctivitis, eye injuries, back injury, sometimes low blood pressure, heart arrhythmia, obesity, pregnancy if new to yoga, brain cancer.
Head to Knee	**Benefits:** Stretches and opens hamstrings, stretches long muscles of the body, massage inner organs, improves lymphatic system, can alleviate some forms of sciatica.
	Contraindications: Acute sciatica, back injury, constipation (do a shorter hold).
King Dancer	**Benefits:** Relieves menstrual cramps, opens chest, increases lung capacity, develops focus and balance, stretches hip flexors, strengthens ankles and feet, increases spinal flexibility, tones kidneys, opens heart, strengthens legs.
	Contraindications: Knee injury, vertigo, lower back injury, ankle injury, high blood pressure, shoulder injury, recent abdominal surgery.
Knee to Chest	**Benefits:** Removes blocks in intestines, massages and nourishes abdominal organs, flexes hips and legs.
	Contraindications: Pregnancy, abdominal surgery, sciatica, prosthetic foot dropping for AK amputees.

Locust   **Benefits:** Lumbar spine strengthener, abdominal strengthener, blood flow to the sacral region, flushes toxins from the kidneys, strengthens abdominal muscles, by releasing venous pressure in the legs cobra can reduce varicose veins, tones endocrine, nervous and digestive system, buttock muscles strengthen, elongates the body to improve posture, energizes the back body.

Contraindications: With weak back muscles do 3-4 repetitions to strengthen, with head and neck problems, place a rolled blanket under the head, not to be done if more than 3 months pregnant, recent abdominal surgery, recent or chronic inflammation or serious injury to the lower back, spine, legs, arms or shoulders.

Lotus   **Benefits:** Lengthens spine, opens hips, stretches ankles, support long sitting in meditation, brings focus to the mind, grounds lower body, increases energy, alleviates menstrual cramps, tones bladder, increases joint mobility, creates a sense of inner and outer balance in the body, calms the mind.

Contraindications: Knee injury, ankle injury, severe tightness in hips, neck injury, sciatica, prosthetic that does not or should not bend.

Mountain   **Benefits:** Corrects bad posture, improves body alignment, counters degenerative effects of aging, tones buttocks, opens the chest, stretches the arches.

Contraindications: Inflammation in knees, shoulders, arms, ankles or neck.

Pigeon   **Benefits:** Energizes entire body, opens hips, stretches hip flexors, opens thighs, chest, shoulders, brings more circulation to lower back, stimulates digestion and reproductive organs, tones thyroid and parathyroid, tones kidneys, relieves headaches, eliminates toxins, increases flexibility in spine and pelvis, increases leg flexibility.

Contraindications: Hip and knee injury, lower back inflammation, shoulder injury, pregnancy.

Plank

Benefits: Develops core strength, increases stamina, increases focus, develops the back body, conditions and tones large muscle groups, and lengthens the spine.

Contraindications: Wrist injury, shoulder injury, recent abdominal surgery, ankle injury, carpal tunnel syndrome, unmedicated high blood pressure.

Relaxation

Benefits: Reduces anxiety, eases tension in the body, relaxes nervous system, lowers blood pressure, cools mind, makes breath easier, helps recovery from long illness.

Contraindications: Lower back injury, pregnancy - practice with caution, PTSD - practice with caution.

Revolved Triangle

Benefits: Reduces hunched shoulders, elasticizes spine, opens hips, improves digestion, improves circulation, strengthens ankles, feet and calves, tones waistline, tones abdominal organs, improves balance, reduces stress, stretches hamstrings, opens throat, opens shoulders, reduces neck tension.

Contraindications: Migraine, insomnia, lower back injury, neck injury, ankle injury, low blood pressure, SI joint injury.

Sage

Benefits: Strengthens wrists, forearms, abdominals, inner thighs and back muscles. Stretches hamstrings, increases focus and coordination opens the heart.

Contraindications: Wrist, elbow and neck injury, recent abdominal surgery, lower back injury. Rotator cuff or other shoulder injury.

Seated Forward Bend

Benefits: Bathes nervous system, gives spine space, increases sexual vitality, calms mind by going inside self to tune out the outer world, relaxes the heart as it is above the head, tones inner organs, opens and releases hips, deep hamstring stretch, helps relieve hemorrhoids and constipation.

Contraindications: Sciatica, recent back surgery, lower back injury, serious hip problems (do in a chair), more than three month's pregnant, weak back.

Seated Twist

Benefits: Prevents spinal curvature, relieves backaches, tones liver, spleen, pancreas, kidneys, makes spine strong and flexible, corrects "slumpasana", improves digestion and circulation, opens hips, opens chest, opens heart.

Contraindications: High or low blood pressure practice with caution, diarrhea, disk injury or recent spinal surgery, lower back injury, headache, menstruation.

Seated Wide Angle

Benefits: Opens hips, lengthens hamstrings, regulates menstruation, relieves sciatica, relieves arthritis in the hips, strengthens lower back, stretches calves, lengthens spine, and stimulates kidneys and liver.

Contraindications: Asthmatics practice with caution against the wall, low blood pressure, low back injury, and groin or hamstring injury.

Side Angle

Benefits: Corrects misalignment of shoulders and shoulder blades, relieves backache and neck sprains, makes spine supple, strengthens the legs, stretches hamstrings, opens hips and hip flexors, tones abdominal and pelvic organs, stimulates digestion, relives acid in the system, relieves sciatica.

Contraindications: Stress related headaches, migraines, osteoarthritis of the knees, rheumatic fever, varicose veins, low BP, chronic fatigue syndrome, diarrhea, psoriasis, insomnia, depression, and bulimia.

Salutation to the Sun

Benefits: Strengthens legs, strengthens ankles, enlivens the spine, support a healthy endocrine system, calms anxiety, regulates blood sugar, detoxifies the body and mind, makes the skin glow, stimulates digestion, helps with hair growth.

Contraindications: Shoulder or back injury, knee injury, neck injury, wrist injury, un-medicated high blood pressure, pregnancy after three months, recent abdominal surgery, during menstruation, hernias.

Side Crow

Benefits: Strengthens the abdominals, wrists and shoulders. Deeply tones the digestive organs, increases focus and coordination.

Contraindications: Wrist or elbow injury, carpal tunnel syndrome, recent abdominal surgery, scar tissue in residual limb that would be pressed in the pose, pregnancy.

Shoulderstand

Benefits: Reduces hypertension, reduces insomnia, balances thyroid and parathyroid, relieves breathlessness, relieves edema, relieves depression, increases blood flow to the brain, scalp, and skin, reduces hemorrhoids. Relieves heart palpitations, stretches hamstrings, and relieves sinus conditions.

Contraindications: Menstruation, high blood pressure, cervical spondylosis, diarrhea, detached retina, neck injury, broken eye capillaries, glaucoma, eye infections, first trimester of pregnancy, chronic thyroid issues, ischemia.

Staff

Benefits: Relieves breath fatigue, relieves asthma, strengthens chest muscles, tones abdominal muscles, lengthens hamstrings, develops focus, and improves muscles in lumbar spine.

Contraindications: Asthmatic attacks, sciatica, sway back, hamstring injury, Achilles tendon injury, neck injury, hyperextended knees (try not to reach the back of the knees to the ground).

Supine Bound Angle

Benefits: Opens hips, tones ovaries, kidneys, bladder, supports healthy menses, can help ease labor, stretches hamstrings and inner thighs, elevates mood, lengthens spine, tones abdominals, increases blood flow to pelvic region, strengthens lower back, relieves sciatica.

Contraindications: Groin injury, knee injury, sexual trauma (proceed with caution), do not practice post-partum or with a prolapsed uterus, neck injuries, serious back injuries, recent shoulder injury.

Supine Hero

Benefits: Energizes fatigued legs, lengthens the quads, improves digestion, stretches the hip flexors, releases emotional trauma in the pelvis, stretches the tops of the feet and arches, reduce menstrual cramps, reduces arthritic symptoms, and opens the hearts and lungs.

Contraindications: Overly tight quads, knee injury or recent knee surgery, ankle issues.

Supine Twist Benefits: Stretches the long muscles of the body, releases tension from the spine, massages the organs, realigns the spine, soothes the spinal nerves.

Contraindications: Spinal or back surgery, weak spinal disks, recent abdominal surgery, shoulder injury.

Triangle Benefits: Relieves gastritis, indigestion, flatulence, acidity, improves spinal flexibility, alleviates backache, corrects alignment of the shoulders, helps treat neck sprains, strengthens ankles, regulates kidney function, firms waistline, and prevents scoliosis tones abdominal muscles.

Contraindications: High blood pressure, nervous disorders, weak back, weak knees, injury or inflammation of knees, pelvis, neck, ankles, shoulders, abdomen, congestive heart disorders.

Tree Benefits: Develops concentration and poise, improves balance and focus, improves circulation and respiration, strengthens arms, legs, abdominals, spine, ankles and knees, improves kidney function, relieves constipation, reduces flat feet.

Contraindications: Inflammation in the knees, ankle injury, high blood pressure (keep arms to the side or at the heart) headache, heart condition, nervous disorders.

Turtle Benefits: Calms the mind, opens hips, stretches inner thighs, stretches hamstrings, lengthens and strengthens spine, improves digestion.

Contraindications: Shoulder or elbow injury, torn groin or ligaments in hips, lower back inflammation, hamstring tear.

Upward Facing Dog Benefits: Strengthens arms and wrists, opens the chest for easier breath, tones the kidneys, tones and strengthens the abdominal muscles, energizes the nervous system, helps tone the uterus and ovaries, relieves menstrual cramps.

Contraindications: Three months or more pregnant, lower back injury, recent abdominal surgery.

Vishnu's Couch **Benefits:** Strengthens back muscles, tones abdominal muscles, develops stability, lengthens hamstrings, stretches side body.

Contraindications: Lower back injury, shoulder injury, groin injury.

Warrior I **Benefits:** Focus, confidence, strength, strengthens ankles, knees, thighs, hips, back, arms, shoulders, neck, abdominals, prevents scoliosis, decongests nervous system, stimulates digestion, improves circulation, muscular endurance.

Contraindications: High BP, weak knees, inflammation in hips, shoulders, ankles, knees, abdomen, cardiac condition, neck injury.

Warrior II **Benefits:** Strengthens legs ankles, knees, helps in treatment of prolapsed disc, alleviates injury to tailbone, relieves lower backache, increases lung capacity, aligns spine, improves focus and balance, improves endurance.

Contraindications: Heart disease, diarrhea, meniscus injury, injury to knees, ankles, lower back, or shoulders, neck injury, high blood pressure.

Warrior III **Benefits:** Strengthens ankles, knees, lower back, improves blood flow to the joints, stretches hips and groins, improves circulation, lengthens and strengthens the spine.

Contraindications: Ankle injury, knee injury, unmedicated high blood pressure.

ANATOMY OF AN AMPUTEE YOGI

What happens with a below knee (BK) amputee who wears a prosthesis?

A below knee amputee who wears a prosthesis has general concerns which can be addressed with yoga. There are knee flexion and contraction issues from a tight posterior knee capsule. Because a below knee amputee is always using the hip flexors, piriformis and gluteus in a more pronounced way, the iliopsoas shortens which affects the way the BK amputee walks. The BK amputee is not able to take a full stride. The opposite leg takes shortened steps which further tighten these muscles while not adequately developing the other muscles. As a BK amputee gets more flexibility in the muscles and strength in the abdominals, she begins to make more efficient strides which use less energy.

A BK amputee with a prosthesis needs to walk on it regularly to increase muscle fiber around the joints and protect the very vulnerable knee. With a BK amputee, the knee wants to buckle as the other leg steps forward. The knee behind the other leg feels safer. Increasing flexibility in the hips while maintaining and strengthening the quads, gastrocnemius, and lower abdominal muscles decreases pressure on the knee and lower back. A BK amputee needs just as much stretch as she does strength. She is already overcompensating with the other leg, so it is important to create a balanced approach, one that addresses both limbs.

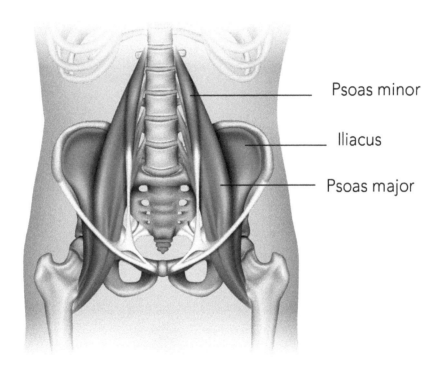

Psoas minor

Iliacus

Psoas major

Muscle groups affected	Pose	Amputee challenge
Hip flexors *Stabilization and range of motion*	Lunge, supine bound angle, frog, childs, bow	Shortened, contracted hip flexor
Piriformis *Pelvic rotation*	Cow, head to knee, tree, pigeon	Out of balance
Obturator internus *Laterally rotates and abducts the thigh, assists in stabilizing the hip joint, when your leg is lifted (hip flexion) this muscle is an essential muscle in abduction. Then the leg is straight this muscle helps with external rotation*	Cow, head to knee, tree, pigeon, lunge,	Shortened, contracted hip flexor
Obturator externus *Lateral rotation and can be affected when wearing prosthesis*	Cow, head to knee, tree, pigeon, lunge,	Shortened, contracted hip flexor
Diaphragm *Muscle that guides inhalation and exhalation*	Bridge, chair, 3-part breath	Kyphosis, weak abdominals
Iliacus *Lifting the leg and aiding forward bending*	Mountain, warrior I, tree, bridge, knee to chest	Weakened due to excess sitting
Psoas *Stabilizes the spine and pelvis, aids twist, flexion and extension of spine and pelvis*	Knee to chest, bridge, easy sitting pose, relaxation	Weakened due to excess sitting
Sartorius *Extends and flexes the pelvis*	Hero, bow, bound angle, warrior II	Weakness

Muscle groups affected	Pose	Amputee challenge
Gluteus Medius *Stabilizes and balances the hips*	Downward dog, tree, locust, frog	Postural control
Hamstrings *Flexion of the knees and hips*	Bound angle, supine padangusthasana, downward dog, gate	Shortened hamstrings
Abductors *Internal and external rotation of the pelvis, leg lifts*	Seated twist, tree, triangle	Weakness
Quadratus Lumborum *Lateral flexion and lower back stabilizer*	Triangle, childs, hero, knee down twist, standing side crescent	Lordosis, weak abdominals
Tensor fascia latae *Knee stabilization, lateral flexion and pelvic stabilization*	Bound angle, supine hero, extended lateral angle	Lateral motion challenges, stability
Quadriceps *Standing, sitting, walking*	Camel, hero, bow, lunge, king dancer	Atrophy
Scalenus *Lift the ribs, involved in inhalation*	Plow, crane, boat, lunge, warrior I, seated twist	Weakness, lordosis, forward head
Sternocleidomastoid *Neck flexion* *Head movement*	Triangle, purvottanasana, jalandhara bandha, seated twist	Shortened psoas, forward head

Bones, Joints, Tendons, Ligaments Affected	Pose	Amputee challenge
Ischial tuberosities *Weight bearing bone*	Mountain, supta padangusthasna, knee down twist	Overuse of remaining limb leads to wear down.
Sacrum *Support to the spine, pubic bone and digestive organs*	Knee/thigh to chest, triangle, legs up the wall, bridge	Asymmetry
SI joint *Weight transference, hip rotation, impact absorption*	King dancer, knee to chest, extended angle, seated twist	Misalignment, weak abdominals
Femoral condyle *Knee articulation* *Shock absorption*	Standing forward bend with bent knees, tiger, staff, warrior II	Pressure from femur, especially if quads aren't stretched and open
Achilles tendon *Attachment between calcaneus and calf aids in walking standing, jumping,* *Foot flexion /extension*	Squat, lunge, half monkey, Vishnu's couch	Shortened hamstrings and quads, hyperextension
Condyles *Links bone to a joint, shock absorption*	Bridge with block between thighs, bound angle, half pike	Lack of suspension, misalignment
Meniscus *Protects the knee joint, shock absorption*	Warrior II, cobra, half locust	Injury, overuse, hyperextension

What happens with an above knee (AK) amputee who wears a prosthesis?

An above knee amputee tends to compensate by lifting the hip up and around then dropping the prosthetic foot. They have no spring system supplied by a knee, so the abdominal muscles can be quite strong. They also often have compensatory scoliosis. They tend to use the upper arms less so there is stagnation in the shoulders, due to lack of swing in the gait unless conscious of practicing the swing. There can also be a tendency to lean slightly away from the prosthetic limb because of the socket. They tend to have loose hamstrings on the residual limb as well as looser hip flexors because there is no knee to bend.

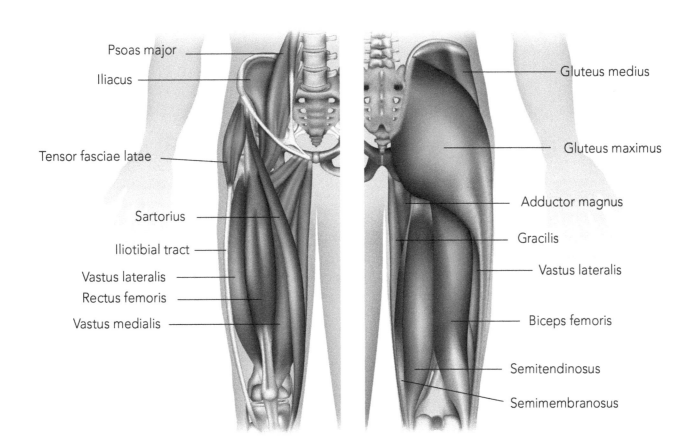

Psoas major
Iliacus
Tensor fasciae latae
Sartorius
Iliotibial tract
Vastus lateralis
Rectus femoris
Vastus medialis

Gluteus medius
Gluteus maximus
Adductor magnus
Gracilis
Vastus lateralis
Biceps femoris
Semitendinosus
Semimembranosus

Muscle groups affected	Pose	Amputee challenge
Quadriceps *Standing, sitting, walking*	Hero, camel, mountain	Atrophy
Piriformis *Hip rotation and extension*	Half lotus, cow, head to knee	Limited range of motion shortened hip psoas
Hip flexors *Stabilization and range of motion*	Lunge, warrior I, parsvokonasana	Shortened hip flexor
Gluteus minimus *Hip rotation*	Bound angle, side angle, triangle	Range of Motion arthritis
Gluteus medius *Hip rotation*	Chair, warrior I, downward facing dog, standing half moon	Range of Motion, arthritis socket fit
Gluteus maximus *Leg abduction* *Hip abduction*	Eagle, goddess, tree	Suspension system, atrophy
Psoas *Stabilizes spine*	Bridge, easy resting pose, extended front stretch, revolved triangle	IT band amputated with no counterbalance to psoas
Diaphragm *Moves the breath*	3-part breath	Suspension system can include a belt that presses on the abdomen
Spinalis *Extension and lateral extensions*	Extended puppy, childs, downward dog, standing forward bend	Atrophy, scoliosis
Gemellus inferior *Hip stabilization, abduction*	Wheel (shortened) double pigeon (lengthened)	Tension in lower back, weak abdominals
Gemellus superior *External rotation of the hip*	Wheel (shortened) double pigeon (lengthened)	Weak abdominals, misaligned prosthetic foot

Muscle groups affected	Pose	Amputee challenge
Obturator internus *Lateral rotation of the thigh*	Eagle, crane, knee down twist, hero	Pistoning in the socket urinary tract infection
Obturator externus Stabilization of the thigh bone Lateral rotation of the thigh	Seated half pigeon, squat, tree	Misalignment of socket, lower back misalignment
Iliacus *Upper leg movement*	Supine bound angle, lunge, boat	Hip flexor contracture, sitting for long periods of time
Quadratus lumborum *Stabilization of the spine* *Lower limb movement*	Crocodile, triangle, revolved triangle	Lordosis, scoliosis, abdominal weakness
Vastus lateralis *Leg extension*	Pigeon, staff, king dancer	Limited range of motion in hip , muscle insertions amputated
Adductor brevis *Stabilization of the trunk* *Adduction of the thigh*	Gate, happy baby, lizard	Loss of leg weight, loss of muscle, shortened psoas
Adductor longus *Leg adduction* *Lateral rotation of the leg*	Frog, seated wide angle, bridge, warrior III	Loss of muscle insertion, socket too tight
Pectineus *Hip flexion* *Adduction of the thigh and hip*	Warrior II, seated wide angle, tree, standing wide angle	Loss of muscle insertion, weak lower back and abdominals
Tensor fasciae latae *Hip rotation*	Warrior II, side angle, chair, squat, cow	Stiff socket, vascular insufficiency

Bones, Joints, Tendons and Ligaments affected	Pose	Amputee challenge
Iliofemoral ligament *Protects hips from overextension*	Knee to chest, extended leg, revolved triangle	Lordosis, lack of stability
Ischiofemoral ligament *Protects hips from over rotation*	Lunge, warrior I, pigeon	Lack of leg weight, overuse
SI joint *Bridge of weight transference between upper and lower body*	Locust, standing forward bend	In an above knee prosthetic wearer, the hip tends to be rotated in
Innominate *Pelvic stabilization*	Downward Dog, knee down twist, supine extended leg	Arthritis Range of motion
Acetebellum *Supports pelvic function*	Chair, half moon, bow	Poor socket fit, lack of leg weight
Obdurator *Thigh rotation*	Cat/Cow, cobra, childs	Pain in the glutes

What happens with an upper extremity (UE) amputee?

Upper extremity amputees are uncommon. Their main issues can be soft tissue damage around the elbow joints, if the elbow is still there. Often there is serious brachial plexus nerve damage, which is below the armpit and acts as a catalyst for upper arm movement. To compensate, shoulders may become frozen. Range of motion can be quite limited. Work is rehabilitative in nature. It is recommended to introduce body mind centering techniques to work from the inside out - lungs, heart, and sternum so exterior muscles can respond.

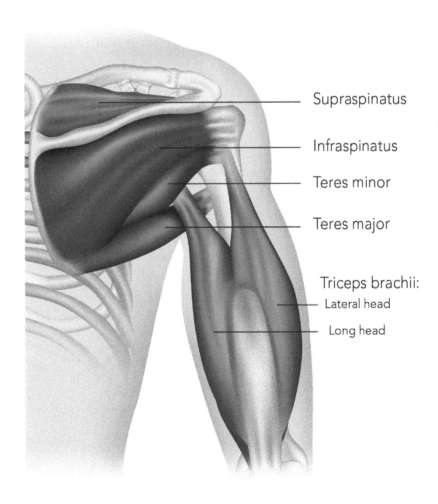

Supraspinatus

Infraspinatus

Teres minor

Teres major

Triceps brachii:
Lateral head
Long head

Muscle groups affected	Pose	Amputee challenge
Supraspinatus *Stabilizes the humerus*	Triangle, Seated Twist, Extended stretch	Overuse/Underuse Thoracic tension
Subscapularis *Moves the humerus*	Gate, Eagle Pose with one arm, Mountain	Arthritis Scar tissue
Infraspinatus *Stabilizes the shoulder socket*	Cobra, Childs, Standing Forward Bend	Prosthetic attachment Limited range of motion
Teres minor *Lateral rotation of the arm* *Stabilization of the shoulder*	Cat/Cow Seated, Warrior II, Eagle with one arm	Lack of insertion point
Coracobrachialis *Flexion and adduction of the upper arm*	Plank at the wall, Chair with available arm reaching back, Bridge	Weakness
Intercostal *Pranayama*	Side Angle, Breath of fire, Standing half moon	Strain
Teres major *Shoulder circles backward*	Side Angle, Reverse table top at the wall, Half cow arms	Limited range of motion Overuse/underuse
Sternocleidomastoid *Head rotation and extension*	Triangle, cat/cow, lunge	Habitual retraction of remaining muscles
Serratus anterior *Arm rotation* *scapular movement*	Downward dog, side plank at the wall, 3- part breath	Tension, spinal misalignment
Serratus posterior superior *Rib movement for pranayama*	Ujjayi breath, shoulder circles, cobra	Tightness in the chest

Muscle groups affected	Pose	Amputee challenge
Scalenus *Lifting the first and second rib*	Head rolls, seated twist, revolved triangle	Overuse, tight jaw
Levator scapulae *Lifting the scapula*	Plow, legs up the wall, warrior I	Anxiety, myofascial pain
Serratus posterior inferior *Lengthening and expanding trunk*	Gate, seated side angle, seated forward bend	Prosthetic strap Lower back pain
Latissimus dorsi *Extension / flexion of the lumbar spine*	Exalted warrior, downward dog, seated staff	Weak abdominals, lower back strain
Trapezius *Movement of the shoulder blade*	Puppy stretch, warrior II, goddess	Weak abdominals, repetitive stress
Diaphragm *Contraction and relaxation of thoracic cavity for pranayama*	Mountain, easy sitting pose, bridge	Weak abdominals, anxiety
Flexor pollicis longus *Thumb flexion*	Seated sage twist, locust, camel	Shortening of connective tissue due to lack of use
Pronator quadratus *Forearm pronation*	Locust, cobra, warrior II	Inability to rotate forearm well.
Extensor carpi ulnaris *Wrist flexion and adduction*	Mountain, eagle, chair	Scattered ulnar nerve
Flexor carpi ulnaris *Wrist flexion and adduction*	Locust, seated sage twist, mountain	Scatted ulnar nerve
Biceps *Lifting the forearm*	Great seal, goddess, side angle	Weak from lack of gripping action
Triceps *Lifting the forearm*	Locust, upward plank on elbows, intense side stretch	Weak from lack of gripping action

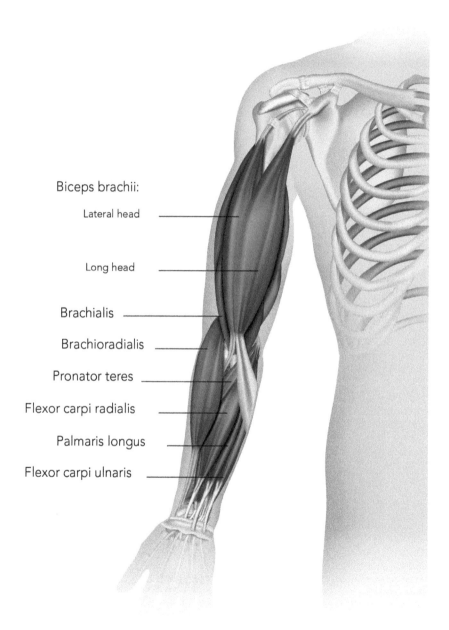

Biceps brachii:

Lateral head

Long head

Brachialis

Brachioradialis

Pronator teres

Flexor carpi radialis

Palmaris longus

Flexor carpi ulnaris

Joints, Tendons and ligaments affected	Pose	Amputee Challenge
Glenohumeral joint *Connects the upper arm to the trunk*	Cow, table with shoulder retraction, cobra	Lack of cushion in the residual limb
Coracohumeral joint *Involved in shoulder movement*	Chair, camel, yoga mudra	Arm rotation challenges
Sternoclavicular joint *Clavicular movement*	Warrior I, five-pointed star, locust	ROM and heaviness of the prosthesis
Acromioclavicular joint *Arm and scapular rotation*	Pigeon, sphinx, mountain	Osteoarthritis
Epicondyles *Attaches muscle and ligament*	Staff, knee to chest, warrior II	Overuse
Elbow *Movement of forearm forward and away from body*	Chair, warrior II, knees to chest	Tennis elbow

The Golgi Tendon

The Golgi tendon organ is located at the meeting point of a tendon and muscle, letting the muscle know when to tense. It responds to muscle contraction, protecting and stretching the tendon nearby. When working with an amputee, the force of pressure in the Golgi tendon organ is different. Body weight is not distributed evenly, and some tendons are over or underused. An amputee must relearn many of their basic motor skills, confusing proprioception as the brain adapts to new neural connections. If there is vascular dysfunction systemically or near the limb, that will influence the Golgi tendon reflex, the "strengthen and relax" neurological muscle message. This whole system must be reprogrammed for amputees. If there has been a cut to the nerve fiber or muscle fiber, those nerves are scarred which affects proprioception. Yoga can be very helpful to re-teach and enhance the proprioception skills of a client..

Additional Amputee Challenges

In addition to the challenges amputees face with joints and muscles, they also deal with skin irritations, infections, prosthetic misalignment, surgical revisions, edema, bone spurs, bursas, and callouses.

Skin irritations can cause great discomfort, often the result of wear and tear on the residual limb in the prosthetic socket. During yoga, some poses may put extra pressure on a skin irritation, so the poses need to be adapted. Normally with skin irritations, less activity until healing occurs is better.

Infections need to be addressed immediately. Because the residual limb is often compressed into the dark moist space of the prosthetic socket, bacteria builds up. Combined with diseases like diabetes, residual limb care, as well as prosthetic care, are a high priority.

Prosthetic misalignment can cause chronic or acute pain, as well as new skin irritations. When practicing yoga, it is better to avoid using the prosthesis until the misalignment has been dealt with.

Surgical revisions happen for many amputees, from bone spurs bursting through skin to myodesis malfunction (skin folds surgically placed to protect the residual bone).

Bursas, fluid filled sacs found at irritated joints, can occur due to constant friction of the residual limb with a prosthesis, as well as overuse of the joint. Often the prosthesis will be adjusted to alleviate the bursa and allow it to heal. Amputees may need to avoid wearing the prosthesis until the residual limb is healed.

TIPS FOR YOGA TEACHERS

1. The student is whole.

2. The student is able.

3. Teach student to move from the center to the periphery.

4. Strengthen the residual limb/s: Chair, Warriors, Mountain.

5. Stretch overused body parts: Twists, Triangle, Forward Bend.

6. Do not tell a new amputee to envision the missing limb.

7. Do abdominal exercises for better stability.

8. Use a lot of props, especially wall.

9. Teach students to use sitz bones if they have them.

10. Teach metta meditation for self-acceptance and self-compassion.

TIPS FOR CLINICIANS

Diagnosis	Evaluation	Yoga Intervention	Outcome	Follow Up
Phantom Pain	Level of pain, location, mental stress, frequency, connection to emotions	Ujjayi breath Joint freeing series Sun salutation	Less phantom pain Better symptom management	30-day home practice with weekly follow up appointments
Balance Issues	Standing, stepping forward, backward, sitting in a chair, getting up from a chair	Core ab exercises Dristi-focused gaze Walking breath meditation with support	Better use of core muscles rather than over/underuse of other muscles Ability to look forward rather than down	Evaluation at 1 month, 3 month and 6 months for changes in balance
Scar tissue	Location of scar tissue, amount of scar tissue, range of motion in joints near or in scar tissue	Hissing breath Slow movements with breath Easy twist	Better awareness of location of scar tissue Learning how to work with and around scar tissue to avoid injury	Daily castor oil packs for one week, then weekly
PTSD	Specific triggers, eye movements, shortness of breath, strong reaction to sudden movements, frozen, tight jaw, disassociation	Deep belly breath Dristi on different spots in the room Seated savasana against the wall with eyes looking toward floor, pillow held at abdomen if arm is available	Better awareness of PTSD symptoms Practice self-regulation yoga tools to handle triggers and symptoms	Daily practice for as long as it takes

Transitions	Standing to sitting Sitting to standing Sitting/standing to floor Floor to sitting	Abdominal crunches If arms available, tricep dips Uddiyana bandha Step process - yoga props such as bolsters, blankets and blocks piled at bottom of chair. Sit at edge of chair and lift off, either reaching for a bar or wall in front to stand, or sliding bottom down to "step" or cushion below	Independence and confidence with transitioning from different movement planes Core strength and abdominal stabilization	Daily practice with clinician nearby until able to do on own.
Nerve Pain	Complete history of pain symptoms, level of pain 1-10, 10 being the worst, how often is the pain, chronic or acute, what time of the day	Shoulder shrugs Chin tilts Mindful slow movement with breath at joints Psoas release exercises Creative visualization	Less pain. More freedom of movement. Less stress. More relaxed mind.	Practice physical exercises every other day for 1-3 months. Practice mindful breathing and creative visualization daily.
Frozen Shoulder	Check range of motion in other shoulder. History and level of discomfort. When did the frozen shoulder begin? Observation of repetitive movement patterns.	Stabilization of scapula with ace bandage. Pranayama sent to the shoulder and surrounding area. Arm raises to the side with mindfulness and breath. Warrior two with armpits turned up.	More self-management of symptoms and commitment to personal health. Slow steady release of frozen shoulder combined with preventative yoga tools.	Practice yoga techniques daily with rest in between each exercise until shoulder begins to release.
Anxiety	History of behaviors such as worry, fear, obsessing, frozen	Ujjayi breath Sniffing breath - 3 sniffs through nose then exhale through the mouth as shoulders release. Forward bend Childs.	Reduction in anxious symptoms, prevention practices for stressful moments, calming yoga breathing techniques	Short breathing practices throughout the day to accustom patient to habitual self-management.

Poor range of motion	Evaluate simple movements at the joints. Watch facial expressions and facial tone for signs of strain.	Six movements of the spine Proprioception exercises, Standing balance-leaning to one side then the other with support of chair and wall Torso circles in both directions	Greater awareness of what is possible with yoga practice. Looser joints with better circulation in and around the joints.	Practice range of motion yoga sequence daily, and weekly with clinician to evaluate progress
Poor circulation	Coolness in extremities, tingling, aching joints, fatigue	Sighing breath Breath of fire Downward dog Hip circles Warrior II Seated wide angle	Better movement in joints, more warmth (not heat which is inflammation) in body, less tingling	Practice hip circles and joint rotation of neck, wrists, knees and ankles, daily

ALTERNATIVE TREATMENTS FOR PHANTOM PAIN

- **Mirror therapy:** The patient watches her remaining limb in a mirror during physical therapy so that the brain to accepts that the limb is no longer there.

- **Brain stimulation:** Small electrodes are surgically placed on the part of the brain affected, sending electric pulses to reduce pain.

- **Nerve stimulation:** A nerve stimulator is placed directly on the nerves that send pain messages to the amputated limb to alleviate pain.

- **Acupuncture:** Small needles are inserted into various meridian points in the body to treat chronic and acute pain.

- **Biofeedback:** Biofeedback therapy is a non-drug treatment in which patients learn to control bodily processes that are normally involuntary, such as muscle tension, blood pressure, or heart rate.

- **Cognitive Behavioral Therapy:** Talk therapy to help amputees change to positive language, thoughts and actions for better means of coping with pain.

- **Virtual reality/ creative visualization:** The practitioner envisions physical and emotional sensations in the body and mind until they become a reality in the physical plane.

- **Nerve block injection:** A physician injects nerve blocking medicine directly into the localized pain source.

RESOURCES

Amputee Organizations and Support

www.amputee-coalition.org

www.oandp.com

www.amplitude-media.com

www.amputeebladerunners.com

www.challengedathletes.org

www.activeamp.org

www.achillesinternational.org

www.opafonline.org

www.teamusa.org

www.yogaforscoliosis.com

www.limbsforlife.org

www.aboutonehandtyping.com

www.nationalamputation.org

www.givenlimb.org

www.limbpower.com

www.thealternativelimbproject.com

www.adaptivesports.org

www.disabledsportsusa.org

www.amputee.ca

www.opcanada.ca

www.amplifyyourself.org

www.amps4ohio.com

Books on Yoga

Feuerstein, Georg. *The Yoga Tradition: Its History, Literature, Philosophy, and Practice.* Prescott, AZ: Hohm, 1998

Iyengar, B. K. S. *Light on Yoga: The Classic Guide to Yoga from the World's Foremost Authority.* London: Thorsons, 2001

Iyengar, B.K.S. *Light on pranayama : the yogic art of breathing.* New York: Crossroad, 1981.

Kaminoff, Leslie. *Yoga Anatomy.* Champaign, IL. Human Kinetics. 2011

McCall, Timothy. *Yoga as Medicine.* NY, NY, Bantam. 2007

Paramahansa Yogananda. *Autobiography of a Yogi.* Rider; UK ed. edition May 4, 1955

Stiles, Mukunda. *Structural Yoga Therapy: Adapting to the Individual.* York Beach, ME: Samuel Weiser, 2000.

Taylor, Matthew. *Yoga Therapy as a Creative Response to Pain.* Philadelphia, PA. Jessica Kingsley Publishers. 2018

The Science of Breath and the Philosophy of the Tatwas. Rama Prasad. The Theophosical Publishing Society, London, 1890

Books on Limb Loss

Burgess, Ernest. *Physical Fitness: A Guide for Individuals with Lower Limb Loss.* Diane Publishing. Darby, PA. 1993

Danzig, Marsha. *From the Roots.* NY, NY. Skyhorse Publishing, 2017

Reinertsen, Sarah. *In a Single Bound: Losing My Leg, Finding Myself, and Training for Life.* Ny, NY. Lyons Press. 2010.

Sabolich, John. *You're Not Alone* Prosthetics, Hanger 1996.

Winchell. Ellen. *Coping with Limb Loss.* Self-published. 1995.

Pain Management Resources

Carolina's Pain Institute http://carolinaspaininstitute.com/

Institute for Pain Management https://www.nopainstl.com/

International Institute for the Study of Pain https://www.iasp-pain.org/

The Pain Institute https://www.thepaininstitute.com/

World Institute of Pain http://wip.agoria.co.uk/

Amputee Rehabilitation

Rehabilitation Institute of Chicago *www.sralab.org*

Kessler Institute for Rehabilitation *www.kessler-rehab.com*

TIRR Memorial Hermann *www.memorialhermann.org*

Mayo Clinic *www.mayoclinic.org*

University of Washington Medical Center *www.uwmedicine.org/uw-medical-center*

Spaulding Rehabilitation Hospital-Massachusetts General Hospital *spauldingrehab.org*

Craig Hospital *craighospital.org*

MossRehab *www.mossrehab.com*

Rusk Rehabilitation at NYU Langone Medical Center *med.nyu.edu/rusk*

Shepherd Center *www.shepherd.org/*

Guttman Institute. www.guttmann.com/en

Veteran Amputees

www.waramps.ca/home.html

www.woundedwarriorproject.org

Yoga Programs for Veterans

www.connectedwarriors.org

www.yogawarriors.com

www.samueliinstitute.org

www.veteransyogaproject.org

www.givebackyoga.org

www.mindfulyogatherapy.org

www.irest.us

www.vetsyoga.com

www.yogaforvets.org

wingsforwarriors.org

www.bootstrapusa.com

Footnotes:

www.dictionary.com

"A divorce is like an amputation; you survive, but there's less of you." Margaret Atwood , Time Magazine, March 19, 1973

www.dalailama.com/messages/compassion

To hear the stories of the amputee yogis in this book, go to www.yogaforamputeesbook.com

Contact

For more information about Yoga for Amputees, go to www.yogaforamputees.com

Author Contact Information

Marsha Therese Danzig

www.marshatheresedanzig.com

Designer Contact Information

Emilia Ryan

www.inspiredcontent.com

Printed in the USA
CPSIA information can be obtained
at www.ICGtesting.com
LVHW071443091023
760568LV00023BA/654